1/13/16
$98.00

ESSENTIALS OF
Geriatric Psychiatry

SECOND EDITION

ESSENTIALS OF
Geriatric Psychiatry

SECOND EDITION

EDITED BY

Dan G. Blazer, M.D., Ph.D.
David C. Steffens, M.D., M.H.S.

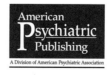

American Psychiatric Publishing
A Division of American Psychiatric Association

Washington, DC
London, England

Note: The authors have worked to ensure that all information in this book is accurate at the time of publication and consistent with general psychiatric and medical standards, and that information concerning drug dosages, schedules, and routes of administration is accurate at the time of publication and consistent with standards set by the U.S. Food and Drug Administration and the general medical community. As medical research and practice continue to advance, however, therapeutic standards may change. Moreover, specific situations may require a specific therapeutic response not included in this book. For these reasons and because human and mechanical errors sometimes occur, we recommend that readers follow the advice of physicians directly involved in their care or the care of a member of their family.

Books published by American Psychiatric Publishing (APP) represent the findings, conclusions, and views of the individual authors and do not necessarily represent the policies and opinions of APP or the American Psychiatric Association.

Copyright © 2012 American Psychiatric Association
ALL RIGHTS RESERVED

Manufactured in the United States of America on acid-free paper
16   15   14   13   12   5   4   3   2   1
Second Edition

American Psychiatric Publishing,
a Division of American Psychiatric Association
1000 Wilson Boulevard
Arlington, VA 22209-3901
www.appi.org

Typeset in Adobe's Bembo and Futura.

Library of Congress Cataloging-in-Publication Data
Essentials of geriatric psychiatry / edited by Dan G. Blazer, David C. Steffens. — 2nd ed.
   p. ; cm.
  Includes bibliographical references and index.
  ISBN 978-1-58562-413-3 (pbk. : alk. paper)
  I. Blazer, Dan G. (Dan German), 1944–   II. Steffens, David C., 1962–
  [DNLM: 1. Mental Disorders. 2. Aged. 3. Aging—physiology. 4. Geriatric Psychiatry—methods.   WT 150]
  618.97′689—dc23
                                   2011043251

British Library Cataloguing in Publication Data
A CIP record is available from the British Library.

CONTENTS

PART I
Basic Science of Geriatric Psychiatry

PART II
Evaluation of Psychiatric Disorders in Late Life

PART III
Presentation of Psychiatric Disorders in Late Life

PART IV
Treatment of Psychiatric Disorders in Late Life

CONTRIBUTORS

Carmen Andreescu, M.D.
Assistant Professor of Psychiatry, University of Pittsburgh Department of Psychiatry, Western Psychiatric Institute and Clinic, Pittsburgh, Pennsylvania

Deborah K. Attix, Ph.D.
Associate Professor of Medical Psychology, Department of Psychiatry and Behavioral Sciences, and Director, Clinical Neuropsychology Service, Division of Neurology, Duke University Medical Center, Durham, North Carolina

John L. Beyer, M.D.
Assistant Professor of Psychiatry, Duke University Medical Center, Durham, North Carolina

Dan G. Blazer, M.D., Ph.D.
J.P. Gibbons Professor of Psychiatry and Behavioral Sciences, Duke University Medical Center, Durham, North Carolina

P. Murali Doraiswamy, M.B.B.S.
Professor of Psychiatry and Chief, Division of Biological Psychiatry, Duke University Medical Center, Durham, North Carolina

Jack D. Edinger, Ph.D.
Senior Psychologist, Durham VA Medical Center; Clinical Professor, Department of Psychiatry and Behavioral Sciences, Duke University Medical Center, Durham, North Carolina

Dawn E. Epstein, B.S.
Department of Psychology and Neuroscience, Duke University, Durham, North Carolina

Harold W. Goforth, M.D.
Assistant Professor of Medicine and Psychiatry, Departments of Internal Medicine and of Psychiatry and Behavioral Sciences, Duke University Medical Center, Durham, North Carolina

Lisa P. Gwyther, M.S.W.
Associate Professor, Department of Psychiatry and Behavioral Sciences, Duke University Medical Center, Durham, North Carolina

Li-Wen Huang, A.B.
Student Intern, Aging Brain Center, Institute for Aging Research, Hebrew SeniorLife, Boston, Massachusetts; and Duke University School of Medicine, Durham, North Carolina

Celia F. Hybels, Ph.D.
Associate Professor, Department of Psychiatry and Behavioral Sciences, Center for the Study of Aging and Human Development, Duke University Medical Center, Durham, North Carolina

Sharon K. Inouye, M.D., M.P.H.
Professor of Medicine, Department of Medicine, Beth Israel Deaconess Medical Center, Harvard Medical School, Boston, Massachusetts; Director and Milton and Shirley F. Levy Family Chair, Aging Brain Center, Institute for Aging Research, Hebrew SeniorLife, Boston, Massachusetts

Dilip V. Jeste, M.D.
Estelle and Edgar Levi Chair in Aging; Director, Sam and Rose Stein Institute for Research on Aging; Distinguished Professor of Psychiatry and Neurosciences, University of California, San Diego; Chief, Division of Geriatric Psychiatry, VA San Diego Healthcare System, San Diego, California

Robert M. Kaiser, M.D., M.H.Sc.
Attending Physician, Geriatrics and Extended Care, and Medical Director, Home-Based Primary Care Program, Washington D.C. Veterans Affairs Medical Center; Associate Professor of Medicine and Associate Director, Fellowship in Geriatric Medicine, George Washington University School of Medicine, Washington, D.C.

Andrew D. Krystal, M.D., M.S.
Director, Sleep Research Laboratory, and Associate Professor, Department of Psychiatry and Behavioral Sciences, Duke University Medical Center, Durham, North Carolina

Nicole M. Lanouette, M.D.
Assistant Clinical Professor, Department of Psychiatry, University of California, San Diego; VA San Diego Healthcare System, San Diego, California

Eric J. Lenze, M.D.
Associate Professor of Psychiatry, Washington University School of Medicine, St. Louis, Missouri

Constantine G. Lyketsos, M.D., M.H.S.
The Elizabeth Plank Althouse Professor and Chair of Psychiatry for Johns Hopkins Bayview, Department of Psychiatry and Behavioral Sciences, Johns Hopkins University School of Medicine, Baltimore, Maryland

Thomas R. Lynch, Ph.D.
Director, Personality and Emotion Biobehavioural Laboratory, School of Psychology, University of Southampton Highfield Campus, Southampton, United Kingdom

Shahrzad Mavandadi, Ph.D.
Investigator, Philadelphia VA Medical Center VISN 4 Mental Illness Research, Education, and Clinical Center; and Adjunct Assistant Professor, Department of Psychiatry, University of Pennsylvania, Philadelphia, Pennsylvania

Diane E. Meglin, M.S.W., L.C.S.W., D.C.S.W.
Associate, Department of Psychiatry and Behavioral Sciences, and Clinical Social Worker, Department of Social Work, Duke University Medical Center, Durham, North Carolina

Benoit H. Mulsant, M.D.
Clinical Director, Geriatric Mental Health Program, and Physician in Chief, Centre for Addiction and Mental Health, Toronto, Ontario, Canada; Professor and Vice-Chair, Department of Psychiatry, University of Toronto, Toronto, Ontario, Canada

David W. Oslin, M.D.
Associate Professor, University of Pennsylvania and Philadelphia VA Medical Center VISN 4 Mental Illness Research, Education, and Clinical Center, Philadelphia, Pennsylvania

Bruce G. Pollock, M.D., Ph.D.
Vice President, Research, Centre for Addiction and Mental Health, Toronto, Ontario, Canada; Professor and Head, Division of Geriatric Psychiatry, Faculty of Medicine, University of Toronto, Toronto, Ontario, Canada

Moria J. Smoski, Ph.D.
Assistant Professor, Department of Psychiatry and Behavioral Sciences, Duke University Medical Center, Durham, North Carolina

David C. Steffens, M.D., M.H.S.
Professor of Psychiatry and Medicine and Head, Division of Geriatric Psychiatry, Duke University Medical Center, Durham, North Carolina

Joel E. Streim, M.D.
Professor of Psychiatry, Department of Psychiatry, University of Pennsylvania; VISN 4 Mental Illness Research, Education, and Clinical Center, Philadelphia VA Medical Center, Philadelphia, Pennsylvania

Mugdha E. Thakur, M.B.B.S.
Assistant Professor of Psychiatry, Duke University Medical Center, Durham, North Carolina

Larry W. Thompson, Ph.D.
Professor, Emeritus, Department of Medicine; Professor, Active Duty, Department of Psychiatry and Behavioral Sciences; Stanford University School of Medicine, Stanford, California

Ipsit V. Vahia, M.D.
Assistant Clinical Professor, Stein Institute for Research on Aging, Department of Psychiatry, University of California, San Diego; VA San Diego Healthcare System, San Diego, California

Richard D. Weiner, M.D., Ph.D.
Professor, Department of Psychiatry and Behavioral Sciences, Duke University Medical School; Chief, Mental Health Service Line, Durham VA Medical Center, Durham, North Carolina

Kathleen A. Welsh-Bohmer, Ph.D.
Professor of Medical Psychology, Department of Psychiatry, and Director, The Joseph and Kathleen Bryan Alzheimer's Disease Research Center, Division of Neurology, Department of Medicine, Duke University Medical Center, Durham, North Carolina

Julie Loebach Wetherell, Ph.D.
Associate Professor of Psychiatry, University of California, San Diego; Staff Psychologist, VA San Diego Healthcare System, San Diego, California

William K. Wohlgemuth, Ph.D.
Research Associate Professor, Departments of Psychology and Neurology, University of Miami, Miami, Florida

Disclosure of Interests

The contributors have declared all forms of support received within the 12 months prior to manuscript submittal that may represent a competing interest in relation to their work published in this volume, as follows:

John L. Beyer, M.D. *Research support:* Astra-Zeneca, Elan/Janssen Pharmaceuticals, Eli Lilly, Forest, Merck, National Institute of Mental Health, Repligen.

P. Murali Doraiswamy, M.B.B.S. *Research grants/Advisory boards:* Alzheimer's Association, Alzheimer's Foundation, Avid Radiopharmaceuticals, Baxter, Bristol-Myers Squibb, Clarimedix, Elan, Eli Lilly, Medivation, Neuronetrix, Neuroptix, Rutgers University, Sonexa, TauRx, University of California. *Speaker's bureau:* AstraZeneca, Labopharm, Lundbeck. *Stockholder:* Clarimedix, Sonexa.

Jack D. Edinger, Ph.D. *Consulting:* Philips Respironics. *Honorarium:* Takeda. *Research support:* Helicor, Philips Respironics. *Speaker's bureau:* Sleep Medicine Education Institute.

Harold W. Goforth, M.D. *Speaker's bureau:* Bristol-Myers Squibb.

Dilip V. Jeste, M.D. *Donations:* AstraZeneca, Bristol-Myers Squibb, Eli Lilly, and Janssen donate medications for our NIMH-funded grant "Metabolic Effects of Newer Antipsychotics in Older Patients." *Research support:* Department of Veterans Affairs, National Institute of Mental Health (grant MH66248).

Andrew D. Krystal, M.D., M.S. *Consulting:* Abbott, Actelion, Arena, Astellas, AstraZeneca, Axiom, Bristol-Myers Squibb, Cephalon, Eli Lilly, GlaxoSmithKline, Jazz, Johnson & Johnson, Kingsdown, Merck, Neurocrine, Neurogen, Novartis, Organon, Ortho-McNeil-Janssen, Pfizer, Philips Respironics, Roche, Sanofi-Aventis, Sepracor, Somaxon, Takeda, Transcept. *Grants/Research support:* Abbott, Astellas, Cephalon, Evotec, GlaxoSmithKline, Kingsdown, Merck, National Institutes of Health, Neurocrine, Neurogen, Pfizer, Philips Respironics, Sepracor, Somaxon, Takeda, Transcept.

Eric J. Lenze, M.D. *Consulting:* Fox Learning Systems. *Research support:* Bristol-Myers Squibb, Forest, National Institute of Mental Health, Pfizer.

Constantine G. Lyketsos, M.D., M.H.S. *Consulting:* Forest, Eli Lilly, Lundbeck, Pfizer, Wyeth. *Research support:* Forest.

Benoit H. Mulsant, M.D. [1999–2006 interests] *Consulting:* AstraZeneca, Bristol-Myers Squibb, Eisai, Eli Lilly, Forest, Fox Learning Systems, GlaxoSmithKline, Janssen, Lundbeck, Pfizer. *Honoraria:* AstraZeneca, Eisai, Forest, Janssen, Lundbeck, GlaxoSmithKline, Pfizer. *Grants/Research support:* AstraZeneca, Bristol-Myers Squibb (current), Canadian Institutes of Health Research (current), Corcept, Eisai, Eli Lilly, Forest, GlaxoSmithKline, Janssen, National Institutes of Health (current), Pfizer, Wyeth (current). *Speaker's bureau:* AstraZeneca, Eisai, Forest, Janssen, Pfizer. *Equities* (as of 2008): AkzoNobel, Alkermes, AstraZeneca, Biogen Idec, Celsion, Elan, Eli Lilly, Forest, General Electric (current), Orchestra Therapeutics, Pfizer. *Other material or financial support:* Forest, Janssen.

Bruce G. Pollock, M.D., Ph.D. *Advisory boards:* Lundbeck Canada (final meeting May 2009); Lundbeck International Neuroscience Foundation (final meeting April 2010). *Consulting:* Wyeth (one-time consultant, October 2008). *Research support:* Canadian Institutes of Health Research, National Institutes of Health.

Joel E. Streim, M.D. *Consulting:* Eisai.

Richard D. Weiner, M.D., Ph.D. *Patent:* Co-inventor of Duke University patent on ECT seizure quality determination; no personal royalties received.

The following authors have no competing interests to report:

Carmen Andreescu, M.D.
Deborah K. Attix, Ph.D.
Dan G. Blazer, M.D., Ph.D.
Dawn E. Epstein, B.S.
Lisa P. Gwyther, M.S.W.
Li-Wen Huang, A.B.
Celia F. Hybels, Ph.D.
Sharon K. Inouye, M.D., M.P.H.
Robert M. Kaiser, M.D., M.H.Sc.
Nicole M. Lanouette, M.D.
Thomas R. Lynch, Ph.D.
Shahrzad Mavandadi, Ph.D.
Diane E. Meglin, M.S.W., L.C.S.W., D.C.S.W.
David W. Oslin, M.D.
Moria J. Smoski, Ph.D.
David C. Steffens, M.D., M.H.S.
Mugdha E. Thakur, M.B.B.S.
Larry W. Thompson, Ph.D.
Ipsit V. Vahia, M.D.
Kathleen A. Welsh-Bohmer, Ph.D.
Julie Loebach Wetherell, Ph.D.
William K. Wohlgemuth, Ph.D.

PREFACE

This second edition of *Essentials of Geriatric Psychiatry* is based on the fourth edition of *The American Psychiatric Publishing Textbook of Geriatric Psychiatry,* published in 2009. (The first edition of the textbook, titled *Geriatric Psychiatry,* was published in 1989; the second edition, retitled *The American Psychiatric Press Textbook of Geriatric Psychiatry,* appeared in 1996; and the third edition was published in 2004.) *Essentials of Geriatric Psychiatry* recognizes the enormous expansion of scientific knowledge about aging and the diseases of late life, as well as the advances in biological psychiatry and neuropsychiatry, that have greatly altered the practice of geriatric psychiatry. A version that captures "the essentials" is specifically designed to provide the clinician with the current state of scientific understanding as well as the practical skills and knowledge base required for dealing with mental disorders in late life.

As in the textbook, the chapters are presented in a sequential and integrated fashion, which we have found enhances the accessibility and usefulness of the information presented. The contributors have a clear ability to make complex material understandable to our readers. We maintained an eclectic orientation regarding theory and practice in geriatric psychiatry. Although most contributors are psychiatrists, we also called on colleagues from relevant biomedical and behavioral disciplines, because of their expertise and their ability to incorporate such knowledge into a comprehensive approach to patient care.

We have targeted this text to psychiatrists and other health professionals who have an interest in and a commitment to the diagnosis, treatment, and long-term management of older adults experiencing psychiatric problems. This book is of particular value to psychiatrists, neurologists, and geriatric psychiatrists sitting for their board examinations, as well as candidates seeking certification in geriatrics from the American Board of Internal Medicine and the American Board of Family Practice. Nonphysicians whose accreditation examinations recognize the critical role of working with the elderly, including psychologists and social workers, will also find this text useful. All of these examinations place considerable emphasis on geriatric psychiatry and the behavioral aspects of aging.

We wish to express our deepest appreciation for the assistance of our staff assistants, Marsha Harrison and Judy Ridley, for their efforts in supporting us.

Dan Blazer and David Steffens
Durham, North Carolina

PART I

Basic Science of Geriatric Psychiatry

CHAPTER 1

DEMOGRAPHY AND EPIDEMIOLOGY OF PSYCHIATRIC DISORDERS IN LATE LIFE

CELIA F. HYBELS, PH.D.
DAN G. BLAZER, M.D., PH.D.

The epidemiology of psychiatric disorders in late life is the study of the distribution of psychiatric disorders and psychiatric symptoms among older adults and the variables that affect the distribution. In this chapter, we review the findings of demographers and epidemiologists as they relate to the care of the psychiatrically impaired older adult.

Demography

In 2008, approximately 38.9 million persons age 65 years and older lived in the United States, accounting for 12.8% of the population. Over the twentieth century, the number of persons in this age group steadily increased, from 3.1 million in 1900 and 12.3 million in 1950 to the current estimate. The size of the elderly population is projected to continue to increase over the next several decades and to reach 72.1 million by the year 2030 and then 88.5 million by 2050. Even more astounding, in 2008, the number of "oldest old," or persons age 85 years and older, was 5.7 million and was projected to reach 19.0 million by 2050. In 2007, 2% of the Medicare population age 65 or older resided in community housing with at least one service available, and 4% resided in long-term care facilities (Federal Interagency Forum on Aging-Related Statistics 2010). Many of these residents are placed in residential care because of psychiatric disorders, especially the behavior problems that result from Alzheimer's disease.

The current older population of the United States is predominantly female and white. In 2008, women accounted for 58% of the population age 65 years and older and 67% of those age 85 and older. The racial and ethnic composition of the older population is projected to change over the next several decades. In 2008, 80.4% of those age 65 or older were non-Hispanic white, 8.5% black, 6.8% Hispanic, 3.3% Asian, and 1.3% other racial/ethnic group. By 2050, the proportion of blacks is projected to be 11.9%, Asians 8.5%, and Hispanics of any race 19.8%, whereas the proportion of non-Hispanic whites is expected to decrease to 58.5% (Federal Interagency Forum on Aging-Related Statistics 2010).

In 1900, life expectancy in the United States was 48.3 years for females and 46.3 years for males, whereas in 2004, the life expectancy at birth was 80.4 years for females and 75.2 years for males. In 2004, a 65-year-old could expect to live an average of 18.7 more years, and a 75-year-old could expect to live 11.9 additional years (National Center for Health Statistics 2006). If an older person develops a psychiatric disorder, the disorder may become chronic, and the person may live many years with a decreased quality of life because of psychiatric morbidity. In addition, the great majority of older persons with psychiatric disorders experience a comorbid physical illness. Currently, the proportion of younger and middle-aged adults with a psychiatric disorder is higher than the proportion of older adults, suggesting that as the younger adults age, the proportion of older adults with a psychiatric disorder also may increase and create a potential crisis in geriatric mental health (Jeste et al. 1999).

Case Identification

Although most epidemiologists and clinicians agree on the core symptoms of psychiatric disorders throughout the life cycle, the absolute distinction between cases and noncases—that is, persons requiring psychiatric attention versus those who do not require such care—is not easily established. Many of the symptoms and signs of a psychiatric disorder in late life may be ubiquitous with the aging process, thus blurring the distinction between cases and noncases. Case identification is also the foundation of descriptive epidemiology: "cases" are the numerator of the equation from which *prevalence* (the proportion of disease that is present in the population during a specified period) and *incidence* (the proportion of new cases that develop in a population at risk over a specified period) estimates are derived in community and clinical samples (the denominator). For most clinicians, the goal of case identification is to identify subjects experiencing uniform underlying psychopathology, as is implicit in DSM-IV and DSM-IV-TR (American Psychiatric Association 1994, 2000).

One method of case identification is the use of diagnostic instruments. These instruments (usually standardized interviews) have been developed and used in community- and clinic-based epidemiological studies to identify persons with symptoms that meet these criteria. The Composite International Diagnostic Interview (CIDI;

World Health Organization 1990), the Structured Clinical Interview for DSM-IV (SCID; First et al. 1997), and the Diagnostic Interview Schedule (DIS; Robins et al. 1981) are examples of these diagnostic interview schedules.

For example, the World Mental Health Survey version of the CIDI was used in the National Comorbidity Survey Replication (NCS-R), which reported that the lifetime prevalence of major depressive disorder was 10.6% among those age 60 years and older compared with 15.4% among those ages 18–29, 19.8% among those ages 30–44, and 18.8% among those ages 45–59 (Kessler et al. 2005). The DIS was used in the landmark Epidemiologic Catchment Area (ECA) study conducted more than 25 years ago, from which a 1-month national estimate of the prevalence of affective disorders in persons age 65 years and older was 2.5% (compared with 6.4% for persons ages 25–44 years) (Regier et al. 1988).

A second approach to case identification is the use of self-administered symptom scales and personality inventories. Frequently used scales in epidemiological surveys include the Center for Epidemiologic Studies—Depression Scale (Radloff 1977) and the Geriatric Depression Scale (Yesavage et al. 1983), which screen for depressive symptoms, and the Short Portable Mental Status Questionnaire (Pfeiffer 1975) and the Mini-Mental State Examination (Folstein et al. 1975), which screen for cognitive impairment. The advantage of these scales is that, unlike diagnostic interviews, they do not subjectively assign patients to a particular diagnostic category; a disadvantage is the lack of diagnostic specificity that can be achieved with their use.

Regardless of the diagnostic system, unusual or borderline cases exist that cannot be clearly placed in a single category. Not infrequently, older adults manifest more than one disease simultaneously (e.g., major depression and dementia). In addition, the prescribed categories of DSM-IV-TR do not always match the symptoms that individuals in this population may be experiencing; generalized anxiety, for instance, is not always disentangled from a major depressive episode in an agitated older adult. Krishnan (2007) suggested that it may be advantageous to separate etiology from clinical manifestation in future classification of disease.

A diagnosis must be reliable and valid for it to be a useful means of communicating clinical information. To pass the test of reliability, a diagnosis must be consistent and repeatable. Standardized or operational methods for identifying psychiatric symptoms and the availability of specific criteria for psychiatric diagnoses have greatly improved the reliability of case identification by psychiatrists and by lay interviewers in psychiatric epidemiological surveys. Reliability, however, does not ensure validity—that is, the test of whether a case identified by a particular method reflects underlying reality (Blazer and Kaplan 2000).

Distribution of Psychiatric Disorders

Epidemiological studies of psychiatric impairment in older adults have generally concentrated on either overall mental health functioning or the distribution of specific psychiatric disorders in the population. Reports from these studies usually begin as general observations of the association of impairment or specific disorders to characteristics such as age, gender, race/

ethnicity, and socioeconomic status. Almost all epidemiological studies provide estimates of prevalence or incidence based on community samples of larger populations. One of the landmark studies of the prevalence of psychiatric disorders in the United States was the ECA survey. The National Institute of Mental Health established the ECA program to determine the prevalence of specific psychiatric disorders in both community and institutional populations (Regier et al. 1984). Data were collected in five communities, and the DIS was used to identify persons who met criteria for specific disorders. DIS diagnoses were based on DSM-III criteria (American Psychiatric Association 1980), the nomenclature in effect at the time the data were collected. More than 18,000 persons were interviewed in the ECA study, including 5,702 persons who were age 65 and older. All disorders, with the exception of cognitive impairment, were more prevalent in younger or middle-aged adults than in older adults. Of those age 65 and older, 12.3% (13.6% of the women and 10.5% of the men) met criteria for one or more psychiatric disorders in the month prior to the interview. The two most prevalent disorders in this age group were any anxiety disorder (5.5%) and severe cognitive impairment (4.9%) (Regier et al. 1988). The original National Comorbidity Survey (NCS) was conducted in a nationally representative sample in the United States from 1990 to 1992, enabling national estimates of the prevalence of DSM-III-R psychiatric disorders (American Psychiatric Association 1987); however, the sample included only people ages 15–54 years.

Two large-scale epidemiological surveys provide more recent estimates of lifetime and current prevalence of psychiatric disorders. The National Epidemiologic Survey on Alcohol and Related Conditions (NESARC) was sponsored by the National Institute on Alcohol Abuse and Alcoholism. From 2001 to 2002, in-person interviews were conducted with 43,093 participants age 18 years and older, and the data were weighted to represent the U.S. population at the time of the 2000 census, enabling national estimates of the prevalence of DSM-IV psychiatric disorders (Grant et al. 2005b). The diagnostic interview used was the Alcohol Use Disorder and Associated Disabilities Interview Schedule—DSM-IV Version (Grant et al. 2001). The World Health Organization (WHO) World Mental Health (WMH) surveys were conducted from 2001 to 2003 in 14 countries, and a total of 60,463 adults were interviewed (WHO World Mental Health Survey Consortium 2004). In the United States, the WMH survey was called the National Comorbidity Survey Replication (NCS-R) and included data from 9,282 adults age 18 years and older (Kessler et al. 2005). These large-scale studies have added to the rich data provided earlier by the ECA surveys and by numerous smaller studies conducted in various geographic locations.

Specific disorders are addressed in detail in subsequent chapters, but Tables 1–1 through 1–5 provide summaries of the prevalence of both psychiatric symptoms and disorders in both community and clinical populations derived from selected studies conducted in the United States and other countries over the last several decades.

The prevalence of cognitive impairment in selected community and institutional populations of older adults is presented in Table 1–1. Although the prevalence of cognitive impairment in community samples

TABLE 1–1. Prevalence of cognitive impairment in community and institutional populations of older adults

Authors	Sample	N	Age (years)	Prevalence
Trollor et al. 2007	Community, Australia	1,792	≥65	7.4%
Di Carlo et al. 2007	Community and institutional, Italy	2,830	65–84	9.5% CIND 16.1% MCI
Ganguli et al. 2004	Community, MoVIES	1,248	Mean age = 74.6	2.9%–4.0% amnestic MCI over 10 years
Lopez et al. 2003	Cardiovascular Health Study—Cognition Study[a]	2,470	≥65	19% MCI <75 years 29% MCI ≥85 years
Busse et al. 2003	Community, Germany	1,045	≥75	3.1% MCI 8.8% age–associated cognitive decline
Graham et al. 1997	Community and institution, Canadian Study of Health and Aging	2,914	≥65	16.8% CIND
Callahan et al. 1995	Primary care patients, Indiana	3,594	≥60	15.7%
Regier et al. 1988	Five U.S. communities, ECA	5,702	≥65	4.9% (2.9% ages 65–74; 6.8% ages 75–84; 15.8% ages ≥85)
Plassman et al. 2008	Community, ADAMS	856	>70	22.2% MCI/CIND

Note. ADAMS=Aging, Demographic and Memory Study; CIND=cognitive impairment, no dementia; ECA=Epidemiologic Catchment Area; MCI= mild cognitive impairment; MoVIES=Monongahela Valley Independent Elders Survey.
[a]Participants in the Cardiovascular Health Study were age 65 or older and were selected from Medicare eligibility lists in four U.S. communities (Fried et al. 1991).

may be as high as 8.8%, the prevalence in primary and residential care may be much higher. Since the late 1990s, much attention has focused on mild cognitive impairment, and studies listed in Table 1–1 report prevalence estimates ranging from 2% to 29% depending on the age group assessed and the research setting (community vs. institutional). Also, as shown in Table 1–1, studies conducted since 2003 have begun to focus on the prevalence of different subtypes of mild cognitive impairment.

Note that the studies in Table 1–1 reporting the prevalence of cognitive impairment measured cognitive function with standardized screening tests. Therefore, these studies do not report the prevalence of dementia or Alzheimer's disease or actual cerebral impairment, although some of the more recent studies have augmented their test results with imaging data (Lopez et al. 2003).

The prevalence of dementia and Alzheimer's disease in both community and institutional samples is shown in Table 1–2. Overall, the prevalence of dementia is lower than that of cognitive impairment or mild cognitive impairment and ranges from less than 1% to more than 17% in the community. The prevalence of dementia in primary care samples is higher than that observed in community samples and lower than that observed in long-term care samples, which often have a higher mean age.

In the East Boston, Massachusetts, Established Populations for Epidemiologic Studies of the Elderly (EPESE), the prevalence of probable Alzheimer's disease increased with age. Specifically, the prevalence was 3.0% in those ages 65–74 years, 18.7% in those ages 75–84 years, and 47.2% in those age 85 years and older (Evans et al. 1989). In recent years, research has focused

more on earlier stages of cognitive decline, such as mild cognitive impairment, than on the prevalence of subtypes of dementia (Panza et al. 2005) assessed with techniques such as imaging data (Feldman and Jacova 2005), resulting in fewer recent studies of the prevalence of Alzheimer's disease.

The prevalence of psychiatric symptoms in community samples of older adults is presented in Table 1–3. The most frequently reported symptoms are generally problems with sleep and feelings of anxiety. Psychotic symptoms are less prevalent in community samples than anxiety symptoms but may be as high as 10% in the oldest old. The prevalence of alcohol use in older adults is low, but the proportion of drinkers who drink in excess is greater than 19% (Saunders et al. 1989).

Numerous studies have reported a high prevalence of depressive symptoms among older adults. As shown in Table 1–3, the prevalence of depressive symptoms may be as high as 25% in community samples. The prevalence is even higher in residential care settings (Anstey et al. 2007) and is generally higher in females than in males (Copeland et al. 1999).

Across the entire life cycle, many psychiatric symptoms, especially hypochondriasis and sleep disorders, have their highest frequencies among elderly adults. A relatively high frequency of certain symptoms in elderly populations, however, does not necessarily signify an increased frequency of specific psychiatric disorders. The paradox of relatively high reports of depressive symptoms and relatively low reports of the prevalence of major depressive episodes illustrates this point (Blazer 1982). Symptoms, the most objective clinical indicators of psychopathology, may reflect more than one diagnostic entity. On the contrary,

TABLE 1–2. Prevalence of dementia and Alzheimer's disease in community and institutional populations

Authors	Sample	N	Age (years)	Prevalence
Stevens et al. 2002	Community, Islington, England	1,085	≥65	9.9% dementia *Among those with dementia:* 31.3% Alzheimer's disease 21.9% vascular dementia 10.9% dementia with Lewy bodies 7.8% frontal lobe dementia
Olafsdottir et al. 2001	Primary care center, Sweden	350	≥70	16.0% dementia
Riedel-Heller et al. 2001	Community, Leipzig, Germany (Leipzig Longitudinal Study of the Aged)	1,692	≥75	17.4% DSM-III-R dementia 12.4% ICD-10 dementia
Canadian Study of Health and Aging Working Group 1994	Canada	10,263	≥65	8.0% dementia 5.1% Alzheimer's disease
Evans et al. 1989	Community, East Boston EPESE	467	≥65	10.3% probable Alzheimer's disease
Bland et al. 1988	Community and institution, Edmonton, AB, Canada	358 community 199 institutional	≥65	*Severe cognitive impairment:* Community: 0.0% Institutional: 42% female; 36.1% male
Rovner et al. 1986	Institution, Maryland	50	Mean age=83	56% primary degenerative dementia 18% multi-infarct dementia 4% Parkinson's dementia
Plassman et al. 2007	Community, ADAMS	856	>70	13.9% dementia

Note. ADAMS = Aging, Demographic and Memory Study; EPESE = Established Populations for Epidemiologic Studies of the Elderly; ICD-10 = International Statistical Classification of Diseases and Related Health Problems, 10th Revision (World Health Organization 1992).

TABLE 1–3. Prevalence of psychiatric symptoms in community populations of older adults

Authors	Sample	N	Age (years)	Symptoms/syndrome	Prevalence
Anstey et al. 2007	Australia	1,116	≥65	Depressive symptoms	14.4% community; 32% institutional
Copeland et al. 1999	EURODEP	13,808	≥65	Cases/subcases of depression	12.3%: 8.6% male; 14.1% female
Black et al. 1998	Hispanic EPESE	2,823	≥65	Depressive symptoms	25.6%: 17.3% male; 31.9% female
Beekman et al. 1995	LASA	3,056	55–85	Minor depression	12.9%
Cornoni-Huntley et al. 1986	New Haven, Connecticut, EPESE	2,811	≥65	Depressive symptoms	15.1%
Ostling and Skoog 2002	Sweden	347	≥85	Psychotic symptoms	10.1% (5.5% delusions; 6.9% hallucinations; 6.9% paranoid ideation)
Livingston et al. 2001	Islington, England	720	≥65	Persecutory symptoms and perceptual disturbance	3.9%
Blazer and Houpt 1979	North Carolina	997	≥65	Hypochondriasis	14%
Cornoni-Huntley et al. 1986	Iowa EPESE	3,673	≥65	Trouble falling asleep Awakening during night Daytime sleepiness	14.1% 33.7% 30.7%
Thomas and Rockwood 2001	Canadian Study of Health and Aging	2,873	≥65	Alcohol abuse Questionable alcohol abuse	8.9% 3.7%
Saunders et al. 1989	Liverpool, England	1,070	≥65	Drinkers exceeding sensible limits	19.6% females; 19.5% males
Forsell and Winblad 1998	Stockholm, Sweden	966	≥78	Feelings of anxiety	24.4%

Note. EPESE = Established Populations for Epidemiologic Studies of the Elderly; EURODEP = European Concerted Action on Depression of Older People; LASA = Longitudinal Aging Studies Amsterdam.

symptoms may not be associated with any disorder of interest to the clinician. For example, decreased appetite can result from several sources. At a given time, grief reactions, more frequent in late life than at other stages of the life cycle, may be virtually indistinguishable from major depressive episodes if appetite alone is considered. Loss of appetite also accompanies major life adjustments such as a forced change of residence or a decline in economic resources. Most commonly, loss of appetite in late life is a result of poor physical health.

The prevalence of selected psychiatric disorders in community populations, shown in Table 1–4, is lower than the prevalence of related psychiatric symptoms (see Table 1–3). The disorder with the highest 12-month prevalence among participants age 65 years and older reported from the NESARC was specific phobia (7.5%; Stinson et al. 2007), whereas the disorder with the highest lifetime prevalence was any alcohol use disorder (16.1%; Hasin et al. 2007). In the NCS-R, the disorder with the highest lifetime prevalence among participants age 60 years or older was major depression (10.6%; Kessler et al. 2005). The presentation of studies in Table 1–4 provides an opportunity to note several important points to consider when comparing prevalence estimates across studies. Lifetime prevalence is generally higher than but can be equal to point prevalence. Similarly, prevalence is dependent on both the incidence and the duration of the disorder within the period of risk, so 12-month prevalence is generally higher than 1-month prevalence. Prevalence estimates also can vary depending on the diagnostic instruments used (which may explain in part the differences between the lifetime prevalence estimates reported in the NCS-R and the NESARC).

As shown in Table 1–4, the current prevalence of major depression reported from these studies ranges from 0.7% reported from the ECA (Regier et al. 1988) to 3% reported from a survey in France (Ritchie et al. 2004) and somewhat higher in the Cache County (Utah) survey (Steffens et al. 2000). Overall, the findings are fairly consistent, with prevalence estimates from the rest of the studies presented falling within that range of 1%–3%. The prevalence is higher in older females than in males (Regier et al. 1988; Steffens et al. 2000). The current prevalence of anxiety disorders is higher than that of major depression, and the estimates depend in part on whether specific phobia is included. As shown in Table 1–4, the prevalence of individual disorders is highest for phobic disorders (3%–10%) and lowest for panic disorder (<1%). The prevalence of generalized anxiety disorder is approximately 1%–2.2%. The prevalence of any anxiety disorder among adults age 65 years or older in the ECA studies was 5.5%, with a higher prevalence in females (6.8%) than in males (3.6%) (Regier et al. 1988). The current prevalence of alcohol abuse or dependence is low (0.1%–1.5%) (Regier et al. 1988; Trollor et al. 2007), with higher lifetime prevalence. Similarly, the 1-month prevalence of schizophrenia among persons age 65 years or older in the ECA was 0.1% (Regier et al. 1988).

Overall, psychiatric disorders are found at a lower prevalence among elderly people than in people at other stages of the life cycle. In the ECA, the 1-month prevalence of any DIS disorder (including cognitive impairment) was 16.9% in those ages 18–24 years, 17.3% in those ages 25–44 years, 13.3% in those ages 45–64 years, and 12.3% in those age 65 years and older (Regier et al.

TABLE 1–4. Prevalence of selected psychiatric disorders in community populations of older adults

Authors	Sample	N	Age	Disorder	Period	Prevalence
Hasin et al. 2007	National Epidemiologic Survey on Alcoholism and Related Conditions	8,205 ≥65 (from total U.S. representative sample of 43,093)	≥65	Alcohol use disorder	12 months Lifetime	1.5% 16.1%
Hasin et al. 2005	National Epidemiologic Survey on Alcoholism and Related Conditions	8,205 ≥65 (from total U.S. representative sample of 43,093)	≥65	Major depression	12 months Lifetime	2.7% 8.2%
Grant et al. 2006	National Epidemiologic Survey on Alcoholism and Related Conditions	8,205 ≥65 (from total U.S. representative sample of 43,093)	≥65	Panic disorder	12 months Lifetime	0.8% 2.8%
Grant et al. 2005a	National Epidemiologic Survey on Alcoholism and Related Conditions	8,205 ≥65 (from total U.S. representative sample of 43,093)	≥65	Social anxiety disorder	12 months Lifetime	1.6% 3.0%
Grant et al. 2005b	National Epidemiologic Survey on Alcoholism and Related Conditions	8,205 ≥65 (from total U.S. representative sample of 43,093)	≥65	Generalized anxiety disorder	12 months Lifetime	1.0% 2.6%
Stinson et al. 2007	National Epidemiologic Survey on Alcoholism and Related Conditions	8,205 ≥65 (from total U.S. representative sample of 43,093)	≥65	Specific phobia	12 months	7.5%

TABLE 1–4. Prevalence of selected psychiatric disorders in community populations of older adults (*continued*)

Authors	Sample	N	Age	Disorder	Period	Prevalence
Trollor et al. 2007	Australian National Mental Health and Well-Being Survey	1,792	≥65	Major depression	1 month	1.2%
				Dysthymia		0.2%
				Panic disorder/agoraphobia		0.3%
				Social phobia		0.1%
				Generalized anxiety disorder		0.8%
				Posttraumatic stress disorder		0.2%
				Alcohol abuse/dependence		0.3%
Kessler et al. 2005	National Comorbidity Survey Replication	1,837 ≥60 (from total U.S. representative sample of 9,282)	≥60	Major depression	Lifetime	10.6%
				Dysthymia		1.3%
				Panic disorder		2.0%
				Agoraphobia without panic		1.0%
				Specific phobia		7.5%
				Social phobia		6.6%
				Generalized anxiety disorder		3.6%
				Posttraumatic stress disorder		2.5%
				Obsessive–compulsive disorder		0.7%
				Alcohol abuse		6.2%
				Alcohol dependence		2.2%
Ritchie et al. 2004	Montpelier district of France	1,873	≥65	Anxiety disorders	Current	14.2%
				Phobia		10.7%
				Major depression		3.0%
				Psychosis		1.7%

TABLE 1–4. Prevalence of selected psychiatric disorders in community populations of older adults (*continued*)

Authors	Sample	N	Age	Disorder	Period	Prevalence
ESEMeD/ MHEDEA 2000 Investigators 2004	European Study of the Epidemiology of Mental Disorders (ESEMeD)	4,401 age ≥65 (from total sample of 21,425)	≥65	Any mood disorder Any anxiety disorder Any alcohol disorder	12 months	3.2% 3.6% 0.1%
Steffens et al. 2000	Cache County (UT) study	4,559	≥65	Major depression	Current	4.4% female; 2.7% male
Beekman et al. 1995	LASA	3,056	55–85	Major depression	Current	2.0%
Blazer et al. 1991	Durham, North Carolina, ECA	784	≥65	Generalized anxiety disorder	12 months	2.2%
Lindesay et al. 1989	Guy's/Age Concern Survey	890	≥65	Phobic disorder	Current	10.0%
Bland et al. 1988	Edmonton, AB, Canada	358	≥65	Major depression Phobic disorder Panic disorder	Current	1.2% 3.0% 0.3%
Regier et al. 1988	ECA in five U.S. communities	5,702 age ≥65 (from total sample of 18,571)	≥65	Major depression Dysthymia Any anxiety disorder Phobic disorder Schizophrenia Alcohol abuse/dependence	1 month	0.7% 1.8% 5.5% 4.8% 0.1% 0.9%

Note.   ECA = Epidemiologic Catchment Area; LASA = Longitudinal Aging Studies Amsterdam.

1988). The virtual absence of alcohol abuse or dependence and of schizophrenia in those age 65 and older may reflect selective mortality. It also may reflect changes in drinking patterns (the lifetime prevalence in the NESARC was 16.1% compared with a 12-month prevalence of 1.5%) (Hasin et al. 2007) or the case finding techniques used because the community data do not include persons in institutions. Another question derives from these data: Do unique late-life symptom presentations render the DSM-IV-TR inadequate as a system of nomenclature? DSM-IV-TR provides age-specific categories for children but not for elderly persons. Yet no compelling evidence exists for developing a new classification specific to older adults. The deficiency inherent in DSM-IV-TR is that it poorly differentiates psychiatric symptoms from symptoms that signify the presence of physical illness and impaired cognition—a situation that also may occur in younger individuals, although it is far more common as a diagnostic problem in late life than in middle life.

The prevalence of psychiatric symptoms and disorders, especially major depression, in treatment settings is presented in Table 1–5. The prevalence of major depression in nursing homes or long-term care facilities is estimated to be 6.0%–14.4%, and the prevalence of minor depression is estimated to be as high as 30.5%. As shown in Table 1–5, the prevalence of major depression in both acute-care hospitals and primary care is higher than that found in the community. Many older adults may be selectively admitted to medical inpatient units or long-term care facilities (because older adults are less likely to use specialty psychiatric care). The lower prevalence in the community, therefore, should not lull clinicians into believing that psychiatric problems are of little consequence to older adults.

Fewer data regarding the incidence of psychiatric disorders in late life are available because most disorders begin early in adulthood. In a study of 875 nondepressed older adults with a mean age of 85 years, the 3-year incidence of depression was 4.1% (Forsell and Winblad 1999). Henderson et al. (1997) reported that the 3- to 6-year incidence of depression in a sample of community-dwelling elders age 70 or older was 2.5%. The 2-year incidence of depression defined by the Geriatric Depression Scale (not necessarily first-onset) was 8.4% in adults age 65 and older in a community sample in London (Harris et al. 2006). Incidence of depression appears to rise with age and differ by gender. In a Swedish population of adults followed up from age 70 to age 85, the incidence of first-onset depression was 12 per 1,000 person-years for men and 30 per 1,000 person-years for women (Palsson et al. 2001). The incidence of schizophrenia among older adults is estimated to be 3 per 100,000 persons per year for new cases (Copeland et al. 1998). The incidence of dementia also increases with age. Bachman et al. (1993) reported from the Framingham data that the 5-year incidence of dementia was 7 per 1,000 in those ages 65–69 and 118 per 1,000 at ages 85–89. A similar increase with age in the 1-year incidence of Alzheimer's disease was reported from the East Boston EPESE: 0.6% in those ages 65–69 years and 8.4% in those age 85 or older (Hebert et al. 1995). The 1-year incidence (per 100 person-years) reported from the ECA among those age 65 years or older was 1.25 for major depression, 0.04 for panic disorder, 4.29 for phobic disorder, and 0.63 for alcohol abuse or dependence (Eaton et al. 1989).

TABLE 1–5. Prevalence of selected psychiatric symptoms and disorders among older adults in selected treatment settings

Authors	Sample	N	Age (years)	Disorder	Prevalence
McCusker et al. 2005	Two acute-care hospitals	380	≥65	Major depression Minor depression	14.2%–44.5% 7.9%–9.4%
Smalbrugge et al. 2005	AGED study nursing home patients on somatic wards	333	≥55	Any anxiety disorder Subthreshold anxiety disorder Anxiety symptoms	5.7% 4.2% 29.7%
Jongenelis et al. 2004	AGED study nursing home patients on somatic wards	333	≥55	Major depression Minor depression Subclinical depression	8.1% 14.1% 24.0%
Sheehan et al. 2003	Primary care	140	≥65	Hypochondriacal neurosis	5.0%
Kvaal et al. 2001	Geriatric inpatients	98	≥70	Anxiety symptoms	47% male; 41% female
Teresi et al. 2001	Nursing homes	319	Mean=84.5	Major depression	14.4%
Lyness et al. 1999	Primary care	224	≥60	Major depression Minor depression	6.5% 5.2%
Parmelee et al. 1989	Nursing homes and congregate housing	708	Mean=84	Major depression Minor depression	12.4% 30.5%
Koenig et al. 1988	Acute-care facility	171	≥70	Major depression Other depressive syndromes	11.5% 23.0%
Rovner et al. 1986	Intermediate-care facility	50	Mean=83	Major depression	6.0%

Note. AGED = Amsterdam Groningen Elderly Depression.

Etiological Studies

Within geriatric psychiatry, it is important to identify factors that can either predispose individuals to developing psychiatric disorders or precipitate recurrence of such disorders. These disorders may have their initial onset in late life, or the disorders may have an early onset and recur later in life. Other factors can be identified that are associated with the prevalence of a disorder, but the antecedent-consequent relation has not been established. For practical purposes in this discussion, we identify all of these as risk factors. These factors generally fall into several categories, including genetic or biological factors, environmental or chemical factors, and social factors. In addition, the presence of a comorbid physical or mental condition or disorder often leads to the development of psychiatric symptoms or another disorder, and these are described in chapters related to specific disorders throughout this textbook.

Genetic research in Alzheimer's disease and dementia, for example, has primarily focused on the ε4 allele of the apolipoprotein E (*APOE*) gene (Evans et al. 1997; Saunders et al. 1993). That is, the ε4 allele is a susceptibility gene in that some (but not all) persons with the allele develop dementia. Some studies also have found a relation between the *APOE*E3 and *APOE*E4 alleles and the onset of late-life depression (Krishnan et al. 1996), whereas other studies did not find a link between genotype and change in the number of depressive symptoms (Mauricio et al. 2000). Current research that focuses on the interaction between genetic and environmental factors and the occurrence of disease (Hernandez and Blazer 2006) can potentially offer new information on the etiology of psychiatric

disorders. One example of a possible gene-environment interaction is evident in Hendrie et al.'s (2004) work in Indianapolis, Indiana, and Ibadan, Nigeria. Hendrie et al. reported a significant association between *APOE*E4 and Alzheimer's disease in African Americans in Indianapolis, but the alleles were not associated with an increased risk for Alzheimer's disease among Yoruba living in Ibadan, suggesting that an interaction between gene and environment may play a role in the etiology of the disease. Gatz et al. (1992) studied genetic and environmental contributions to self-reported depressive symptoms in older adults in a sample of twin pairs. Genetic influence accounted for 16% of the variance in depression scores and 19% of the variance in psychomotor and somatic complaints; however, heritability was minimal for depressed mood and well-being. Although shared experiences contributed to the variance, the most important correlate of late-life depressive symptoms was nonshared experiences.

Environmental or chemical factors also may lead to cognitive problems and other psychiatric symptoms. For example, epidemiological studies have suggested that head trauma or elevated levels of aluminum and other metals such as copper, zinc, and iron in the brain may be risk factors for the development or progression of Alzheimer's disease (Mortimer et al. 1991; Shcherbatykh and Carpenter 2007), whereas the use of estrogen has been shown to be protective (Kawas et al. 1997).

By far, the most frequently investigated environmental factors associated with psychiatric disorders are social factors. Many investigators believe that the changing roles and circumstances of older adults can cause stress and thereby contribute to the onset of psychiatric disorders and cognitive difficulties. In a study of 986 community-dwelling older adults, Blazer (1980) found a twofold risk for mental health impairment given the recent experience of life events. In a study of individuals age 55 years and older, Murrell et al. (1983) found that social factors, including widowhood, divorce, separation, and decreased income, were related to depressive symptomatology in the community. In the Hispanic EPESE, economic stressors and conditions such as chronic financial strain were associated with depressive symptoms in Mexican American elders (Black et al. 1998).

In the Longitudinal Aging Study Amsterdam, major depression was associated with unmarried status, functional limitation, perceived loneliness, internal locus of control, poorer self-perceived health, and lack of instrumental social support (Beekman et al. 1995). In the Duke ECA study, recent negative life events and poor social support were associated with major depression (Blazer et al. 1987). Perceived health and loneliness were also some of the correlates of depressive symptoms in the Leiden 85-plus study (Stek et al. 2004). Depression also has been linked with variables suggesting increased dependency (Anstey et al. 2007). Impairment or dissatisfaction with one's social network has been reported to be associated with anxiety symptoms in late life (Forsell and Winblad 1998). Nevertheless, the study of social factors in relation to psychiatric disorders must not be viewed simplistically. The mitigating effect of social support, the perception of a stressful life event (as well as the actual occurrence of the event), the expectancy of an event, and the perceived importance of an event all may contribute to the effect of environmental stress on the older adult.

Epidemiological research also has focused on the effect of contextual factors such as the poverty level or residential stability of the neighborhood and the prevalence of psychiatric disorders. More than 70 years ago, Faris and Dunham (1939) looked at the addresses of psychiatric patients and found that patients with schizophrenia and substance use disorders tended to have addresses in areas within Chicago, Illinois, that were more deteriorated and disorganized than the neighborhoods of those patients with affective disorders. But these and similar findings were subject to "ecologic fallacy" or drawing conclusions about individuals from group data. Improved statistical software has made the process of separating individual and contextual effects easier, and more recent studies have explored the association between neighborhood characteristics and psychiatric symptoms in older adults. For example, on the basis of data from the New Haven EPESE, Kubzansky et al. (2005) reported that living in a poor neighborhood increased the risk of depressive symptoms beyond that attributed to individual vulnerabilities and that the presence of more older adults in the neighborhood was protective.

From these examples, it is clear that both psychiatric disorders and psychiatric symptoms in late life can have multiple causes and that these factors may interact with one another to produce adverse outcomes. Skoog (2004) suggested that the science of epidemiology has much to contribute to increased knowledge of the etiology of mental disorders in older adults and that to maximize that contribution, future population studies should be longitudinal and should include assessments of psychosocial risk factors and biological markers such as brain imaging, neurochemical analyses, and genetic information.

Health Service Use

Community-based epidemiological studies provide an opportunity not only to estimate the prevalence of psychiatric disorders but also to examine service use among those with psychiatric symptoms or disorders. In the NCS-R, participants age 60 years and older were less likely than those in younger age groups to receive any mental health treatment in the last 12 months. Among those who received treatment, those age 60 years and older were less likely to receive treatment in the health care setting and, among those who did receive treatment in the health care setting, less likely to receive treatment in a mental health specialty (Wang et al. 2005b). Being in an older cohort was also associated with failure to make initial contact for mental health treatment after initial onset of the disorder and with delay among those who eventually made treatment contact (Wang et al. 2005a). One study reported that older adults who met criteria for a psychiatric disorder were less likely than younger adults to perceive a need for mental health care, to receive specialty mental health care or counseling, and to receive referrals from primary care to mental health specialty care (Klap et al. 2003). Older patients seen in primary care who receive a diagnosis of depression are more likely to have increased total ambulatory costs, tests, and consultations than are older primary care patients without this diagnosis (Luber et al. 2001).

In contrast to less treatment use by older adults than younger adults, the use of psychotropic drugs is high among older adults. Hanlon et al. (1992) found that 12.5% of community-dwelling persons older than 65 years during 1986 were taking central nervous system drugs, and psychotropic medications were the second most frequently used therapeutic class of medication. Even though a high proportion of older adults uses psychotropic medications, their disorders, such as depression, remain untreated. Unutzer et al. (2000) found in a study of health maintenance organization enrollees that 4%–7% of the older adults received treatment for depression but that most individuals with probable depression did not receive treatment. Similarly, Steffens et al. (2000) found in the Cache County study that only 35.7% of the older adults with major depression were taking antidepressants, and 27.4% of those with major depression were taking sedative-hypnotic medications.

By sampling elderly community-dwelling populations, researchers can collect data on the proportion of older adults with impairment, those with a need or a perceived need for services, and the current use of services. This information can be used by government and private agencies to chart effective assessment, treatment, and prevention patterns. This development is especially relevant to the care of older adults because they tend to be isolated, their psychiatric impairment may be masked, and they are less active advocates for their mental health needs than are younger persons. In summary, community studies of older adults have shown that the prevalence rates of psychiatric disorders and psychiatric symptoms in older adults are significant, and this has implications for all types of health service use.

Key Points

- The proportion of older adults in the United States is expected to increase dramatically over the next 50 years and to be accompanied by an increase in the number of older adults with psychiatric disorders.

- The prevalence of clinically significant psychiatric symptoms is generally higher than the prevalence of psychiatric disorders, and the prevalence of both symptoms and disorders is higher in clinical samples than in community samples. Psychiatric syndromes, rather than disorders, are the more realistic diagnostic entities in geriatric psychiatry.

- Alzheimer's disease is the most prevalent form of dementia, and its prevalence increases with age.

- Sleep problems, anxiety symptoms, and depressive symptoms are the most prevalent psychiatric symptoms among older adults.

- Besides dementia, anxiety disorders (particularly phobic disorders) are the most prevalent psychiatric disorders in older adults in community samples.

- Genetic, environmental, and social factors, as well as their interaction, can predispose individuals to psychiatric disorders in late life or be risk factors for the recurrence of psychiatric symptoms.

- Older adults are less likely than younger adults to seek treatment for mental health problems, and if treatment is sought, it is likely to be within the primary care setting.

- Even though a high proportion of older adults uses psychotropic medications, psychiatric disorders, particularly depression, are generally untreated in older persons.

References

American Psychiatric Association: Diagnostic and Statistical Manual of Mental Disorders, 3rd Edition. Washington, DC, American Psychiatric Association, 1980

American Psychiatric Association: Diagnostic and Statistical Manual of Mental Disorders, 3rd Edition, Revised. Washington, DC, American Psychiatric Association, 1987

American Psychiatric Association: Diagnostic and Statistical Manual of Mental Disorders, 4th Edition. Washington, DC, American Psychiatric Association, 1994

American Psychiatric Association: Diagnostic and Statistical Manual of Mental Disorders, 4th Edition, Text Revision. Washington, DC, American Psychiatric Association, 2000

Anstey KJ, von Sanden C, Sargent-Cox K, et al: Prevalence and risk factors for depression in a longitudinal, population-based study including individuals in the community and residential care. Am J Geriatr Psychiatry 15:497–505, 2007

Bachman DL, Wolf PA, Linn RT, et al: Incidence of dementia and probable Alzheimer's disease in a general population: the Framingham study. Neurology 43:515–519, 1993

Beekman ATF, Deeg DJH, van Tilberg T, et al: Major and minor depression in later life: a study of prevalence and risk factors. J Affect Disord 36:65–75, 1995

Black SA, Markides KS, Miller TQ: Correlates of depressive symptomatology among older community-dwelling Mexican Americans: the Hispanic EPESE. J Gerontol B Psychol Sci Soc Sci 53B:S198–S208, 1998

Bland RC, Newman SC, Orn H: Prevalence of psychiatric disorders in the elderly in Edmonton. Acta Psychiatr Scand 77 (suppl 338):57–63, 1988

Blazer DG: Life events, mental health functioning and the use of health care services by the elderly. Am J Public Health 70:1174–1179, 1980

Blazer DG: The epidemiology of late life depression. J Am Geriatr Soc 30:587–592, 1982

Blazer DG, Houpt JL: Perception of poor health in the healthy older adult. J Am Geriatr Soc 27:330–334, 1979

Blazer D, Kaplan B: Controversies in community-based psychiatric epidemiology. Arch Gen Psychiatry 57:227–228, 2000

Blazer D, Hughes DC, George LK: The epidemiology of depression in an elderly community population. Gerontologist 27:281–287, 1987

Blazer D, Hughes D, George L: Generalized anxiety disorder, in Psychiatric Disorders in America: The Epidemiologic Catchment Area Study. Edited by Robins L, Regier D. New York, Free Press, 1991, pp 180–203

Busse A, Bischkopf J, Riedel-Heller SG, et al: Mild cognitive impairment: prevalence and incidence according to different diagnostic criteria: results of the Leipzig Longitudinal Study of the Aged (LEILA 75+). Br J Psychiatry 182:449–454, 2003

Callahan CM, Hendrie HC, Tierney WM: Documentation and evaluation of cognitive impairment in elderly primary care patients. Ann Intern Med 122:422–429, 1995

Canadian Study of Health and Aging Working Group: Canadian Study of Health and Aging: study methods and prevalence of dementia. CMAJ 150:899–913, 1994

Copeland JRM, Dewey ME, Scott A, et al: Schizophrenia and delusional disorder in older age: community prevalence, incidence, comorbidity, and outcome. Schizophr Bull 24:153–161, 1998

Copeland JRM, Beekman ATF, Dewey ME, et al: Depression in Europe: geographic distribution among older people. Br J Psychiatry 174:312–321, 1999

Cornoni-Huntley J, Brock D, Ostfeld A, et al: Established Populations for Epidemiologic Studies of the Elderly: Resource Data Book (NIH Publ No 86-2443). Bethesda, MD, National Institutes of Health, 1986

Di Carlo A, Lamassa M, Baldereschi M, et al: CIND and MCI in the Italian elderly: frequency, vascular risk factors, progression to dementia. Neurology 68:1909–1916, 2007

Eaton WW, Kramer M, Anthony JC, et al: The incidence of specific DIS/DSM-III mental disorders: data from the NIMH Epidemiologic Catchment Area program. Acta Psychiatr Scand 79:163–178, 1989

ESEMeD/MHEDEA 2000 Investigators: Prevalence of mental disorders in Europe: results from the European Study of the Epidemiology of Mental Disorders (ESEMeD) project. Acta Psychiatr Scand 109 (suppl 420):21–27, 2004

Evans DA, Funkenstein HH, Albert MS, et al: Prevalence of Alzheimer's disease in a community population of older persons: higher than previously reported. JAMA 262:2551–2556, 1989

Evans DA, Beckett LA, Field T, et al: Apolipoprotein E ε4 and incidence of Alzheimer's disease in a community population of older persons. JAMA 277:822–824, 1997

Faris RE, Dunham HW: Mental Disorders in Urban Areas: An Ecological Study of Schizophrenia and Other Psychoses. Chicago, IL, University of Chicago Press, 1939

Federal Interagency Forum on Aging-Related Statistics: Older Americans Update 2010: Key Indicators of Well-Being. Washington, DC, U.S. Government Printing Office, 2010

Feldman HH, Jacova C: Mild cognitive impairment. Am J Geriatr Psychiatry 13:645–655, 2005

First MB, Spitzer RL, Gibbon M, et al: Structured Clinical Interview for DSM-IV Axis I Disorders, Research Version. Washington, DC, American Psychiatric Association, 1997

Folstein MF, Folstein SE, McHugh P: "Mini-mental state": a practical method for grading the cognitive state of patients for clinicians. J Psychiatr Res 12:189–198, 1975

Forsell Y, Winblad B: Feelings of anxiety and associated variables in a very elderly population. Int J Geriatr Psychiatry 13:454–458, 1998

Forsell Y, Winblad B: Incidence of major depression in a very elderly population. Int J Geriatr Psychiatry 14:368–372, 1999

Fried LP, Borhani NO, Enright P, et al: The Cardiovascular Health Study: design and rationale. Ann Epidemiol 1:263–276, 1991

Ganguli M, Dodge HH, Shen C, et al: Mild cognitive impairment, amnestic type: an epidemiologic study. Neurology 63:115–121, 2004

Gatz M, Pedersen N, Plomin R, et al: Importance of shared genes and shared environments for symptoms of depression in older adults. J Abnorm Psychol 101:701–708, 1992

Graham JE, Rockwood K, Beattie BL, et al: Prevalence and severity of cognitive impairment with and without dementia in an elderly population. Lancet 349:1793–1796, 1997

Grant BF, Dawson DA, Hasin DS: The Alcohol Use Disorder and Associated Disabilities Interview Schedule DSM-IV. Bethesda, MD, National Institute on Alcohol Abuse and Alcoholism, 2001

Grant BF, Hasin DS, Blanco C, et al: The epidemiology of social anxiety disorder in the United States: results from the National Epidemiologic Survey on Alcohol and Related Conditions. J Clin Psychiatry 66:1351–1361, 2005a

Grant BF, Hasin DS, Stinson FS, et al: Prevalence, correlates, co-morbidity, and comparative disability of DSM-IV generalized anxiety disorder in the USA: results from the National Epidemiologic Survey on Alcohol and Related Conditions. Psychol Med 35:1747–1759, 2005b

Grant BF, Hasin DS, Stinson FS, et al: The epidemiology of DSM-IV panic disorder and agoraphobia in the United States: results from the National Epidemiologic Survey on Alcohol and Related Conditions. J Clin Psychiatry 67:363–374, 2006

Hanlon JT, Fillenbaum GG, Burchett B, et al: Drug-use patterns among black and non-black community-dwelling elderly. Ann Pharmacother 26:679–685, 1992

Harris T, Cook DG, Victor C, et al: Onset and persistence of depression in older people: results from a 2-year community follow-up study. Age Ageing 35:25–32, 2006

Hasin DS, Goodwin RD, Stinson FS, et al: Epidemiology of major depressive disorder: results from the National Epidemiologic Survey on Alcohol and Related Conditions. Arch Gen Psychiatry 62:1097–1106, 2005

Hasin DS, Stinson FS, Ogburn E, et al: Prevalence, correlates, disability, and comorbidity of DSM-IV alcohol abuse and dependence in the United States: results from the National Epidemiologic Survey on Alcohol and Related Conditions. Arch Gen Psychiatry 64:830–842, 2007

Hebert LE, Scherr PA, Beckett LA, et al: Age-specific incidence of Alzheimer's disease in a community population. JAMA 273:1354–1359, 1995

Henderson AS, Korten AE, Jacomb PA, et al: The course of depression in the elderly: a longitudinal community-based study in Australia. Psychol Med 27:119–129, 1997

Hendrie HC, Hall KS, Ogunniyi A, et al: Alzheimer's disease, genes, and environment: the value of international studies. Can J Psychiatry 49:92–99, 2004

Hernandez LM, Blazer DG: Beyond the Nature/Nurture Debate: Connecting Genes, Behavior, and the Social Environment. Washington, DC, National Academies Press, 2006

Jeste DV, Alexopoulos GS, Bartels SJ, et al: Consensus statement on the upcoming crisis in geriatric mental health. Arch Gen Psychiatry 56:848–853, 1999

Jongenelis K, Pot AM, Eisses AMH, et al: Prevalence and risk indicators of depression in elderly nursing home patients: the AGED study. J Affect Disord 83:135–142, 2004

Kawas C, Resnick S, Morrison A, et al: A prospective study of estrogen replacement therapy and the risk of developing Alzheimer's disease: the Baltimore Longitudinal Study of Aging. Neurology 48:1517–1521, 1997

Kessler RC, Berglund P, Demler O, et al: Lifetime prevalence and age-of-onset distributions of DSM-IV disorders in the National Comorbidity Survey Replication. Arch Gen Psychiatry 62:593–602, 2005

Klap R, Unroe KT, Unutzer J: Caring for mental illness in the United States: a focus on older adults. Am J Geriatr Psychiatry 11:517–524, 2003

Koenig HG, Meador KG, Cohen HJ, et al: Depression in elderly hospitalized patients with medical illness. Arch Intern Med 148:1929–1936, 1988

Krishnan KRR: Concept of disease in geriatric psychiatry. Am J Geriatr Psychiatry 15:1–11, 2007

Krishnan KRR, Tupler LA, Ritchie JC, et al: Apolipoprotein E ε4 frequency in geriatric depression. Biol Psychiatry 40:69–71, 1996

Kubzansky LD, Subramanian SV, Kawachi I, et al: Neighborhood contextual influences on depressive symptoms in the elderly. Am J Epidemiol 162:253–260, 2005

Kvaal K, Macijauskiene J, Engedal K, et al: High prevalence of anxiety symptoms in hospitalized geriatric patients. Int J Geriatr Psychiatry 16:690–693, 2001

Lindesay J, Briggs K, Murphy E: The Guy's/Age Concern Survey: prevalence rates of cognitive impairment, depression and anxiety in an urban elderly community. Br J Psychiatry 155:317–329, 1989

Livingston G, Kitchen G, Manela M, et al: Persecutory symptoms and perceptual disturbance in a community sample of older people: the Islington study. Int J Geriatr Psychiatry 16:462–468, 2001

Lopez OL, Jagust WJ, DeKosky ST, et al: Prevalence and classification of mild cognitive impairment in the Cardiovascular Health Study Cognition Study. Arch Neurol 60:1385–1389, 2003

Luber MP, Meyers BS, Williams-Russo PG, et al: Depression and service utilization in elderly primary care patients. Am J Geriatr Psychiatry 9:169–176, 2001

Lyness JM, King DA, Cox C, et al: The importance of subsyndromal depression in older primary care patients: prevalence and associated functional disability. J Am Geriatr Soc 47:647–652, 1999

Mauricio M, O'Hara R, Yesavage JA, et al: A longitudinal study of apolipoprotein-E genotype and depressive symptoms in community-dwelling older adults. Am J Geriatr Psychiatry 8:196–200, 2000

McCusker J, Cole M, Dufouil C, et al: The prevalence and correlates of major and minor depression in older medical inpatients. J Am Geriatr Soc 53:1344–1353, 2005

Mortimer JA, van Duijn CM, Chandra V, et al: Head trauma as a risk factor for Alzheimer's disease: a collaborative re-analysis of case-control studies: EURODEM Risk Factors Research Group. Int J Epidemiol 20 (suppl 2):S28–S35, 1991

Murrell SA, Himmelfarb S, Wright K: Prevalence of depression and its correlates in older adults. Am J Epidemiol 117:173–185, 1983

National Center for Health Statistics: Health, United States 2006 With Chartbook on Trends in the Health of Americans. Hyattsville, MD, National Center for Health Statistics, 2006

Olafsdottir M, Marcusson J, Skoog I: Mental disorders among elderly people in primary care: the Linkoping study. Acta Psychiatr Scand 104:12–18, 2001

Ostling S, Skoog I: Psychotic symptoms and paranoid ideation in a nondemented population-based sample of the very old. Arch Gen Psychiatry 59:53–59, 2002

Palsson SP, Ostling S, Skoog I: The incidence of first-onset depression in a population followed from the age of 70 to 85. Psychol Med 31:1159–1168, 2001

Panza F, D'Introno A, Colacicco AM, et al: Current epidemiology of mild cognitive impairment and other predementia syndromes. Am J Geriatr Psychiatry 13:633–644, 2005

Parmelee PA, Katz IR, Lawton MP: Depression among institutionalized aged: assessment and prevalence estimation. J Gerontol A Biol Sci Med Sci 44:M22–M29, 1989

Pfeiffer E: A short portable mental status questionnaire for the assessment of organic brain deficit in elderly patients. J Am Geriatr Soc 23:433–441, 1975

Plassman BL, Langa KM, Fisher GG, et al: Prevalence of dementia in the United States: the Aging, Demographics, and Memory Study. Neuroepidemiology 29:125–132, 2007

Plassman BL, Langa KM, Fisher GG, et al: Prevalence of cognitive impairment without dementia in the United States. Ann Intern Med 148:427–434, 2008

Radloff LS: The CES-D scale: a self-report depression scale for research in the general population. Applied Psychological Measurement 1:385–401, 1977

Regier DA, Myers JK, Kramer M, et al: The NIMH Epidemiologic Catchment Area Program: historical context, major objectives and study population characteristics. Arch Gen Psychiatry 41:934–941, 1984

Regier DA, Boyd JH, Burke JD, et al: One-month prevalence of mental disorders in the United States. Arch Gen Psychiatry 45:977–986, 1988

Riedel-Heller SG, Busse A, Aurich C, et al: Prevalence of dementia according to DSM-III-R and ICD-10. Br J Psychiatry 179:250–254, 2001

Ritchie K, Artero S, Beluche I, et al: Prevalence of DSM-IV psychiatric disorder in the French elderly population. Br J Psychiatry 184:147–152, 2004

Robins LN, Helzer JE, Croughan J, et al: National Institute of Mental Health Diagnostic Interview Schedule: its history, characteristics, and validity. Arch Gen Psychiatry 38:381–389, 1981

Rovner BW, Kafonek S, Filipp L, et al: Prevalence of mental illness in a community nursing home. Am J Psychiatry 143:1446–1449, 1986

Saunders AM, Schmader K, Breitner J, et al: Apolipoprotein E ε4 allele distributions in late-onset Alzheimer's disease and in other amyloid-forming diseases. Lancet 342:710–711, 1993

Saunders PA, Copeland JRM, Dewey ME, et al: Alcohol use and abuse in the elderly: findings from the Liverpool Longitudinal Study of Continuing Health in the Community. Int J Geriatr Psychiatry 4:103–108, 1989

Shcherbatykh I, Carpenter DO: The role of metals in the etiology of Alzheimer's disease. J Alzheimers Dis 11:191–205, 2007

Sheehan B, Bass C, Briggs R, et al: Somatization among older primary care attenders. Psychol Med 33:867–877, 2003

Skoog I: Psychiatric epidemiology of old age: the H70 study—the NAPE Lecture 2003. Acta Psychiatr Scand 109:4–18, 2004

Smalbrugge M, Pot AM, Jongenelis K, et al: Prevalence and correlates of anxiety among nursing home patients. J Affect Disord 88:145–153, 2005

Steffens DC, Skoog I, Norton M, et al: Prevalence of depression and its treatment in an elderly population: the Cache County study. Arch Gen Psychiatry 57:601–607, 2000

Stek ML, Gussekloo J, Beekman ATF, et al: Prevalence, correlates and recognition of depression in the oldest old: the Leiden 85-plus study. J Affect Disord 78:193–200, 2004

Stevens T, Livingston G, Kitchen G, et al: Islington study of dementia subtypes in the community. Br J Psychiatry 180:270–276, 2002

Stinson FS, Dawson DA, Chou SP, et al: The epidemiology of DSM-IV specific phobia in the USA: results from the National Epidemiologic Survey on Alcohol and Related Conditions. Psychol Med 37:1047–1059, 2007

Teresi J, Abrams R, Holmes D, et al: Prevalence of depression and depression recognition in nursing homes. Soc Psychiatry Psychiatr Epidemiol 36:613–620, 2001

Thomas VS, Rockwood KJ: Alcohol abuse, cognitive impairment, and mortality among older people. J Am Geriatr Soc 49:415–420, 2001

Trollor JN, Anderson TM, Sachdev PS, et al: Prevalence of mental disorders in the elderly: the Australian National Mental Health and Well-Being Survey. Am J Geriatr Psychiatry 15:455–466, 2007

Unutzer J, Simon G, Belin T, et al: Care for depression in HMO patients aged 65 or older. J Am Geriatr Soc 48:871–878, 2000

Wang PS, Berglund P, Olfson M, et al: Failure and delay in initial treatment contact after first onset of mental disorders in the National Comorbidity Survey Replication. Arch Gen Psychiatry 62:603–613, 2005a

Wang PS, Lane M, Olfson M, et al: Twelve-month use of mental health services in the United States. Arch Gen Psychiatry 62:629–640, 2005b

WHO World Mental Health Survey Consortium: Prevalence, severity, and unmet need for treatment of mental disorders in the World Health Organization World Mental Health Surveys. JAMA 291:2581–2590, 2004

World Health Organization: Composite International Diagnostic Interview, Version 1.0. Geneva, World Health Organization, 1990

World Health Organization: International Statistical Classification of Diseases and Related Health Problems, 10th Revision. Geneva, World Health Organization, 1992

Yesavage JA, Brink TL, Rose TL, et al: Development and validation of a geriatric depression screening scale. J Psychiatr Res 17:37–49, 1983

Suggested Readings

Beekman ATF, Deeg DJH, van Tilberg T, et al: Major and minor depression in later life: a study of prevalence and risk factors. J Affect Disord 36:65–75, 1995

Blazer DG: Psychiatry and the oldest old. Am J Psychiatry 157:1915–1924, 2000

Jeste DV, Alexopoulos GS, Bartels SJ, et al: Consensus statement on the upcoming crisis in geriatric mental health. Arch Gen Psychiatry 56:848–853, 1999

Kessler RC, Berglund P, Demler O, et al: Lifetime prevalence and age-of-onset distributions of DSM-IV disorders in the National Comorbidity Survey Replication. Arch Gen Psychiatry 62:593–602, 2005

Krishnan KRR: Concept of disease in geriatric psychiatry. Am J Geriatr Psychiatry 15:1–11, 2007

Wang PS, Lane M, Olfson M, et al: Twelve-month use of mental health services in the United States. Arch Gen Psychiatry 62:629–640, 2005b

CHAPTER 2

PHYSIOLOGICAL AND CLINICAL CONSIDERATIONS OF GERIATRIC PATIENT CARE

ROBERT M. KAISER, M.D., M.H.SC.

The retirement of the generation born after World War II, the baby boomers, has begun. People older than 65 years constitute one of the fastest-growing segments of the U.S. population, with a baby boomer now turning 65 every 8 seconds (Fried 2000; Hobbs 2001; O'Connor et al. 2010). Individuals are living longer, and the numbers of elderly grow with each passing year. The average life span has lengthened significantly (Fried 2000; Hall 1997; Vaillant and Mukamal 2001).

The hallmarks of physiological change in elderly people are twofold: impaired homeostasis (also called *homeostenosis*) and increased vulnerability because of decreased reserve capacity (Armbrecht 2001; Taffet 1999). Homeostasis—that is, the ability of the organism to maintain a steady state—lessens with time. Altered physiology leads

the elderly patient to be more susceptible to harm. As time passes, none of us can expect—like an aspiring Olympic athlete—to run faster, throw farther, and leap higher. Age brings with it expected decrements in function. In this chapter, I detail the various physiological changes that occur with "normal" aging—in other words, those progressive changes that take place over time but not as a result of disease.

Physiological Changes in Major Organ Systems

Sensory Systems: Vision and Hearing

Older adults develop significant age-related changes in the eye. The weakening of the ciliary muscle, combined with decreased curvature of the lens, results in a loss of accommodation; therefore, it becomes difficult for an individual to focus on near objects, and bifocals may be needed. It is also difficult for elderly people to adapt to light because of rigidity of the pupil and increasing size and opacity of the lens. With age, the lens opacifies (i.e., becomes less transparent as a result of protein aggregations), and a cataract can form. Elderly patients are also at risk for age-related macular degeneration, which causes loss of central vision when drusen (yellowish-white deposits) accumulate in the retina. Age-related macular degeneration is the most common cause of blindness in elderly people (Haegerstrom-Portnoy and Morgan 2007; Harvey 2003).

Older adults can also expect alterations in the ear, which may lead to hearing loss in both high and low frequencies. In the inner ear, the degeneration of the organ of Corti is associated with high-frequency sensorineural hearing loss, whereas atrophy of the stria vascularis may cause hearing loss across all frequencies. The stiffening of the basilar membrane and atrophy of the spiral ligament both can result in loss of speech discrimination (Mills 2003; Taffet 1999).

Cardiovascular System

The heart and blood vessels of aging people undergo significant anatomical alterations and lead to changes in function. Age-associated changes occur in the autonomic nervous system and in the response of the cardiovascular system. The ability of the heart to beat faster and pump efficiently and the ease with which blood vessels dilate or constrict are markedly affected. Both cardiac output and cardiac reserve decrease (O'Rourke and Hashimoto 2006; Seals and Esler 2000).

With age, human blood vessels stiffen. The vessels are thicker and less distensible. Higher pressures can increase the load on the heart and lead to left ventricular enlargement as well as increased left ventricular oxygen requirements, thereby increasing the risk of congestive heart failure. Increased pressures also can result in damage to the endothelium and media in the microcirculation of the brain and kidneys and may be connected with organ dysfunction (O'Rourke and Hashimoto 2006).

Age-related changes in the sympathetic nervous system affect the adaptability of the heart and blood vessels to stress. Sympathetic nervous activity rises in elderly patients. The β-adrenergic response of the heart during exercise is attenuated; a lower maximum heart rate and decreased force of contraction are the result. Similarly, large arteries do not respond as well to β-adrenergic stimulation, and their ability to dilate is reduced (Lakatta 1999; Seals and Esler 2000).

Respiratory System

As individuals age, the chest wall becomes stiffer and less compliant. When an older adult generates a breath, the relative contribution of the diaphragm and abdominal muscles is increased compared with the thoracic muscles, as a result of decreased chest wall compliance. Respiratory muscle function also declines because of changes in the rib cage, decreased chest wall compliance, and decreased elastic recoil of the lung. Respiratory muscles weaken with age, as a result of nutritional deficiencies, anatomical changes in skeletal muscle, and physiological decline (Janssens 2005). Changes in the lung itself and in the control of breathing negatively affect the respiratory system. A loss of elastic tissue in the lung occurs, with a loss of elastic recoil, and the alveolar ducts and respiratory bronchioles enlarge. This enlargement leads to a loss of alveolar surface area; less tissue is available for gas exchange, and partial pressure of oxygen decreases with age, but the decline is not uniform. The diffusing capacity of the lung also declines. In older individuals, the lung is less able to guard itself against infection. The mucociliary tree lining the respiratory tract is slower in ridding the lung of invading particles and microorganisms. With age, the person's ability to generate a sufficiently strong cough declines. The development of higher closing volumes further complicates defense against infection by making it more difficult to expel secretions from the lower areas of the lungs (Taffet 1999).

Gastrointestinal System

As people age, numerous anatomical changes take place throughout the gastrointestinal tract (Firth and Prather 2002; Hall and Wiley 2003; Majumdar et al. 1997; Taffet 1999). The production of saliva is generally maintained. The strength of esophageal contractions is diminished, but food nonetheless traverses the length of the esophagus uneventfully. The production of acid and pepsin by the stomach is mostly preserved. Both the stomach and the small intestine do not dilate as easily as a bolus of food enters, and transit through the large bowel may be slower. The small bowel is less effective at absorbing vitamins and minerals (such as vitamin D, calcium, and iron) and sugars (such as xylose and lactose). The motor function of the colon is not significantly affected by aging. The liver, gallbladder, and pancreas continue to function well in elderly patients (Hall and Wiley 2003; Majumdar et al. 1997; Oskvig 1999; Taffet 1999). The liver's ability to manufacture

binding proteins and metabolize drugs is stable. Few significant anatomical changes occur in the gallbladder, and its function remains intact. In the aging pancreas, there is no impairment in the synthesis of pancreatic enzymes and bicarbonate. The role of the pancreas in digestive function is therefore unaffected.

Endocrine System
Prolactin

Levels of prolactin in aging women have been reported to increase, decrease, or remain the same, whereas prolactin levels in aging men are slightly increased. None of these changes is believed to have an effect on normal function (Gruenewald and Matsumoto 2003).

Antidiuretic Hormone

Aging causes significant changes in antidiuretic hormone (ADH) and the body's response to it, which alter the older patient's ability to excrete free water—resulting in hyponatremia—or to prevent losses in volume—resulting in dehydration. Basal levels of ADH are normal to increased in older adults; because renal free water clearance decreases with age, hyponatremia can more easily occur. However, when volume loss takes place, with subsequent hypotension, less ADH is released in older individuals (Gruenewald and Matsumoto 2003; Oskvig 1999; Perry 1999).

Corticotropin and Cortisol

Basal corticotropin levels are normal in elderly individuals. Stimulation of the hypothalamic-pituitary-adrenal (HPA) axis by exogenous corticotropin produces the expected cortisol response, but the cortisol secretion rate actually declines. Cortisol levels remain the same because of a decrease in the cortisol metabolic clearance rate. When subjected to stress, the HPA axis produces higher peak cortisol levels, which then dissipate more slowly; this occurs because the negative feedback of cortisol on the HPA axis is less effective (Gruenewald and Matsumoto 2003).

Adrenal Androgens

Both dehydroepiandrosterone (DHEA) and dehydroepiandrosterone sulfate (DHEA-S) decrease significantly in older adults. Production of DHEA peaks at age 20 and then declines (Fried and Walston 2003; Gruenewald and Matsumoto 2003).

Adrenal Medulla and Sympathetic Nervous System

In older people, secretion of norepinephrine increases and clearance decreases; plasma levels therefore increase. Epinephrine secretion and clearance both increase with age, so the level of epinephrine does not change. The level of sympathetic nervous system activity is increased in older individuals, but both α-adrenergic and β-adrenergic receptors are less sensitive to stimulation (Gruenewald and Matsumoto 2003; Oskvig 1999; Seals and Esler 2000).

Renin, Angiotensin, and Aldosterone

An age-related decrease in plasma renin activity leads to reduced aldosterone secretion; aldosterone levels are thus reduced significantly. The rise in natriuretic hormone secretion in older adults also serves to decrease aldosterone levels; higher levels of natriuretic hormone suppress renin secretion, plasma renin activity, and angiotensin II, further lowering aldosterone secretion. In addition, natriuretic hormone itself can inhibit aldosterone secretion. The overall decrease in aldosterone adversely affects sodium retention in the kidney and predisposes elderly people to dehydration. Another consequence of lower aldosterone levels is an increased likelihood of hyperkalemia (Gruenewald and Matsumoto 2003).

Growth Hormone

Growth hormone levels peak at puberty and then decrease by 14% per decade. Both a decrease in growth hormone–releasing hormone secretion and an increase in somatostatin are responsible for the decline in growth hormone. Insulinlike growth factor (IGF-1), which is produced by the liver and mediates the actions of growth hormone in the body, also diminishes gradually, at a rate of 7%–13% per decade. The decline in growth hormone with age may result in a decrease in both lean body mass and bone mass (Gruenewald and Matsumoto 2003; Perry 1999).

Parathyroid Hormone, Vitamin D, and Calcium Regulation

Older adults generally consume insufficient calcium in their diet; calcium is also less efficiently absorbed in the small intestine. Vitamin D is essential to that absorption, and levels of vitamin D, 25-hydroxy (25,D) and vitamin D, 1,25-dihydroxy (1,25D) both decrease as a result of several factors, including 1) decreased sunlight exposure and less efficient photoconversion in the skin of 2-dehydrocholesterol to vitamin D_3; 2) insufficient dietary intake of vitamin D; 3) intestinal malabsorption of, or resistance to, vitamin D; 4) decreased 1-α-hydroxylase activity in the kidney; and 5) the use of medications that cause the liver to break down vitamin D.

The decline in both serum calcium and 1,25D levels triggers a compensatory increase in parathyroid hormone (PTH). PTH then 1) stimulates osteoclasts to resorb bone and 2) acts on the renal distal tubule to promote calcium reabsorption, thereby increasing serum calcium levels. PTH levels are higher in elderly individuals because of increased secretion and decreased renal clearance. This is thought to represent a form of secondary, rather than primary, hyperparathyroidism and can have a deleterious effect on bone mass in older patients (Perry 1999; Prestwood and Duque 2003).

Testosterone

As men age, the number of Leydig cells in the testis declines and testosterone secretion gradually decreases. The overall decline in testosterone causes a decrease in both the number of Sertoli's cells and daily sperm production; the sperm produced may have defects in motility as well as chromosomal abnormalities. The changes in testosterone secretion are common but not universal, and some men have normal serum testosterone levels as they age (Gruenewald and Matsumoto 2003; Perry 1999). Testing for testosterone deficiency is generally recommended only for those patients with clinical symptoms of hypogonadism (Bhasin et al. 2006; Sadovsky et al. 2007). Screening all patients with erectile dysfunction for testosterone deficiency is not universally endorsed by experts; only 2% of men with erectile dysfunction have an endocrine disorder (Sadovsky et al. 2007). The Endocrine Society has established clinical practice guidelines for testosterone replacement (Bhasin et al. 2006). Replacement has several potential benefits, including improved libido, sexual functioning, and sense of well-being, as well as increased muscle mass and strength and better physical functioning (Matsumoto 2002).

Estrogen

Estrogen declines precipitously with menopause. The loss of estrogen affects bone mass and places women at risk for osteoporosis. Women also lose the beneficial effects of estrogen on lipids, with rising low-density lipoprotein levels, and are at higher risk for cardiovascular disease. The lack of estrogen causes atrophy of the vaginal endothelium; the endothelium thins, less lubrication occurs with intercourse, and dyspareunia can result (Gruenewald and Matsumoto 2003; Perry 1999; Taffet 1999). The results of a widely cited randomized clinical trial, the Women's Health Initiative, indicated that estrogen replacement in postmenopausal women did not produce the expected reductions in cardiovascular events, stroke, fractures, and dementia that had been anticipated based on previous observational studies (Grimes and Lobo 2002; Nelson et al. 2002). Some obstetricians and gynecologists have nonetheless suggested that estrogen can be safely prescribed, at lower doses than those given in the Women's Health Initiative trial, for the relief of common postmenopausal symptoms such as hot flashes (Grimes and Lobo 2002).

Thyroid

Although age-related changes in the thyroid gland occur, these changes have no corresponding effect on thyroid function. The renal and thyroidal iodide clearance rate declines in older persons. Although the thyroid continues to make sufficient amounts of thyroxine (T_4), it fails to metabolize T_4 as well. The synthesis of T_4 actually declines, but its level is unchanged. Peripheral deiodination of T_4 to triiodothyronine (T_3) also decreases, and the level of T_3 declines by 10%–20% in elderly people. Reverse T_3 levels do not change. T_4-binding globulin levels remain normal with age (Hassani and Hershman 2003; Perry 1999).

Insulin

Elderly patients have a tendency toward hyperglycemia. Circulating insulin levels may rise but are less efficiently used. Although insulin secretion by the pancreatic β cells is preserved with age, insulin clearance declines and insulin levels increase. Peripheral uptake of insulin is affected by insulin resistance in peripheral tissues; some of these tissues, particularly adipocytes, have fewer receptors, thereby decreasing their sensitivity to insulin.

Elderly patients have decreased muscle mass and a higher percentage of fat and therefore an increased number of adipocytes. These notable changes in insulin secretion and tissue sensitivity in the periphery may lead to observed increases in fasting glucose level in older adults. IGF-1, which acts at insulin receptors to promote glucose uptake, is less abundant in older adults (Halter 2003; Perry 1999; Rizvi 2007; Taffet 1999). Several other factors contribute to the increased prevalence of glucose intolerance and type 2 diabetes mellitus in elderly people, including changes in body composition, a reduction in physical activity, and increased comorbid illness and medication use. According to estimates of the Centers for Disease Control and Prevention, 10.3 million (20.9%) people ages 60 years and older in the United States have diabetes (Rizvi 2007).

Musculoskeletal System

In general, elderly people are weaker and less muscular. In the fourth decade, both muscle mass and strength begin to decrease. There are smaller numbers of type II fast-twitch fibers and fewer motor units and synapses; slow muscle fibers predominate. Exercise may modify age-associated changes in muscle mass and strength. Decreased muscle mass places older people at risk for significant physical disability and a decline in their ability to perform activities of daily living and may ultimately undermine their ability to live independently.

Elderly people also develop demonstrable changes in cartilage, tendons, and ligaments. Cartilage becomes less cellular with age. Older tendons and ligaments may be stiffer. These alterations may make them less able to withstand mechanical stress and more susceptible to fatigue, and they may decrease the range of motion of joints in older adults and make them more prone to tendonitis, ligament tears, and ligament ruptures (Loeser and Delbono 2003; Taffet 1999).

Age-related changes in the structure of both cortical and trabecular bone occur. Cortical bone becomes thinner and more porous; trabecular bone also thins, and whole trabeculae are lost. Bones are therefore weaker. Mechanical strain, an important stimulus to bone formation, has less of an effect in older people, and less bone is made. Older individuals are at increased risk for bone loss. Without estrogen replacement, women can lose significant bone mass after menopause. Elderly men with testosterone deficiency also may develop osteoporosis. Other factors that contribute to bone loss in both men and women include low peak bone density, poor calcium intake, secondary hyperparathyroidism (as discussed earlier), and insufficient exercise (Prestwood and Duque 2003).

Hematological and Immune Systems

Despite a decrease in bone marrow mass, the aging adult does not lose the ability to produce normal numbers of red blood cells, white blood cells, and platelets; however, when challenged to produce more red blood cells by the occurrence of blood loss or by the presence of hypoxic conditions, the bone marrow is less able to respond quickly. Red blood cells and white blood cells retain normal function. Platelets, however, may be more sensitive to substances that trigger them to form blood clots (Chatta and Lipschitz 2003; Taffet 1999).

When confronted with a new infection, older people are less able to mount an adequate cell-mediated response. With age, the thymus decreases in size, the number of T lymphocytes is diminished, and the person's capacity to respond is adversely affected. The humoral, or antibody, response in elderly people is also impaired. Older adults respond less vigorously to the first presentation of an antigen as well as to the reintroduction of antigen. These decreased primary and secondary responses may explain why older adults respond less well to vaccination (Aw et al. 2007; Miller 1999; Taffet 1999).

The body's primary defenses against infection are also affected by age. The thinner skin of elderly people is more vulnerable to injury; when compromised, surface bacteria may enter, resulting in cellulitis or a potentially serious bacteremia. The mucous membranes of the genitourinary and respiratory tracts of elderly people may become more easily colonized with gram-negative organisms, thereby serving as a potential source of infection. In urine, the amount, concentration, and acidity of urea are decreased, depriving the urine of an intrinsic defense against possible bacterial infection. Elderly patients with swallowing dysfunction may subsequently aspirate bacteria from the oral cavity, or those unable to produce an adequate cough will leave infectious material in the airways (Taffet 1999).

Renal System

As a person ages, the size of the kidney progressively decreases as a result of fatty infiltration, fibrosis, and the dropout of cortical nephrons. The rate of decline of nephrons is 0.5%–1.0% per year; by age 60, 30%–50% of functioning glomeruli have been eliminated. Cortical nephrons become diffusely sclerotic. Decreased reserve capacity does predispose the kidney to possible dysfunction or failure. Creatinine clearance declines 7.5%–10.0% per decade (Oskvig 1999; Taffet 1999).

These anatomical changes have important physiological consequences, including the decreased ability of the kidney to acidify urine or to excrete an acid or a water load. Renin activity declines, and less renin is produced in the face of decreased intravascular volume or a depletion of salt. The kidney is able to maintain its output of erythropoietin, but the hydroxylation of vitamin D declines. The kidney less reliably metabolizes hormones such as glucagon, calcitonin, and PTH; drug metabolism is also significantly affected (Oskvig 1999; Taffet 1999), as discussed in the following section, "Considerations in Geriatric Prescribing: Effects of Aging on Pharmacokinetics and Pharmacodynamics."

Considerations in Geriatric Prescribing: Effects of Aging on Pharmacokinetics and Pharmacodynamics

The effect of aging on pharmacokinetics (absorption, volume of distribution, clearance rate, and elimination half-life) and pharmacodynamics (the effect of a drug at a given dose) is crucial to understanding how drugs should be prescribed in the elderly patient (Schwartz 1999; Semla and Rochon 2006).

Pharmacokinetics

Age has no significant effect on *absorption*. The *volume of distribution* is significantly affected by the changes in body mass and total body water that occur with aging. Older patients, with decreased lean body mass and total body water, have a smaller volume of distribution. Frail elderly patients may have significant decreases in albumin levels, which affect the binding of potentially harmful drugs such as warfarin, which must be vigilantly titrated. With age, renal mass and renal blood flow are decreased, resulting in a decline in glomerular filtration rate and *creatinine clearance*. This decrease in clearance can alter the rate at which drugs are excreted, and dosages must be appropriately adjusted. Certain drugs, such as nonsteroidal anti-inflammatory drugs and angiotensin converting enzyme inhibitors, also may alter renal blood flow and thereby depress kidney function. *Hepatic drug clearance* is decreased by an age-related decline in hepatic blood flow; oxidative metabolism in the cytochrome P450 system is slower, thereby affecting elimination, but conjugation is not. Underlying hepatic disease and drug interactions also may significantly affect the metabolism of drugs by the liver. The *elimination half-life*—the time required for the drug concentration to decrease by half—of certain drugs increases in older adults. This may require adjustment of the drug dosing interval. For example, aspirin, certain antibiotics (e.g., vancomycin), digoxin, and the calcium channel blockers (diltiazem, felodipine, and nifedipine) all have higher elimination half-lives, and the dosages must be adjusted downward.

Pharmacodynamics

The pharmacodynamic effects of drugs in elderly patients also must be considered. Frequently, older adults are more sensitive to medications, and drugs must be given in lower doses. For example, because their response to anticholinergic drugs is increased, elderly patients develop side effects, including constipation, urinary retention, and delirium, more frequently than do younger patients. Other notable examples of drugs with enhanced pharmacodynamic effects in elderly people include diazepam, morphine, and theophylline.

Chronic Disease in Older Adults

Some chronic diseases are more prevalent in older people, and these predominantly occur as a result of "usual aging." The cumulative effect of environment and heredity on the individual over time makes these diseases more common, and they account for significant morbidity and mortality. Among the most formidable and omnipresent are cardiovascular disease, cerebrovascular disease, and cancer. Hypercholesterolemia and hypertension are frequently diagnosed. As people age, weight and the incidence of obesity increase; patients are at higher risk for the development of type 2 diabetes mellitus. Aging also leads to an increased occurrence of joint problems, particularly osteoarthritis, which can result in chronic pain and the need for joint replacement. Elderly people can develop cataracts and macular degeneration and therefore impaired vision; hearing loss in the elderly, caused by either previous noise exposure or age-related anatomical changes in the ear, is also prevalent. Postmenopausal women and some hypogonadal elderly men are prone to develop osteoporosis. Benign prostatic hypertrophy, often with resultant urinary frequency and nocturia, becomes more of a clinical problem as men age. Polymyalgia rheumatica and temporal arteritis are collagen vascular diseases that occur often in elderly patients. The increasing prevalence of multisystem disease in the older patient can impose a substantial burden on the individual; in the face of already diminished physiological reserves, such an individual is considerably more vulnerable to declining health (Fried 2000).

Geriatric Syndromes

Memory Loss and Dementia

Various studies have documented a decline in cognitive function with age. Such decline may occur in several areas, including intelligence, ability to maintain attention, language, memory, learning, visuospatial function, and psychomotor function. These deficits do not occur uniformly across all areas and do not occur in every person. Visuospatial tasks are more difficult, and both motor speed and response times decline with aging. Some evidence suggests that executive function, or the ability to conceive, organize, and carry out a plan or activity, may remain intact in the elderly (Craft et al. 2003).

Dementia is defined as the development of significant deficits in two or more areas of cognition—an impairment of memory and at least one other area, such as abstract thinking, judgment, language, or visuospatial ability—that are severe enough to affect the individual's day-to-day functioning (Nyenhuis and Gorelick 1998). With the inevitable decline in intellectual functioning and in

the ability to perform activities of daily living that occurs, dementia poses particular challenges for the clinician and special burdens for caregivers.

Two-thirds of all dementia is caused by Alzheimer's disease. Alzheimer's disease is present in about 5% of the population older than 65, and beyond that age, the prevalence of the disease doubles every 5 years (Klafki et al. 2006). Vascular dementia accounts for 15%–25% of dementia (Gomez-Tortosa et al. 1998), and Lewy body dementia constitutes 10%. The natural history and symptomatology of dementia vary according to its etiology (Marin et al. 2002).

The accurate diagnosis of dementia requires a comprehensive assessment by the clinician, including a detailed history; thorough physical, neurological, and mental status examinations; and a depression screen. The evaluating clinician should order laboratory studies to rule out vitamin B_{12} deficiency, syphilis, and hypothyroidism and should examine the patient for evidence of anemia, electrolyte abnormalities, renal failure, and liver dysfunction. This laboratory evaluation enables the clinician to detect reversible causes of dementia and uncover evidence of metabolic abnormalities that might point to a diagnosis of delirium rather than dementia (Marin et al. 2002). In 2010, an expert panel convened by the National Institute on Aging and the Alzheimer's Association called for changes in diagnostic criteria for Alzheimer's disease that would lead to earlier and more precise detection of disease (Alzheimer's Association 2011).

Above all, the treatment of dementia involves the building of a proper support system for the patient. Pharmacological treatment of Alzheimer's disease may be appropriate in some cases. Acetylcholinesterase inhibitors, including donepezil, galantamine, and rivastigmine, have shown some effectiveness in clinical trials of patients with mild to moderate disease, with documented improvements in the Alzheimer's Disease Assessment Scale Cognitive Subscale score (Clark and Karlawish 2003; Frisoni 2001; Klafki et al. 2006; Sramek et al. 2001), although the overall effects of these drugs may be modest (Raina et al. 2008). Patients with moderate to severe Alzheimer's disease who took memantine, an N-methyl-D-aspartate (NMDA) receptor inhibitor, in randomized clinical trials showed a benefit in measures of cognition and function (Klafki et al. 2006; McShane et al. 2006; Tariot et al. 2004).

Falls

Falls are a common phenomenon in older patients; every year, one-half of all nursing home residents and one-third of all community-dwelling elderly have a fall. These falls produce notable morbidity: 2% cause hip fractures, 5% cause other fractures, and 10% cause head injuries or other significant injuries. In the aftermath of falls, disability may result. Those people who fall frequently are at risk for a decline in their instrumental activities of daily living and their activities of daily living (assessment of such functions is discussed later in this chapter in "Fundamentals of Geriatric Assessment"). A decline in these functions can ultimately undermine independence and also might result in hospitalization (Fried 2000; King and Tinetti 1995; Rubenstein and Josephson 2006; Rubenstein et al. 1994).

Falls are generally multifactorial and are caused by 1) intrinsic factors: disease-specific deficits in an individual patient, including neurological problems (central, neuromuscular, vestibular, visual, and proprioceptive) and systemic illness; 2) situational factors re-

lated to the particular activity that is taking place; 3) extrinsic factors related to the demands and hazards of a particular environment; and 4) medications, which can adversely affect mental status, cognition, balance, circulation, and neuromuscular function (Alexander 1999; King and Tinetti 1995).

The proper evaluation of a fall requires 1) taking a detailed history and review of systems and 2) performing a thorough physical examination and neurological examination (Rubenstein and Josephson 2006). The prevention of falls focuses on altering both intrinsic and extrinsic factors (Gillespie et al. 2003; King and Tinetti 1995; Rubenstein and Josephson 2006). With regard to intrinsic factors, one could 1) prescribe medication appropriately, 2) optimally treat disease, 3) improve balance and gait through physical therapy, and 4) improve conditioning and strength through exercise. With regard to extrinsic factors, one could 1) improve the environment by reducing or eliminating hazards, 2) monitor patients more carefully by increasing staff supervision and using motion detection, 3) eliminate restraints and the risk of injury they pose, 4) encourage patients to wear hip protectors, and 5) install protective flooring. Preventing falls ultimately requires multiple steps to produce successful results.

A meta-analysis of five randomized clinical trials suggested that vitamin D supplementation may reduce the risk of falls in ambulatory or institutionalized older individuals by more than 20% (Bischoff-Ferrari et al. 2004).

Urinary Incontinence

Urinary incontinence is a prevalent condition in older adults that causes significant morbidity and affects quality of life (Du-

Beau 2006; Tannenbaum et al. 2001). One-half of all nursing home residents and up to one-third of persons older than 65 years who reside in the community carry the diagnosis. It is a condition with multiple causes, including age-related changes, genitourinary tract abnormalities, and coexisting illnesses. Incontinence can ultimately have harmful medical consequences, including pressure ulcers, cellulitis, falls, and fractures. It can interfere with sleep. It can also result in sexual dysfunction and depression. The proper treatment of incontinence is therefore important and can yield significant benefits.

Urinary incontinence can be classified into two main categories: 1) transient incontinence and 2) established incontinence.

Transient incontinence is reversible and can be easily treated. Transient incontinence could be a consequence of an acute urinary tract infection, inadequately controlled diabetes mellitus, or a recent prescription of a diuretic and will resolve with the correction of those conditions.

Established incontinence is further subdivided into the following three subcategories:

1. *Urge incontinence.* This is the most prevalent form. It results from detrusor overactivity and sometimes impaired contractility. Detrusor overactivity is more common with aging but can occur for other reasons, including neurological dysfunction (e.g., stroke) or irritation of the bladder (secondary to cancer, urolithiasis, or infection); it can also occur in elderly patients without other illnesses. Patients usually complain of a sudden urge to urinate. They also classically have urinary frequency and nocturia. They experience varying amounts of leakage.

2. *Stress incontinence.* Stress incontinence occurs when increased abdominal pressure, triggered by cough or sneezing, results in urinary leakage. It happens commonly in women with weak pelvic muscles, although it also may occur as a consequence of failed anti-incontinence surgery or vaginal mucosal atrophy in women or prostatectomy in men. It is a frequent form of incontinence among elderly women, ranking second in prevalence.

3. *Overflow incontinence.* Detrusor underactivity and bladder outlet obstruction can both produce overflow incontinence. Detrusor underactivity can be caused by fibrosis of the detrusor muscle, peripheral neuropathy, disc herniation, or spinal stenosis. Detrusor underactivity is an infrequent cause of urinary incontinence in older adults. Urethral strictures, benign prostatic hypertrophy, and prostate cancer can cause bladder outlet obstruction in elderly men; this form of incontinence is the second most prevalent in this population. Bladder outlet obstruction in women occurs much less frequently; the etiology is either the presence of a large cystocele or a history of anti-incontinence surgery.

In general, the treatment of incontinence in elderly people begins with behavioral interventions, which are followed by medical treatment. Surgery is considered the last option and is appropriate only for stress incontinence or outlet obstruction. Because urinary incontinence in the elderly is invariably the result of more than one cause, clinicians must appreciate that a single intervention may not be effective. Medications must be reviewed to determine whether they are contributing to incontinence. Patients must be cautioned against intake of fluids such as alcohol, coffee, tea, and soft drinks, which stimulate urination. Fluid restriction at bedtime may be appropriate to decrease nocturia.

Polypharmacy

Defined as the simultaneous use of multiple medications or the prescribing of more medications than is clinically appropriate, *polypharmacy* is a common problem in older adults (Hanlon et al. 2001; Stewart 2001). Polypharmacy carries with it certain consequences, including adverse drug reactions, drug interactions, and patient noncompliance, and also increases the incidence of geriatric syndromes such as urinary incontinence, falls, cognitive impairment, and delirium.

Clinicians should take several steps to ensure that medicines are prescribed appropriately. They should take a careful, comprehensive medication history, including allergies and adverse drug reactions. Current use of alcohol, tobacco, and recreational drugs should be documented. Medicines should be prescribed only if they have a known benefit, and they should be given at the lowest effective dose. Instructions about medication use should be communicated clearly to patients. Patients taking medication should be carefully monitored for therapeutic effectiveness and for side effects (Semla and Rochon 2006). A systematic review of 14 clinical trials on optimizing prescribing in older patients reported that certain clinical interventions, including geriatric medicine services, the participation of a pharmacist in clinical care, and computerized decision support, had beneficial effects on prescribing (Spinewine et al. 2007).

Frailty

The sum effect of physiological decline in the older patient, combined with the cumulative and simultaneous burden of chronic disease, may result in the geriatric syndrome known as frailty (Cohen 2000; Hamerman 1999; Morley et al. 2006). *Frailty* has been defined by Fried and Walston (2003) as "a state of age-related physiologic vulnerability resulting from impaired homeostatic mechanisms and a reduced capacity of the organism to withstand stress" (p. 1489). Older patients have less pulmonary, cardiac, and renal reserve. They are less able to mount an effective immune response. They also have higher sympathetic nervous tone, which may increase cortisol production and further impair the immune system. In older patients, cortisol also may have catabolic effects on bone and muscle and result in insulin resistance. These patients also may have higher levels of circulating cytokines—such as interleukin-6, interleukin-1B, and tumor necrosis factor-α—which also may have deleterious catabolic effects on muscle. Changes in neuroendocrine function—the decline in sex steroids, growth hormone, and DHEA—can have corresponding negative effects on the size and strength of muscle and, in the case of estrogen and testosterone, on bone mass. The frail older individual is characteristically weak as a result of declining muscle and bone mass; a tendency toward a sedentary state may lead to deconditioning, further weakness, and fatigue. Poor oral intake may lead to weight loss and nutritional compromise, adding even more to the tendency to tire easily. Progressive weakness may adversely affect balance and the ability to ambulate. Ultimately, the frail older patient loses the capacity to function independently and may require skilled assistance in a facility outside the home. Frailty also carries a higher risk of medical illness and mortality (Fried and Walston 2003).

Fundamentals of Geriatric Assessment

The effective evaluation and treatment of the geriatric patient—from the fully functioning community-dwelling older adult to the frail older adult in decline—require a global approach that includes, but reaches beyond, a consideration of the patient's medical problems. Reuben (2003) defined *geriatric assessment* as a comprehensive patient evaluation, conducted by an individual clinician or an interdisciplinary team, which considers the effect of key medical, social, psychological, and environmental factors on health and pays careful attention to patient functioning. During the medical assessment, the clinician performs a complete history and physical examination. He or she reviews the medication list for appropriateness and evidence of polypharmacy; checks for deficits in vision, hearing, ambulation, and balance; and screens for common geriatric problems such as falling, incontinence, and malnutrition. Vision is tested with Snellen's eye chart. Hearing is screened with the "whispering voice test" or a handheld audiometer. The patient's weight and height are measured, and the body mass index is calculated. In addition to the standard neurological examination, the patient's mobility and balance can be determined through use of a "get up and go" test; the patient is asked to stand, walk 10 feet, turn around, return, and be seated. The task is timed; a time greater than 20 seconds suggests that more extensive evaluation is needed.

Cognitive assessment is performed with the Mini-Mental State Examination (Folstein et al. 1975). The Geriatric Depression Scale (Yesavage and Brink 1983) is used to screen for depression. Fundamental day-to-day functioning is determined by documenting activities of daily living—bathing, dressing, toileting, feeding, and transferring—and instrumental activities of daily living—driving, shopping, cooking, housekeeping, using the telephone, and managing finances. The clinician also must gather other important information about function: 1) the extent, strength, and reliability of the patient's social support system (most often the patient's family); 2) the patient's economic resources; and 3) the safety of the patient's home and its proximity to medical care and other essential services. The patient's spiritual preferences and needs are also assessed. After the assessment is completed, recommendations are developed and a care plan is implemented.

Although the results across clinical trials have not been consistent, the effectiveness of comprehensive geriatric assessment and management has been validated in several studies. Increased diagnostic accuracy has been noted. Patients have shown significant improvements in functional status. Affect and cognition have improved. The use of health care services, as measured by nursing home days, hospital services, and medical costs, has been reduced. The use of medications has improved, with fewer drugs being prescribed (Hanlon et al. 2001; Reuben 2003; Spinewine et al. 2007; Stuck et al. 1993). In-home geriatric assessment of older patients may postpone the onset of disability, as well as reduce the number of patients requiring permanent placement in nursing homes (Stuck et al. 1995). A multi-institutional randomized controlled trial of geriatric evaluation and management units in the Veterans Affairs Health Care System showed a positive effect on functional status and quality of life for inpatients and on mental health and quality of life for outpatients, with overall costs equivalent to those for usual care, but no effect on morbidity or mortality (Cohen et al. 2002). As suggested by the evidence, comprehensive geriatric assessment and management may serve as a useful tool for the diagnosis and the care of older patients, and the geriatrician has a valuable and essential role in the evaluation and treatment of this population.

Key Points

- People older than 65 years constitute one of the fastest-growing segments of the U.S. population, and the average life span has lengthened significantly.

- The hallmarks of physiological change in older adults are twofold: impaired homeostasis (also called homeostenosis) and increased vulnerability because of decreased reserve capacity.

- The time needed for older adults to learn new information increases, and they may have more difficulty accessing data from long-term memory.

- Older persons develop significant age-related changes in vision—including decreases in accommodation, ability to adapt to light, color discrimination, and visual acuity—and in hearing, with loss of hearing ability in both high and low frequencies.

- Aging results in arterial stiffening and subsequent increased systolic blood pressure and aortic pulse pressure, with resultant susceptibility to left ventricular hypertrophy, cardiac ischemia, left ventricular failure, cerebrovascular ischemia, and renal dysfunction.

- The immune response of the older individual is less vigorous, with decreased cell-mediated response, impaired humoral response, and increased susceptibility to infection.

- The decline in renal clearance and the increase in the elimination half-life in elderly people may require adjustment of the dosing interval of medications; because older adults are more sensitive to medications, drugs often must be given in lower doses.

- Some chronic diseases are more prevalent in older adults, predominantly occurring as a result of "usual aging"; these include obesity, hypertension, hypercholesterolemia, type 2 diabetes mellitus, osteoarthritis, cerebrovascular disease, cardiovascular disease, and cancer.

- Several common syndromes—known generally as geriatric syndromes—are found more frequently in older patients, including dementia, falls, urinary incontinence, polypharmacy, and frailty.

- The effectiveness of comprehensive geriatric assessment and management has been validated in several large randomized studies, and the geriatrician has a valuable and essential role in the evaluation and treatment of this population.

References

Alexander NB: Falls and gait disturbances, in Geriatrics Review Syllabus: A Core Curriculum in Geriatric Medicine. Edited by Cobbs E, Duthie EH, Murphy JB. Dubuque, IA, Kendall/Hunt, 1999, pp 145–149

Alzheimer's Association: Publication of New Criteria and Guidelines for Alzheimer's Disease Diagnosis, April 2011. Available at: http://www.alz.org/documents_custom/Alz_Diag_Criteria_FAQ.pdf. Accessed October 19, 2011.

Armbrecht HJ: The biology of aging. J Lab Clin Med 138:220–225, 2001

Aw D, Silva AB, Palmer DB: Immunosenescence: emerging challenges for an ageing population. Immunology 120:435–446, 2007

Bhasin S, Cunningham GR, Hayes FJ, et al: Testosterone deficiency in men with androgen deficiency syndromes: an Endocrine Society clinical practice guideline. J Clin Endocrinol Metab 91:1995–2010, 2006

Bischoff-Ferrari HA, Dawson-Hughes B, Willett WC, et al: Effect of vitamin D on falls: a meta-analysis. JAMA 291:1999–2006, 2004

Chatta GS, Lipschitz DA: Aging of the hematopoietic system, in Principles of Geriatric Medicine and Gerontology, 5th Edition. Edited by Hazzard WR, Blass JP, Halter JB, et al. New York, McGraw-Hill, 2003, pp 763–770

Clark CM, Karlawish JH: Alzheimer disease: current concepts and emerging diagnostic and therapeutic strategies. Ann Intern Med 138:400–410, 2003

Cohen HJ: In search of underlying mechanisms of frailty. J Gerontol A Biol Sci Med Sci 55:M706–M708, 2000

Cohen HJ, Feussner JR, Weinberger M, et al: A controlled trial of inpatient and outpatient geriatric evaluation and management. N Engl J Med 346:905–912, 2002

Craft S, Cholerton B, Reger M: Aging and cognition: what is normal?, in Principles of Geriatric Medicine and Gerontology, 5th Edition. Edited by Hazzard WR, Blass JP, Halter JB, et al. New York, McGraw-Hill, 2003, pp 1355–1372

DuBeau CW: Urinary incontinence, in Geriatrics Review Syllabus: A Core Curriculum in Geriatric Medicine, 6th Edition. Edited by Pompei P, Murphy JB. New York, American Geriatrics Society, 2006, pp 184–195

Firth M, Prather CM: Gastrointestinal motility problems in the elderly patient. Gastroenterology 122:1688–1700, 2002

Folstein MF, Folstein SE, McHugh PR: "Mini-mental state": a practical method for grading the cognitive state of patients for the clinician. J Psychiatr Res 12:189–198, 1975

Fried LP: Epidemiology of aging. Epidemiol Rev 22:95–106, 2000

Fried LP, Walston J: Frailty and failure to thrive, in Principles of Geriatric Medicine and Gerontology, 5th Edition. Edited by Hazzard WR, Blass JP, Halter JB, et al. New York, McGraw-Hill, 2003, pp 1487–1502

Frisoni GB: Treatment of Alzheimer's disease with acetylcholinesterase inhibitors: bridging the gap between evidence and practice. J Neurol 248:551–557, 2001

Gillespie LD, Gillespie WJ, Robertson MC, et al: Interventions for preventing falls in elderly people. Cochrane Database of Systematic Reviews 2003, Issue 4. Art. No.: CD000340. DOI: 10.1002/14651858.CD000340

Gomez-Tortosa E, Ingraham AO, Irizarry MC, et al: Dementia with Lewy bodies. J Am Geriatr Soc 46:1449–1458, 1998

Grimes DA, Lobo RA: Perspectives on the Women's Health Initiative trial of hormone replacement therapy. Obstet Gynecol 100:1344–1353, 2002

Gruenewald DA, Matsumoto AM: Aging of the endocrine system, in Principles of Geriatric Medicine and Gerontology, 5th Edition. Edited by Hazzard WR, Blass JP, Halter JB, et al. New York, McGraw-Hill, 2003, pp 819–836

Haegerstrom-Portnoy G, Morgan MW: Normal age-related vision changes, in Rosenbloom and Morgan's Vision and Aging. Edited by Rosenbloom AA Jr. St. Louis, MO, Elsevier, 2007, pp 31–48

Hall KE, Wiley JW: Age-associated changes in gastrointestinal function, in Principles of Geriatric Medicine and Gerontology, 5th Edition. Edited by Hazzard WR, Blass JP, Halter JB, et al. New York, McGraw-Hill, 2003, pp 593–600

Hall WJ: Update in geriatrics. Ann Intern Med 127:557–564, 1997

Halter JB: Diabetes mellitus, in Principles of Geriatric Medicine and Gerontology, 5th Edition. Edited by Hazzard WR, Blass JP, Halter JB, et al. New York, McGraw-Hill, 2003, pp 855–874

Hamerman D: Toward an understanding of frailty. Ann Intern Med 130:945–950, 1999

Hanlon JT, Schmader KE, Ruby CM, et al: Suboptimal prescribing in older inpatients and outpatients. J Am Geriatr Soc 49:200–209, 2001

Harvey PT: Common eye diseases of elderly people: identifying and treating causes of vision loss. Gerontology 48:1–11, 2003

Hassani S, Hershman JM: Thyroid diseases, in Principles of Geriatric Medicine and Gerontology, 5th Edition. Edited by Hazzard WR, Blass JP, Halter JB, et al. New York, McGraw-Hill, 2003, pp 837–854

Hobbs FB: The elderly population. U.S. Census Bureau, Population Division and Housing and Household Economic Statistics Division, 2001. Available at: http://www.census.gov/population/www/pop-profile/elderpop.html. Accessed February 2, 2008

Janssens JP: Aging of the respiratory system: impact on pulmonary function tests and adaptation to exertion. Clin Chest Med 26:469–484, 2005

King MB, Tinetti ME: Falls in community-dwelling older persons. J Am Geriatr Soc 43:1146–1154, 1995

Klafki HW, Staufenbiel S, Kornhuber J, et al: Therapeutic approaches to Alzheimer's disease. Brain 129:2840–2855, 2006

Lakatta EG: Cardiovascular aging research: the next horizons. J Am Geriatr Soc 47:613–625, 1999

Loeser RF, Delbono O: Aging and the musculoskeletal system, in Principles of Geriatric Medicine and Gerontology, 5th Edition. Edited by Hazzard WR, Blass JP, Halter JB, et al. New York, McGraw-Hill, 2003, pp 905–918

Majumdar AP, Jaszewski R, Dubick MA: Effect of aging on gastrointestinal tract and the pancreas. Proc Soc Exp Biol Med 215:134–144, 1997

Marin DB, Sewell MC, Schlecter A: Alzheimer's disease: accurate and early diagnosis in the primary care setting. Geriatrics 57:36–40, 2002

Matsumoto AM: Andropause: clinical implications of the decline in serum testosterone levels with aging in men. J Gerontol A Biol Sci Med Sci 57:M76–M99, 2002

McShane R, Areosa Sastre A, Minakaran N: Memantine for dementia. Cochrane Database of Systematic Reviews 2006, Issue 2. Art. No.: CD003154. DOI: 10.1002/14651858.CD003154.pub5

Miller RA: The biology of aging and longevity, in Principles of Geriatric Medicine and Gerontology. Edited by Hazzard WR, Blass JP, Ettinger WH, et al. New York, McGraw-Hill, 1999, pp 3–19

Mills JH: Age-related changes in the auditory system, in Principles of Geriatric Medicine and Gerontology, 5th Edition. Edited by Hazzard WR, Blass JP, Halter JB, et al. New York, McGraw-Hill, 2003, pp 1239–1251

Morley JE, Haren MT, Rolland YR, et al: Frailty. Med Clin North Am 90:837–847, 2006

Nelson HD, Humphrey LL, Nygren P, et al: Postmenopausal hormone replacement therapy: scientific review. JAMA 288:872–881, 2002

Nyenhuis DL, Gorelick PB: Vascular dementia: a contemporary review of epidemiology, diagnosis, prevention and treatment. J Am Geriatr Soc 46:1437–1448, 1998

O'Connor SD, Prusiner S, Dychtwald K: The age of Alzheimer's. New York Times, October 27, 2010. Available at: http://www.nytimes.com/2010/10/28/opinion/28oconnor.html. Accessed October 19, 2011.

O'Rourke MF, Hashimoto J: Mechanical factors in arterial aging: a clinical perspective. J Am Coll Cardiol 50:1–13, 2006

Oskvig RM: Special problems in the elderly. Chest 155(suppl):158S–164S, 1999

Perry HM: The endocrinology of aging. Clin Chem 45:1369–1376, 1999

Prestwood K, Duque G: Osteoporosis, in Principles of Geriatric Medicine and Gerontology, 5th Edition. Edited by Hazzard WR, Blass JP, Halter JB, et al. New York, McGraw-Hill, 2003, pp 973–985

Raina P, Santaguida P, Ismaila A, et al: Effectiveness of cholinesterase inhibitors and memantine for treating dementia: evidence review for a clinical practice guideline. Ann Intern Med 148:379–397, 2008

Reuben DB: Principles of geriatric assessment, in Principles of Geriatric Medicine and Gerontology, 5th Edition. Edited by Hazzard WR, Blass JP, Halter JB, et al. New York, McGraw-Hill, 2003, pp 99–110

Rizvi AA: Management of diabetes in older adults. Am J Med Sci 333:35–47, 2007

Rubenstein LZ, Josephson KR: Falls and their prevention in elderly people: what does the evidence show? Med Clin North Am 90:807–824, 2006

Rubenstein LZ, Josephson KR, Robbins AS: Falls in the nursing home. Ann Intern Med 121:442–451, 1994

Sadovsky R, Dhindsa S, Margo K: Testosterone deficiency: which patients should you screen and treat? J Fam Pract 56 (5 Suppl Testosterone):S1–S20, 2007

Schwartz JB: Clinical pharmacology, in Principles of Geriatric Medicine and Gerontology, 4th Edition. Edited by Hazzard WR, Blass JP, Ettinger WH, et al. New York, McGraw-Hill, 1999, pp 303–332

Seals DR, Esler MD: Human ageing and the sympathoadrenal system. J Physiol 528:407–417, 2000

Semla TP, Rochon PA: Pharmacotherapy, in Geriatrics Review Syllabus: A Core Curriculum in Geriatric Medicine, 6th Edition. Edited by Pompei P, Murphy JB. New York, American Geriatrics Society, 2006, pp 72–80

Spinewine A, Schmader KE, Barber N, et al: Appropriate prescribing in elderly people: how well can it be measured and optimised? Lancet 370:173–184, 2007

Sramek JJ, Alexander BD, Cutler NR: Acetylcholinesterase inhibitors for the treatment of Alzheimer's disease. Annals of Long Term Care 9(10):15–22, 2001

Stewart RB: Drug use in the elderly, in Therapeutics in the Elderly, 3rd Edition. Edited by Delafuente JC, Stewart RB. Cincinnati, OH, Harvey Whitney, 2001, pp 235–256

Stuck AE, Siu AL, Wieland GD, et al: Comprehensive geriatric assessment: a meta-analysis of controlled trials. Lancet 342:1032–1036, 1993

Stuck AE, Aronow HU, Steiner A, et al: A trial of annual in-home comprehensive geriatric assessments for elderly people living in the community. N Engl J Med 333:1184–1189, 1995

Taffet GE: Age-related physiologic changes, in Geriatrics Review Syllabus: A Core Curriculum in Geriatric Medicine, 5th Edition. Edited by Cobbs E, Duthie EH, Murphy JB. Dubuque, IA, Kendall/Hunt, 1999, pp 10–23

Tannenbaum C, Perrin L, DuBeau CE, et al: Diagnosis and management of urinary incontinence in the older patient. Arch Phys Med Rehabil 82:134–138, 2001

Tariot PN, Farlow MR, Grossberg GT, et al: Memantine treatment in patients with moderate to severe Alzheimer's disease already receiving donepezil: a randomized controlled trial. JAMA 291:317–324, 2004

Vaillant GE, Mukamal K: Successful aging. Am J Psychiatry 158:839–847, 2001

Yesavage JA, Brink TL: Development and validation of a geriatric depression screening scale: a preliminary report. J Psychiatr Res 17:37–49, 1983

Suggested Readings

Cohen HJ, Feussner JR, Weinberger M, et al: A controlled trial of inpatient and outpatient geriatric evaluation and management. N Engl J Med 346:905–912, 2002

Fried LP: Epidemiology of aging. Epidemiol Rev 22:95–106, 2000

Raina P, Santaguida P, Ismaila A, et al: Effectiveness of cholinesterase inhibitors and memantine for treating dementia: evidence review for a clinical practice guideline. Ann Intern Med 148:379–397, 2008

Rubenstein LZ, Josephson KR: Falls and their prevention in elderly people: what does the evidence show? Med Clin North Am 90:807–824, 2006

Spinewine A, Schmader KE, Barber N, et al: Appropriate prescribing in elderly people: how well can it be measured and optimised? Lancet 370:173–184, 2007

Vaillant GE, Mukamal K: Successful aging. Am J Psychiatry 158:839–847, 2001

PART II

Evaluation of Psychiatric Disorders in Late Life

CHAPTER 3

THE PSYCHIATRIC INTERVIEW OF OLDER ADULTS

DAN G. BLAZER, M.D., PH.D.

The foundation of the diagnostic workup of the older adult experiencing a psychiatric disorder is the diagnostic interview. Unfortunately, in this age of increasing technology in the laboratory and standardization of interview techniques, the art of the clinical interview has suffered. Also, time pressures limit clinicians' ability to perform a thorough diagnostic workup. Nevertheless, such a workup will save valuable time over the course of an older adult's illness. In fact, there is no substitute, even with modern technologies, for a thorough initial assessment of the older adult. In this chapter, I review the core of the psychiatric interview, including history taking, assessment of the family, and the mental status examination; describe structured interview schedules and

rating scales that are of value in the assessment of older adults; and outline techniques for communicating effectively with older adults.

History

The elements of a diagnostic workup of the elderly patient are presented in Table 3–1. To obtain historical information, the clinician should first interview the patient, if that is feasible, and then ask the patient's permission to interview family members. Members from at least two generations, if available for interview, can expand the perspective on the older adult's impairment. If the patient has difficulty providing an accurate or understandable history, the clinician

TABLE 3–1. Diagnostic workup of the elderly patient

History
    Current illness
    Past history
    Family history
    Context
    Medication history
    Medical history
Family assessment
Mental status examination

should concentrate especially on eliciting the symptoms or problems that the patient perceives as being most disabling, then fill the historical gap with data from the family.

Current Illness

DSM-IV-TR (American Psychiatric Association 2000) provides the clinician with a useful catalogue of symptoms and behaviors of psychiatric interest that are relevant to the diagnosis of the current illness. Symptoms are bits of data—the most visible part of the clinical picture and generally the part most easily agreed on among clinicians. Symptoms should be defined in such a way that if multiple clinicians each obtain equivalent information, they would have minimal disagreement about the presence or absence of a symptom. The decision about whether those symptoms form a syndrome or derive from a particular etiology must be determined independently of the data collection on symptoms.

Even so, the clinical interaction may be confounded by bias when a clinician communicates with an older adult about psychiatric symptoms. During the process of becoming a patient, the older adult, usually with the advice of others, forms a self-diag-

nosis of his or her problem and makes a judgment about the degree of ill-being perceived. For these reasons, the clinician must take care to avoid accepting the patient's explanation for a given problem or set of problems. Statements such as "I guess I'm just getting old, and there's nothing really to worry about" or "Most people slow down when they get to be my age" can lull the clinician into complacency about what may be a treatable psychiatric disorder. On the contrary, the advent of new and disturbing symptoms in an older adult between office visits can exhaust the clinician's patience, thereby derailing pursuit of the problem. For example, the older adult with hypochondriasis whose awakenings during the night are increasing may insist that this symptom be treated with a sedative and plead with the clinician not to allow continual suffering. In the clinician's view, however, the symptom is a normal accompaniment of old age and therefore should be accepted. Distress over changes in functioning, such as sexual functioning, may overwhelm the older adult patient and, especially if the clinician is perceived as unconcerned, may precipitate self-medication or even a suicide attempt.

To prevent attitudinal biases when eliciting reports by the older adult (which may result in missing the symptoms and signs of a treatable psychiatric disorder), the clinician must include in the initial interview a review of the more important psychiatric symptoms in a relatively structured format. Common symptoms that should be reviewed include excessive weakness or lethargy; depressed mood or "the blues"; memory problems; difficulty concentrating; feelings of helplessness, hopelessness, and uselessness; isolation; suspicion of others; anxiety and agitation; sleep problems; and appetite problems and weight loss. Critical symptoms that should be reviewed include the presence or absence of suicidal thoughts, profound anhedonia, impulsive behavior ("I can't control myself"), confusion, and delusions and hallucinations.

The review of symptoms is most valuable when considered in the context of symptom presentation: When did the symptoms begin? How long have they lasted? Has their severity changed over time? Are there physical or environmental events that precipitate the symptoms? What steps, if any, have been taken to try to correct the symptoms? Have any of these interventions proved successful? Do the symptoms vary during the day (diurnal variation)? Do they vary during the week or with seasons of the year? Do the symptoms form clusters—that is, are they associated with one another? Which symptoms appear ego-syntonic, and which appear ego-dystonic? As symptoms are reviewed, a specific time frame facilitates focus on the current illness. Having a 1-month or 6-month window enables the patient to review symptoms and events temporally—an approach not usually taken by distressed elders, who tend to concentrate on their immediate sufferings.

Critical to the assessment of the current illness is an assessment of function and change in function. The two parameters that are most important (and not included in usual assessments of physical and psychiatric illness) are social functioning and activities of daily living (ADLs). Questions should be asked about the social interaction of the older adult, such as the frequency of his or her visits outside the home, telephone calls, and visits from family and friends. Many scales have been developed to assess ADLs; however, in the interview, the clinician can simply ask about the pa-

tient's ability to get around (e.g., walk inside and outside the house), to perform certain physical activities independently (e.g., bathe, dress, shave, brush teeth, and select clothes), and to perform instrumental activities (e.g., cook, maintain a bank account, shop, and drive). It is also important to assess how often the elder actually engages in these activities; for example, the ability to walk outside does not always translate to outside exercise.

Past History

Next, the clinician must review the history of symptoms and episodes. Has the patient had similar episodes in the past? How long did the episodes last? When did they occur? How many times in the patient's lifetime have such episodes occurred? Unfortunately, the older adult may not equate present distress with past episodes that are symptomatically similar, so the perspective of the family is especially valuable in the attempt to link current and past episodes.

Other psychiatric and medical problems should be reviewed as well, especially medical illnesses that have led to hospitalization and the use of medication. Not infrequently, an older adult has experienced a major illness or trauma in childhood or as a younger adult but views this information as being of no relevance to the current episode and therefore dismisses it. Probes to elicit these data are essential. Older adults may ignore or even forget past psychiatric difficulties, especially if these difficulties were disguised. For example, mood swings in early or middle life may have occurred during periods of excessive and productive activity, episodes of excessive alcohol intake, or periods of vague, undiagnosed physical problems. Previous periods of overt disability in usual activities may flag those episodes. An older person sometimes becomes angry or irritated when the clinician continues to probe. Reassurance regarding the importance of obtaining this information will generally suffice, except when dealing with a patient who cannot tolerate the discomfort and distress, even for brief periods. Older persons who have chronic and moderately severe anxiety or a histrionic personality style, as well as distressed Alzheimer's patients, tolerate their symptoms poorly.

Family History

The distribution of psychiatric symptoms and illnesses in the family should be determined next. The older person with symptoms consistent with senile dementia or primary degenerative dementia is likely to have a family history of dementia. A history should be obtained about institutionalization, significant memory problems in family members, hospitalization for a nervous breakdown or depressive disorder, suicide, alcohol abuse and dependence, electroconvulsive therapy, long-term residence in a mental health facility (and possibly a diagnosis of schizophrenia), and use of mental health services by family members (Blazer 1984).

Of relevance to the pharmacological treatment of certain disorders—especially depression—in older adults is the tendency of individuals in a family to respond therapeutically to the same pharmacological agent. If the older adult has a depressive disorder and if depression has been treated effectively in biological relatives, the clinician should determine what pharmacological agent was used to treat the depression. Accurate genetic information can be better obtained when family members from more than one generation are interviewed. Many

psychiatric disorders are characterized by a variety of symptoms, so asking the patient or one family member for a history of depression is insufficient.

Context

Psychiatric disorders occur in a biomedical and psychosocial context. Although the clinician will try to determine what medical problems the patient has experienced, it is possible to overlook a variation in the relative contribution of these medical disorders to psychopathology or to overlook the psychosocial contribution to the onset and continuance of the problem. Has the spouse of the older adult undergone a change? Are the middle-aged children managing high stress, such as simultaneously caring for an emotionally disturbed child and the loss of employment? Are the grandchildren placing emotional stress on the elderly patient, perhaps by requesting money? Has the economic status of the older adult deteriorated? Has the availability of medical care changed? Although many psychiatric disorders are biologically driven, they do not occur in a psychosocial vacuum. Environmental precipitants remain important in the web of causation leading to the onset of an episode of emotional distress and are critical to the assessment of the older adult.

Medication History

Evaluating the medication history of the older adult is essential. A careful review of current and past medications by the clinician, a nurse, or a physician's assistant is essential. The older person should be asked to bring to the appointment all pill bottles, a list of medications taken, and the dosage schedule. A comparison between the written schedule and the pill containers will frequently expose some discrepancy. Both prescription medications and over-the-counter drugs, such as laxatives and vitamins, should be recorded. The clinician can then identify the medications that are potentially critical in terms of drug-drug interactions and ask about them during subsequent patient visits.

Older persons are less likely than younger persons to abuse alcohol, but a careful history of alcohol intake is essential to the diagnostic workup. Although older persons do not usually volunteer information about their alcohol intake, they are generally forthcoming when asked about their drinking habits. Substance abuse beyond alcohol and prescription drugs is rare in older adults but not entirely absent.

Medical History

Given the high likelihood of comorbid medical problems associated with psychiatric disorders in late life, a comprehensive medical history is essential. Most older persons see a primary care physician regularly (although decreasing payments from Medicare render this assumption less accurate each year). The geriatric psychiatrist should obtain medical records, if possible. Major illnesses should be recorded. A brief telephone call to the primary care physician can be extremely useful.

Family Assessment

Clinicians working with older adults must be equipped to evaluate the family—both its functionality and its potential as a resource for the older adult. Geriatric psychiatry, almost by definition, is family psychiatry.

A primary goal of the clinician, as advocate for the older adult with psychiatric disturbance, is to facilitate family support for the elder during a time of disability. At least four parameters of support are important for the clinician to evaluate as the treatment plan evolves: 1) the availability of family members to the older person over time; 2) the tangible services provided by the family to the older person; 3) the perception of family support by the older patient (and therefore the willingness of the patient to cooperate and accept support); and 4) tolerance by the family of specific behaviors that derive from the psychiatric disorder.

The clinician should ask the older person, "If you become ill, is there a family member who will take care of you for a short time?" Next, the availability of family members who can care for the older adult over an extended period should be determined. If a particular member is designated as the primary caregiver, plans for respite care should be discussed. Given the increased focus on short hospital stays and the documented higher levels of impairment on discharge, the availability of family members becomes essential to the effective care of the older adult after hospitalization for a psychiatric disorder or a combined medical and psychiatric disorder.

What specific, tangible services can be provided to the older adult by family members? Even the most devoted spouse can be limited in the delivery of certain services because, for example, he or she does not drive a car, and therefore cannot provide transportation, or is not physically strong enough to provide certain types of nursing care. Generic services of special importance in at-home support of the older adult with psychiatric impairment include transportation; nursing services (e.g., administering medications at home); physical therapy; checking on or continuous supervision of the patient; homemaker and household services; meal preparation; administrative, legal, and protective services; financial assistance; living quarters; and coordination of the delivery of services. These services are considered generic because they can be defined in terms of their activities, regardless of who provides each service. Assessing the range and extent of service delivery by the family to the older person with functional impairment provides a convenient barometer of the economic, social, and emotional burdens placed on the family.

Family tolerance of specific behaviors may not correlate with overall support. Every person has a level of tolerance for specific behaviors that are especially difficult. Sanford (1975) found that the following behaviors were tolerated by families of older persons with impairments (in decreasing percentages): incontinence of urine (81%), personality conflicts (54%), falls (52%), physically aggressive behavior (44%), inability to walk unaided (33%), daytime wandering (33%), and sleep disturbance (16%). This frequency may appear counterintuitive because incontinence is generally considered particularly aversive to family members. However, the outcome of incontinence can be corrected easily enough, but a few nights of no sleep can easily extend family members beyond their capabilities for serving a parent, sibling, or spouse.

Mental Status Examination

Physicians and other clinicians are at times hesitant to perform a structured mental status examination, fearing that the effort will insult or irritate the patient or that the patient will view the examination as a waste of time. Nevertheless, the mental status examination of the older psychiatric patient is central to the diagnostic workup. Many as-

pects of this examination can be assessed during the history-taking interview.

Appearance may be affected by the older patient's psychiatric symptoms (e.g., the depressed patient may neglect grooming), cognitive status (e.g., the patient with dementia may not be able to match clothes or even put on clothes appropriately), and environment (e.g., a nursing home patient may not be groomed as well as a patient living at home with a spouse).

Affect and mood usually can be assessed by observing the patient during the interview. *Affect* is the feeling tone that accompanies the patient's cognitive output (Linn 1980). Affect may fluctuate during the interview; however, the older person is more likely to have a constriction of affect. *Mood,* the state that underlies overt affect and is sustained over time, is usually apparent by the end of the interview. For example, the affect of a depressed older adult may not reach the degree of dysphoria seen in younger persons (as evidenced by crying spells or protestations of uncontrollable despair), yet the depressed mood is usually sustained and discernible from beginning to end.

Psychomotor activity may be agitated or retarded. Psychomotor retardation or underactivity is characteristic of major depression and severe schizophreniform symptoms, as well as of some variants of primary degenerative dementia. Psychiatrically impaired older persons, except some who have advanced dementia, are more likely to show hyperactivity or agitation. Those who are depressed will appear uneasy, move their hands frequently, and have difficulty remaining seated through the interview. Patients with mild to moderate dementia, especially those with vascular dementia, will be easily distracted, rise from a seated position, and/or walk around the room or even out of the room. Pacing is often observed when the older adult is admitted to a hospital ward. Agitation usually can be distinguished from anxiety—the agitated individual does not complain of a sense of impending doom or dread. In patients with psychomotor dysfunction, movement generally relieves the immediate discomfort, although it does not correct the underlying disturbance. Occasionally, the older adult with motor retardation may actually be experiencing a disturbance in consciousness and may even reach an almost stuporous state. The patient may not be easily aroused, but when aroused, he or she will respond by grimacing or withdrawal.

Perception is the awareness of objects in relation to each other and follows stimulation of peripheral sense organs (Linn 1980). Disturbances of perception include hallucinations—that is, false sensory perceptions not associated with real or external stimuli. For example, a paranoid older person may perceive invasion of his or her house at night by individuals who disarrange belongings and abuse him or her sexually. Hallucinations often take the form of false auditory perceptions, false perceptions of movement or body sensation (e.g., palpitations), and false perceptions of smell, taste, and touch. The older patient who is severely depressed may have frank auditory hallucinations that condemn or encourage self-destructive behavior.

Disturbances in thought content are the most common disturbances of cognition noted in older patients with psychosis. The depressed patient often develops beliefs that are inconsistent with the objective information obtained from family members about the patient's abilities and social resources. Even after elderly persons recover from depression, they may still experience periodic

recurrences of delusional thoughts, which can be most disturbing to otherwise rational older adults. Older patients appear less likely to experience delusional remorse, guilt, or persecution.

Even if delusions are not obvious, preoccupation with a particular thought or idea is common among depressed elderly persons. Such preoccupation is closely associated with obsessional thinking or irresistible intrusion of thoughts into the conscious mind. Although the older adult rarely acts on these thoughts compulsively, the guilt-provoking or self-accusing thoughts may occasionally become so difficult to bear that the person considers, attempts, or succeeds in committing suicide.

Disturbances of thought progression accompany disturbances of content. Evaluation of the content and process of cognition may uncover disturbances such as problems with the structure of associations, the speed of associations, and the content of thought. Thinking is a goal-directed flow of ideas, symbols, and associations initiated in response to environmental stimuli, a perceived problem, or a task that requires progression to a logical or reality-based conclusion (Linn 1980). The older adult who is compulsive or has schizophrenia may pathologically repeat the same word or idea in response to a variety of probes, as may the patient who has primary degenerative dementia. Some older adults with dementia have circumstantiality—that is, the introduction of many apparently irrelevant details to cover a lack of clarity and memory problems. Interviews with patients who have this problem can be most frustrating because they proceed at a very slow pace. On other occasions, elderly patients may appear incoherent, with no logical connection to their thoughts, or they may produce irrelevant answers. The intrusion of thoughts from previous conversations into a current conversation is a prime example of the disturbance in association found in patients with primary degenerative dementia (e.g., Alzheimer's disease). This symptom is not typical of other dementias, such as the dementia of Huntington's disease. However, in the absence of dementia, even paranoid older adults do not generally show a significant disturbance in the structure of associations.

Suicidal thoughts are critical to assess in the elderly patient with psychiatric impairment. Although thoughts of death are common in late life, spontaneous revelations of suicidal thoughts are rare. A stepwise probe is the best means of assessing the presence of suicidal ideation (Blazer 1982). First, the clinician should ask the patient if he or she has ever thought that life was not worth living. If so, has the patient considered acting on that thought? If so, how would the patient attempt to inflict such self-harm? If the patient has definite plans, the clinician should probe further to determine whether the implements for a suicide attempt are available. For example, if a patient has considered shooting himself, the clinician should ask, "Do you have a gun available and loaded at home?" Suicidal ideation in an older adult is always of concern, but intervention is necessary when suicide has been considered seriously and the implements are available.

Assessment of memory and cognitive status is most accurately performed through psychological testing. However, the psychiatric interview of the older adult must include a reasonable assessment of these domains. Although older adults may not complain of memory dysfunction, they are more likely than younger patients to have problems with memory, concentration, and intellect. A brief, informal means of testing cognitive functioning should be included in the diagnostic workup. The clinician proceeding through an evaluation of memory and intellect also must remember that poor performance may reflect psychic distress or a lack of education, as opposed to mental retardation or dementia. In addition, to rule out the potential confounding of agitation and anxiety, testing can be performed on more than one occasion.

Testing of memory is based on three essential processes: 1) registration (the ability to record an experience in the central nervous system), 2) retention (the persistence and permanence of a registered experience), and 3) recall (the ability to summon consciously the registered experience and report it) (Linn 1980). *Registration,* apart from recall, is difficult to evaluate directly. Occasionally, events or information that the older adult denies remembering will appear spontaneously during other parts of the interview. Registration usually is not impaired except in patients with one of the more severely dementing illnesses.

Retention, on the other hand, can be blocked by both psychic distress and brain dysfunction. Lack of retention is especially relevant to the unimportant data often asked for on a mental status examination. For example, requesting the older adult to remember three objects for 5 minutes will frequently identify a deficit if the older adult has little motivation to attempt the task.

Disturbances of *recall* can be tested directly in several ways. The most common are tests of orientation to time, place, person, and situation. Most individuals continually orient themselves through radio, television, and reading material, as well as through conversations with others. Some elderly individuals may be isolated through sensory impairment or lack of social contact; poor orientation in these patients may represent deficits in the physical and social environment rather than brain dysfunction. *Immediate recall* can be tested by asking the older person to repeat a word, phrase, or series of numbers, but it can also be tested in conjunction with cognitive skills by requesting the individual to spell a specific word backwards or to recall elements of a story.

During the mental status examination, intelligence can be assessed only superficially. Tests of simple arithmetic calculation and fund of knowledge, supplemented by portions of well-known psychiatric tests, are helpful. The classic test for calculation is to ask a patient to subtract 7 from 100 and to repeat this operation on the succession of remainders. Usually, five calculations are sufficient to determine the older adult's ability to complete this task. If the older adult fails the task, a less exacting test is to request the patient to subtract 3 from 20 and to repeat this operation on the succession of remainders until 0 is reached. These examinations must not be rushed, for older persons may not perform as well when they perceive time pressure. A capacity for abstract thinking is often tested by asking the patient to interpret a well-known proverb, such as "A rolling stone gathers no moss." A more accurate test of abstraction, however, is classifying objects in a common category. For example, the patient is asked to state the similarity between an apple and a pear. Whereas naming objects from a category (such as fruits) is retained despite moderate and sometimes marked declines in cognition, the opposite process of classifying two different objects in a common category is not retained as well.

Rating Scales and Standardized Interviews

Rating scales and standardized or structured interviews have progressively been incorporated into the diagnostic assessment of the elderly psychiatric patient. Such rating procedures have increased in popularity as the need has increased for systematic, reproducible diagnoses for third-party carriers (part of the impetus for the dramatic change in nomenclature evidenced in DSM-IV-TR) and for a standard means of assessing change in clinical status. A thorough review in this chapter of all instruments that are used is not possible. Therefore, selected instruments are presented and evaluated in this section, chosen either because they have special relevance to the geriatric patient or because they are widely used.

Cognitive Dysfunction and Dementia Schedules

Several standardized assessment methods for delirium have emerged. Perhaps the best and the most easily used is the Confusion Assessment Method (Inouye 1990). The scale assesses nine characteristics of delirium, including acute onset (evidence of such onset), fluctuating course (behavior change during the day), inattention (trouble in focusing), disorganized thinking (presence of rambling or irrelevant conversations and illogical flow of ideas), and altered level of consciousness (rated from alert to comatose). Diagnosis of delirium according to DSM-IV-TR criteria can be derived from the scale.

Two interviewer-administered cognitive screens for dementia have been popular in both clinical and community studies. The first is the Short Portable Mental Status Questionnaire (SPMSQ; Pfeiffer 1975), a derivative of the Mental Status Questionnaire developed by Kahn et al. (1960). The SPMSQ consists of 10 questions designed to assess orientation, memory, fund of knowledge, and calculation. For most community-dwelling older adults, two or fewer errors indicate intact functioning; three or four errors, mild impairment; five to seven errors, moderate impairment; and eight or more errors, severe impairment. The ease of administration of this instrument and its reliability as supported by accumulated epidemiological data make it useful for both clinical and community screens.

The Mini-Mental State Examination (Folstein et al. 1975) is a 30-item screening instrument that assesses orientation, registration, attention and calculation, recall, and language. It requires 5–10 minutes to administer and includes more items of clinical significance than does the SPMSQ. Seven to 12 errors suggest mild to moderate cognitive impairment, and 13 or more errors indicate severe impairment. This instrument is perhaps the most frequently used standardized screening instrument in clinical practice.

A dementia scale for assessing the probability that a patient's dementia is a vascular dementia was suggested by Hachinski et al. (1975). In their study, cerebral blood flow in patients with primary degenerative dementia was compared with that in patients who had vascular dementia. Certain clinical features were determined to be more associated with multi-infarct dementia, and each of these features was assigned a score. Those clinical features, along with their scores, are as follows: abrupt onset = 2, stepwise deterioration = 1, fluctuating course = 2, nocturnal confusion = 1, relative preservation of personality = 1, depression = 1, somatic complaints = 1, emotional incontinence = 1, history of hypertension = 1, history of strokes = 2, evidence of associated atherosclerosis = 1, focal neurological symptoms = 2, and focal neurological signs = 2. A score of 7 or greater was highly suggestive of multi-infarct dementia. However, given the frequent overlap of multiple small infarcts and primary degenerative dementia, as well as the difficulty of assessing these items effectively, most investigators have ceased to rely on the Hachinski scale for clinical use.

Depression Rating Scales

Several self-rating depression scales have been used to screen for depression in patients at all stages of the life cycle; most of these scales have been studied in older populations. The most widely used of the current instruments in community studies is the Center for Epidemiologic Studies Depression Scale (CES-D; Radloff 1977). The scale consists of 20 behaviors and feelings, and the patient indicates how frequently each was experienced over the past week (from no days to most days). In a factor-analytic study of the CES-D in a community population, four factors were identified: somatic symptoms, positive affect, negative affect, and interpersonal relationships (Ross and Mirowsky 1984). The disaggregation of these factors and the exploration of their interaction are significant steps forward in understanding the results derived from symptom scales such as the CES-D in older populations. For example, the somatic items (e.g., loss of interest, poor appetite) are more likely to be associated with a course of depressive episodes similar to that described for major depression with melancholia, and the positive-affect items are more likely to be associated with life satisfaction scores.

The Geriatric Depression Scale (GDS) was developed because the scales discussed earlier present problems for older individuals who have difficulty in selecting one of four forced-response items (Yesavage et al. 1983). The 30-item GDS permits patients to rate items as either present or absent; it includes questions about symptoms such as cognitive complaints, self-image, and losses. Items selected were thought to have relevance to late-life depression. The GDS has not been used extensively in community populations and is not as well standardized as the CES-D, but its yes/no format is preferred to the CES-D by many clinicians.

Of the scales used by interviewers to rate patients, the Hamilton Rating Scale for Depression (Ham-D; Hamilton 1960) is by far the most commonly used. The advantage of having ratings based on clinical judgment has made the Ham-D a popular instrument for rating outcome in clinical trials. For example, a reduction in the score to one-half the initial score or to a score below a certain value would indicate partial or complete recovery from an episode of depression.

A scale that has received considerable attention clinically, having been standardized in clinical but not community populations, is the Montgomery-Åsberg Rating Scale for Depression (Montgomery and Åsberg 1979). This scale follows the pattern of the Ham-D and concentrates on 10 symptoms of depression; the clinician rates each symptom on a scale of 0–6 (for a range of scores between 0 and 60). The symptoms include apparent sadness, reported sadness, inattention, reduced sleep, reduced appetite, concentration difficulties, lassitude, inability to feel, pessimistic thoughts, and suicidal thoughts. Theoretically, this scale is an improvement over the Ham-D in that it appears to better differentiate between responders and nonresponders to intervention for depression. The Montgomery-Åsberg scale does not include many somatic symptoms that tend to be more common in older adults, and therefore it may be of greater value in tracking the symptoms of depressive illness that would be expected to change with therapy.

General Assessment Scales

Several general assessment scales of psychiatric status (occasionally combined with functioning in other areas) have been found to be useful in both community and clinical populations. One of the more frequently used scales is the Global Assessment of Functioning Scale (American Psychiatric Association 2000). On this scale, the rater makes a single rating, from 0 to 100, that best describes—on the basis of his or her clinical judgment—the lowest level of the subject's functioning in the week before the rating. The Global Assessment of Functioning Scale has not been standardized for older adults, but its common use in psychiatric studies suggests the need for standardization. The scale was incorporated as Axis V in DSM-IV-TR to measure overall functioning. Newer scales have been planned for DSM-5.

The Older Americans Resources and Services (OARS) Multidimensional Functional Assessment Questionnaire (Duke University Center for the Study of Aging and Human Development 1978), administered by a lay interviewer, produces functional impairment ratings in five dimensions: mental health, physical health, social functioning, economic functioning, and

ADLs. In one community survey that used OARS (Blazer 1978a), 13% of the persons in the community were found to have mental health impairment. The OARS instrument was developed to integrate functional measures across a series of parameters relevant to older adults; it has been used widely in both community and clinical surveys. With the recent emphasis on discrete psychiatric disorders, however, the instrument has not been as widely used by mental health workers as it might otherwise have been.

Structured Diagnostic Interviews

Several structured interview schedules are available for both clinical and community diagnosis. These interview schedules have allowed increased reliability of the identification of particular symptoms and psychiatric diagnoses; however, if one adheres closely to the structured interview, the richness inherent in the unstructured interview tends to be lost. Comments made by the patient during the evaluation that could be used to trace relevant associations must be ignored to push through the interview schedule. Most of these interviews require more time than the traditional unstructured first session with the patient.

The most frequently used instrument in the United States is the Structured Clinical Interview for DSM-IV (SCID; First et al. 1997). This instrument is easily adaptable to the Research Diagnostic Criteria (RDC) and DSM-IV-TR. Although specific questions are suggested for probing most areas of interest, the interviewer using the SCID has the flexibility to ask additional questions and can use any available data to assign a diagnosis. The interviewer must have clin-ical training but does not have to be a psychiatrist. Many of the symptoms may not be relevant to older adults (especially the extensive probes for psychotic symptoms), and the interview frequently takes 2.5 to 3 hours to administer. Nevertheless, the experience gained by the clinician in using this instrument can contribute to a more effective clinical practice.

The Diagnostic Interview Schedule (DIS; Robins et al. 1981) is a highly structured, computer-scored interview that can be administered by a lay interviewer and allows psychiatric diagnoses to be made according to DSM-III criteria, Feighner criteria (Feighner et al. 1972), and RDC. The DIS questions probe for the presence or absence of symptoms or behaviors relevant to a series of psychiatric disorders, the severity of the symptoms, and the putative cause of the symptoms. Diagnoses of cognitive impairment, schizophrenia or schizophreniform disorder, major depression, generalized anxiety disorder, panic disorder, agoraphobia, obsessive-compulsive disorder, dysthymic disorder, somatization disorder, alcohol abuse and/or dependence, and other substance abuse and/or dependence can be made from Axis I of DSM-III. A diagnosis of antisocial personality disorder (Axis II) also can be made. The instrument has proved reasonably reliable in clinical populations for both current and lifetime diagnoses.

The range of disorders probed by the DIS questions, coupled with the instrument's relative ease of administration (it generally takes 45–90 minutes to administer to an older adult), has made it popular for use in clinical studies. In addition, community-based comparative data are available on a large sample from the Epidemiologic Catchment Area study (Myers et al. 1984;

Regier et al. 1984). The DIS can be supplemented with additional questions to probe for specific symptoms, such as melancholic symptoms, and additional data on sleep disorders for depressed older adults. No problems have arisen when the instrument is used among older adults in the community. In general, the memory decay that occurs in elderly persons causes no more of a performance problem on this instrument than on others. Nevertheless, the DIS is of less value in the study of institutional populations and in reconstruction of lifetime history regardless of setting because memory problems cannot be circumvented by clinical judgment. Supplementary data can be added to the instrument for developing a standardized diagnosis. A shortened version of the DIS, which has been used in epidemiological surveys, is the Composite International Diagnostic Interview (World Health Organization 1989).

Effective Communication With the Older Adult

The clinician who works with the older adult should be cognizant of factors relating to both the patient and the clinician that may produce barriers to effective communication (Blazer 1978b). Many older persons experience a relatively high level of anxiety yet do not complain of this symptom. Stress deriving from a new situation, such as visiting a clinician's office or being interviewed in a hospital, may intensify such anxiety and subsequently impair effective communication. Perceptual problems, such as hearing and visual impairment, may exacerbate disorientation and complicate the communication of problems to the clinician. Elderly persons are more likely to withhold information than

to hazard answers that may be incorrect—in other words, older persons tend to be more cautious. Elderly persons frequently take longer to respond to inquiries and resist the clinician who attempts to rush through the history-taking interview.

The elderly patient may perceive the physician unrealistically, on the basis of previous life experiences (i.e., transference may occur). Although the older patient will sometimes accept the role of child, viewing the physician as parent, the patient is initially more likely to view the clinician as the idealized child who can provide reciprocal care to the previously capable but now impaired parent. Splitting between the physician (idealized) and the children of the patient (devalued) may subsequently occur. Also, the clinician may perceive the older adult patient incorrectly because of fears of aging and death or because of previous negative experiences with his or her own parents. In order for a clinician to work effectively with older adults, these personal feelings should be discussed during training—and afterward.

Once physician and patient attitudes have been recognized and acknowledged, certain techniques have generally proved to be valuable in communicating with the elderly patient. These techniques should not be implemented indiscriminately, however, for the variation in the population of older adults is significant. First, the older person should be approached with respect. The clinician should knock before entering a patient's room and should greet the patient by surname (e.g., Mr. Jones, Mrs. Smith) rather than by a given name, unless the clinician also wishes to be addressed by a given name.

After taking a position near the older person—near enough to reach out and touch the patient—the clinician should speak clearly and slowly and use simple sentences in case the person's hearing is impaired. Because of hearing problems, older patients may understand conversation better over the telephone than in person. By placing the receiver against the mastoid bone, the patient with otosclerosis can take advantage of preserved bone conduction.

The interview should be paced so that the older person has enough time to respond to questions. Most elders are not uncomfortable with silence because it gives them an opportunity to formulate their answers to questions and elaborate certain points they wish to emphasize. Nonverbal communication is frequently a key to effec-tive communication with elderly persons because they may be reticent about revealing affect verbally. The patient's facial expressions, gestures, postures, and long silences may provide clues to the clinician about issues that are unspoken.

One key to successful communication with an older adult is a willingness to continue working as a professional with that person. Older adults—possibly unlike some of their children and grandchildren—place a great deal of stress on loyalty and continuity. Most elderly patients do not require large amounts of time from clinicians, and those who are more demanding can usually be controlled through structure in the interview.

Key Points

- The diagnostic interview is the cornerstone of assessment and treatment assignment for the older adult with psychiatric impairment.

- A thorough medication history, although it takes time to obtain, saves valuable time and complications in the treatment of psychiatric disorders in older adults.

- Functional status (i.e., the ability to perform usual activities of daily living) is often as important as diagnosis in tracking the progress of treatment of psychiatric disorders in older adults.

- Geriatric psychiatry is family psychiatry.

- What is gained in reliability by using a structured diagnostic interview is offset by the loss of valuable information about the subjective feelings of the older adult and the context of the emergence of symptoms.

- The clinician should speak clearly and slowly but not in a patronizing way to the older adult, who might have a hearing impairment.

References

American Psychiatric Association: Diagnostic and Statistical Manual of Mental Disorders, 4th Edition, Text Revision. Washington, DC, American Psychiatric Association, 2000

Blazer DG: The OARS Durham surveys: description and application, in Multidimensional Functional Assessment: The OARS Methodology—A Manual, 2nd Edition. Durham, NC, Duke University Center for the Study of Aging and Human Development, 1978a, pp 75–88

Blazer DG: Techniques for communicating with your elderly patient. Geriatrics 33:79–80, 83–84, 1978b

Blazer DG: Depression in Late Life. St Louis, MO, CV Mosby, 1982

Blazer DG: Evaluating the family of the elderly patient, in A Family Approach to Health Care in the Elderly. Edited by Blazer D, Siegler IC. Menlo Park, CA, Addison-Wesley, 1984, pp 13–32

Duke University Center for the Study of Aging and Human Development: Multidimensional Functional Assessment: The OARS Methodology—A Manual, 2nd Edition. Durham, NC, Duke University Center for the Study of Aging and Human Development, 1978

Feighner JP, Robins E, Guze SB, et al: Diagnostic criteria for use in psychiatric research. Arch Gen Psychiatry 26:57–63, 1972

First MB, Spitzer RL, Gibbon M: Structured Clinical Interview for DSM-IV. Washington, DC, American Psychiatric Press, 1997

Folstein MF, Folstein SE, McHugh PR: "Mini-Mental State": a practical method for grading the cognitive state of patients for the clinician. J Psychiatr Res 12:189–198, 1975

Hachinski VC, Iliff LD, Zilhka E, et al: Cerebral blood flow in dementia. Arch Neurol 32:632–637, 1975

Hamilton M: A rating scale for depression. J Neurol Neurosurg Psychiatry 23:56–62, 1960

Inouye SK: Clarifying confusion: the Confusion Assessment Method—a new method for detection of delirium. Ann Intern Med 113:941–950, 1990

Kahn RL, Goldfarb AI, Pollack M, et al: Brief objective measures for the determination of mental status in the aged. Am J Psychiatry 117:326–328, 1960

Linn L: Clinical manifestations of psychiatric disorders, in Comprehensive Textbook of Psychiatry, 3rd Edition, Vol 1. Edited by Kaplan HI, Freedman AM, Sadock BJ. Baltimore, MD, Williams & Wilkins, 1980, pp 990–1034

Montgomery SA, Åsberg M: A new depression scale designed to be sensitive to change. Br J Psychiatry 134:382–389, 1979

Myers JK, Weissman MM, Tischler GL, et al: Six-month prevalence of psychiatric disorders in three communities: 1980 to 1982. Arch Gen Psychiatry 41:959–967, 1984

Pfeiffer E: A Short Portable Mental Status Questionnaire for the assessment of organic brain deficit in elderly patients. J Am Geriatr Soc 23:433–441, 1975

Radloff LS: The CES-D Scale: a self-report depression scale for research in the general population. Applied Psychological Measurement 1:385–401, 1977

Regier DA, Myers JK, Kramer M, et al: The NIMH Epidemiologic Catchment Area program: historical context, major objectives, and study population characteristics. Arch Gen Psychiatry 41:934–941, 1984

Robins LN, Helzer JE, Croughan J, et al: National Institute of Mental Health Diagnostic Interview Schedule: its history, characteristics, and validity. Arch Gen Psychiatry 38:381–389, 1981

Ross CE, Mirowsky J: Components of depressed mood in married men and women: the CES-D. Am J Epidemiol 119:997–1004, 1984

Sanford JRA: Tolerance of debility in elderly dependents by supporters at home: its significance for hospital practice. BMJ 3:471–473, 1975

World Health Organization: Composite International Diagnostic Interview. Geneva, Switzerland, World Health Organization, 1989

Yesavage JA, Brink TL, Rose TL, et al: Development and validation of a geriatric depression screening scale: a preliminary report. J Psychiatr Res 17:37–49, 1983

Suggested Readings

Blazer DG: Techniques for communicating with your elderly patient. Geriatrics 33:79–80, 83–84, 1978

Folstein MF, Folstein SE, McHugh PR: "Mini-Mental State": a practical method for grading the cognitive state of patients for the clinician. J Psychiatr Res 12:189–198, 1975

Inouye SK: Clarifying confusion: the Confusion Assessment Method: a new method for detection of delirium. Ann Intern Med 113:941–950, 1990

Othmer E, Othmer SC, Othmer JP: Psychiatric interview, history and mental status examination, in Kaplan and Sadock's Comprehensive Textbook of Psychiatry, Vol 1. Edited by Sadock BJ, Sadock VA. Philadelphia, PA, Lippincott Williams & Wilkins, 2005, pp 794–826

CHAPTER 4

Use of the Laboratory in the Diagnostic Workup of Older Adults

Mugdha E. Thakur, M.B.B.S.

P. Murali Doraiswamy, M.B.B.S.

Laboratory testing is an essential component of the psychiatric evaluation of elderly individuals, who often present with comorbid medical illnesses. Because of the significant growth in the number of diagnostic tests available, it is essential to balance what we *can* do with what we *should* do, as guided by our clinical judgment and evidence-based assessment of cost-effectiveness. It is also important for clinicians to realize that many, if not most, normative laboratory values have been derived from studies in 20- to 50-year-old Caucasian adults, which may not be optimal for the elderly. In this chapter, we summarize selected tests of high relevance to the clinician.

Hematological Tests

A complete blood cell (CBC) count screens for multiple problems, including infections and anemia. Anemia in elderly psychiatric patients may signal a selective serotonin reuptake inhibitor (SSRI)–associated gastrointestinal blood loss or vitamin or mineral deficiencies. A platelet count is important to monitor for psychiatric medications associated with thrombocytopenia, such as divalproex sodium or carbamazepine because the risk of drug-induced thrombocytopenia may increase with age (Trannel et al. 2001). Lithium, in contrast, may result in mild leukocytosis. Because of the risk of agranulocytosis, CBC testing is required weekly or biweekly for patients taking clozapine and may be needed more frequently if the patient develops signs of infection. Mirtazapine can also rarely cause agranulocytosis, and although routine CBC monitoring is not indicated, it should be pursued if a patient develops sore throat, fever, stomatitis, or other signs of infection.

Chemistry Tests

Measures of serum sodium, potassium, and other electrolytes can help in the workup of confusional states and help monitor drug side effects. Hyponatremia is a common side effect of SSRIs in the elderly (Jacob and Spinler 2006). Potassium abnormalities may result in severe cardiac arrhythmias. Abnormal calcium and magnesium levels may result in paranoid ideation or frank psychosis. Any or all of these results may be abnormal in patients receiving hemodialysis or in the intensive care unit (ICU).

Diabetes can be diagnosed from a random plasma glucose level greater than 200 mg/dL with symptoms of diabetes or a fasting glucose level greater than 126 mg/dL (Dagogo-Jack 2001). Because second-generation antipsychotic drugs can lead to weight gain and diabetes, a new set of guidelines has been proposed to screen and monitor patients who are started on these drugs for risk of metabolic dysregulation (American Diabetes Association et al. 2004) (Table 4–1). In patients who develop abdominal pain while taking atypical antipsychotic medications or valproic acid, amylase and lipase levels should be checked to rule out pancreatitis, given that several cases have been reported. Liver function test results should be monitored periodically in patients

receiving valproic acid and in patients receiving venlafaxine and duloxetine who develop symptoms of liver disease, because both of these medications have been associated with elevated hepatic enzymes. Suspicion of alcohol abuse should likewise trigger a liver workup.

Serum urea nitrogen and creatinine levels will be elevated in kidney failure and in hypovolemic states such as dehydration. These tests also must be performed before initiating lithium therapy because of lithium's potential for nephrotoxicity. Paroxetine, venlafaxine, risperidone, and ziprasidone are some other psychotropics whose kinetics may be altered significantly in renal failure.

Serologic Tests for Syphilis and Other Infections

Currently, unless a patient has some specific risk factor (e.g., another sexually transmitted disease, evidence of prior syphilitic infection, or residence in a high-risk geographic zone), screening for syphilis in patients with dementia is not justified (Knopman et al. 2001). The Venereal Disease Research Laboratory and the rapid plasmin reagin tests, which are screening tools for infection with *Treponema pallidum,* the cause of syphilis, are nonspecific. More specific tests, the fluorescent treponemal antibody and the microhemagglutination–*Treponema pallidum,* may distinguish false-positive from true-positive results and may aid in diagnosing late syphilis when blood and even cerebrospinal fluid (CSF) reagin test results are negative. Herpes encephalitis, meningitis, and rickettsial fever are other conditions that might present with neuropsychiatric sequelae and necessitate serologic confirmation.

TABLE 4–1. Guidelines for screening and monitoring of patients started on second-generation antipsychotic agents[a]

Assessment	Frequency
Personal and family history[b]	At baseline and annually
Weight	At baseline, every 4 weeks for 12 weeks, then quarterly
Waist circumference[c]	At baseline and annually
Blood pressure	At baseline, at 12 weeks, and annually
Fasting plasma glucose	At baseline, at 12 weeks, and annually
Fasting lipid profile	At baseline, at 12 weeks, and every 5 years

[a]More frequent assessments may need to be done based on clinical status.

[b]Personal and family history includes obesity, diabetes, dyslipidemia, hypertension, or cardiovascular disease.

[c]Waist circumference is measured at umbilicus.

Source.   American Diabetes Association, American Psychiatric Association, American Association of Clinical Endocrinologists, North American Association for the Study of Obesity: "Consensus Development Conference on Antipsychotic Drugs and Obesity and Diabetes." *Diabetes Care* 27:596–601, 2004.

HIV Testing

From 1990 to the end of 2001, the cumulative number of AIDS cases reported to the Centers for Disease Control and Prevention in adults age 50 years or older increased fivefold, from 16,288 to 90,513 (Mack and Ory 2003). It is advisable to screen for risk factors, such as a history of sexually transmitted diseases, intravenous drug use, risky sexual behavior, or a history of blood transfusions, particularly if they occurred prior to the early 1990s. We recommend HIV testing in individuals who have these risk factors or those who present with atypical neuropsychiatric symptoms.

Thyroid Function Tests

A serum thyroid-stimulating hormone (TSH) test is the most frequently used screen for thyroid disease; it is an excellent screening test because of its high negative predictive value

(Klee and Hay 1997). However, many medications may result in increased TSH levels (amiodarone, estrogens) or decreased TSH levels (glucocorticoids, phenytoin) (Kaplan 1999), and altered thyrotropin levels also may be seen in patients with acute nonthyroidal illness or systemic stress. A physical examination and measurement of thyroxine, triiodothyronine, and thyroxine-binding globulin may be required for a definitive diagnosis of thyroid disease (Table 4–2). TSH testing should be done in all older adults presenting with neuropsychiatric symptoms because hypothyroidism may cause symptoms of depression, fatigue, and impaired cognition, and hyperthyroidism can cause symptoms of anxiety or even psychosis. Older women in particular have a high prevalence of hypothyroidism. Patients receiving lithium treatment should have their TSH level checked every 6 months. Hashimoto's thyroiditis, which mimics mood disorders or dementia, is recognized by antithyroid antibodies.

TABLE 4–2. Patterns of thyroid function tests

TSH	Free thyroxine	Triiodothyronine	Suggested diagnosis
Normal	Normal	Normal	Euthyroid
High	Low	Low or normal	Primary hypothyroidism
High	Normal	Normal	Subclinical hypothyroidism
Low	High or normal	High	Hyperthyroidism

Note. TSH = thyroid-stimulating hormone.

Vitamin B$_{12}$, Folate, and Homocysteine

The prevalence of B$_{12}$ deficiency increases with age; the deficiency is present in up to 15% of the elderly population (Stabler et al. 1997). Although macrocytic anemia is a well-known sign of B$_{12}$ deficiency, it is a later presentation in most cases, with neuropsychiatric symptoms presenting much earlier.

B$_{12}$ and folate deficiencies may result in neuropsychiatric disturbances, including depression, psychosis, or cognitive deficits. Studies in populations with dementia report that B$_{12}$ deficiencies often result in delirium or disorientation (Carmel et al. 1995; Cunha et al. 1995). Low levels of these vitamins also may result in visuospatial and word fluency deficits (Robins Wahlin et al. 2001) and even greater behavioral disturbances in Alzheimer's disease (Meins et al. 2000).

Serum homocysteine levels may serve as a functional indicator of B$_{12}$ and folate status (Selhub et al. 2000) because both vitamins are needed to convert homocysteine to methionine in one-carbon metabolism in brain tissue. Hyperhomocysteinemia is prevalent in elderly persons, and high serum levels of homocysteine can be attributed to an inadequate supply of B$_{12}$ and folate, even in the presence of low normal serum levels (Selhub et al. 2000). Results on whether vitamin supplementation to reduce plasma homocysteine levels leads to improved cognition are mixed, with some studies showing benefit (Durga et al. 2007; Nilsson et al. 2001) and others showing no benefit despite lowered homocysteine levels (McMahon et al. 2006).

Plasma Amyloid Testing

Plasma amyloid measurement has emerged as a promising biomarker, with lower amyloid beta (Aβ)$_{42}$ and A$\beta_{42/40}$ levels demonstrating an association with increased risk of developing Alzheimer's disease (Graff-Radford et al. 2007). Furthermore, lower plasma A$\beta_{42/40}$ is shown to be associated with greater cognitive decline among elderly persons without dementia over 9 years, and this association is stronger among those with low measures of cognitive reserve (Yaffe et al. 2011).

Toxicology and Drug and Alcohol Use

In addition to liver function (e.g., γ-glutamyl transferase) and blood alcohol, two recent tests, NailStat and HairStat, are now available to detect ethyl glucuronide, a marker of alcohol abuse, over the preceding 90 days. Because of their high sensitivity, these tests may produce false-positive results because of exposure to alcohol in cosmetics or household items (www.usdtl.com). When an acute change in an individual's mental status occurs, an investigation of the cause of the change must include considering the possibility of ingestion of a substance. If the individual is taking medications such as lithium, phenytoin, tricyclic antidepressants (TCAs), or any medication that requires monitoring of blood levels, those levels should be checked. Likewise, levels for common over-the-counter medications such as acetaminophen and salicylates can be tested. Concomitantly, a serum alcohol level also should be drawn. Depending on the individual's history, even a negative result may be critical if withdrawal is possible. Finally, urine can be tested for prescription medications, such as benzodiazepines, barbiturates, and opioids, as well as illicit substances, such as cocaine and marijuana. Advanced age does not preclude addiction. One must bear in mind that several prescription drugs (e.g., bupropion, antipsychotics, stimulants, TCAs) may produce a false-positive drug screen.

Urinalysis

A urinalysis is an inexpensive, noninvasive test that provides a significant amount of information. It determines the urine's specific gravity, which may indicate dehydration, and also tests for glucose and ketones, important in the evaluation of diabetic patients. In the elderly population, the most important use of urinalysis may be as a screening tool for urinary tract infections (UTIs). A urine culture is a definitive means of diagnosing a UTI and will identify the infecting organism and its susceptibility to antimicrobial treatments.

Cerebrospinal Fluid Analysis

Although the lumbar puncture is known to be useful in the workup of suspected central nervous system infections, such as meningitis, CSF analysis has only recently become part of the assessment of patients with dementia.

Hsich et al. (1996) described an immunoassay for the detection of the 14-3-3 protein in CSF that had a specificity of 99% and a sensitivity of 96% for the diagnosis of Creutzfeldt-Jakob disease (CJD) among patients with dementia. The American Academy of Neurology recommends testing for CSF 14-3-3 protein for confirming or rejecting the diagnosis of CJD in clinically appropriate circumstances (Knopman et al. 2001).

CSF $A\beta_{42}$, total tau protein, and tau phosphorylated at position threonine 181 (P-tau) recently have been shown to predict incipient Alzheimer's disease in individuals with mild cognitive impairment over a 2-year period (Mattsson et al. 2009).

Electrocardiogram

In psychiatry, the most important applications of the electrocardiogram (ECG) include screening for cardiovascular disease that may preclude the use of specific medications and monitoring for drug-induced electrocardiographic changes either from standard doses or from overdose. Electrocardiographic changes associated with specific psychotropic medications are summarized in Table 4–3.

TABLE 4–3. Common electrocardiographic abnormalities associated with psychotropic medications

Medication	Electrocardiographic change
Antipsychotics (typical or atypical agents)	Increased QTc interval Potential for torsades de pointes
β-Blockers	Bradycardia
Lithium	Sick sinus syndrome Sinoatrial block
Tricyclic antidepressants	Increased PR, QRS, or QT intervals Atrioventricular block

The TCAs are well known to be cardiotoxic in overdose; even at therapeutic doses, their use is considered unsafe in patients with cardiovascular disease, particularly ischemic disease (Roose 2000). TCAs have the same pharmacological properties as type IA antiarrhythmics, such as quinidine and procainamide. TCAs slow conduction at the bundle of His; individuals with preexisting bundle branch block who take TCAs are at increased risk for atrioventricular block. If TCAs are used, baseline and frequent follow-up ECGs should be obtained.

Lithium appears to most affect the sinus node, and even at therapeutic levels, it may result in sick sinus syndrome or sinoatrial block, either of which may occur early or later in treatment. At higher levels, there have been reports of sinus arrest and asystole. An ECG is recommended prior to starting lithium treatment and regularly during therapy.

Antipsychotics can cause prolongation of the QT interval (when corrected for heart rate, the QTc interval) and may contribute to potentially fatal ventricular arrhythmias, particularly torsades de pointes. QTc values are typically around 400 ms; 500 ms is frequently used as a cutoff (Glassman and Bigger 2001). QTc prolongation is more likely to be seen with thioridazine and haloperidol among typical antipsychotics and with ziprasidone among atypical antipsychotics (Glassman and Bigger 2001). Unfortunately, there are currently concerns about QTc prolongation for all atypical antipsychotic agents.

With few exceptions, an ECG should always be obtained in cases of potential medication overdose because medications may affect heart rhythm in overdose when they would not do so at usual doses. Also, suicidal patients often do not report all the medications that they have used to overdose.

Imaging Studies

Although plain film radiographs are essential for screening comorbid lung and bone diseases, computed tomography (CT), magnetic resonance imaging (MRI), and single-photon emission computed tomography (SPECT) and positron emission tomography (PET) are of growing interest in psychiatric diagnostics.

Computed Tomography

CT is particularly useful for demonstrating bone abnormalities (such as skull fractures),

TABLE 4–4. Neuroimaging in geriatric psychiatry

Suspected condition	Preferred neuroimaging study
Sudden loss of consciousness	Noncontrast CT scan
Pituitary tumor (hyperprolactinemia)	MRI
Old vs. new lacunar infarct	Diffusion weighted imaging
Hippocampal atrophy	Coronal thin slice MRI
Wernicke's encephalopathy	MRI to rule out midbrain hemorrhage

Note. CT = computed tomography; MRI = magnetic resonance imaging.

areas of hemorrhage (such as a subdural hematoma, acute stroke), and the mass effect from various lesions. It can also show atrophy or ventricular enlargement. However, CT is not very useful for visualizing posterior fossa or brain stem structures because of surrounding bone, and its resolution is less than that of MRI. CT scans expose patients to radiation (Nickoloff and Alderson 2001) but produce less claustrophobia than MRI does.

Magnetic Resonance Imaging

MRI has advantages and disadvantages when compared with CT imaging. MRI produces higher-resolution images and can obtain good detail in regions (such as the posterior fossa) that are poorly visualized on CT. Additionally, no radiation is involved. Unfortunately, the procedure is more grueling than CT because the patient must remain motionless for a longer time in a smaller, enclosed space. Additionally, the magnetic device must be housed in an area devoid of iron, and staff and patients must not carry or wear certain metals or have them embedded in their bodies. Moreover, MRI tends to be more costly than CT imaging in most institutions. Hearing loss concerns can be minimized with in-ear headphones.

In the psychiatric workup of a geriatric patient (Table 4–4), MRI should be considered when the clinician suspects small lesions in regions difficult to visualize—for example, to obtain evidence of midbrain hemorrhage in a patient with suspected Wernicke's encephalopathy or to confirm a suspected pituitary tumor in a patient with hyperprolactinemia, which may be seen in association with risperidone and other high-potency antipsychotic agents. MRI also can easily identify vascular pathology, including lacunar infarcts, and it is better than CT for defining exact anatomical localization.

The American Academy of Neurology recommends routine use of structural neuroimaging (noncontrast head CT or MRI) in the initial evaluation of all patients with dementia (Knopman et al. 2001).

A limitation of both CT and routine MRI is that they cannot differentiate between acute and chronic lesions. Diffusion-weighted imaging (DWI) overcomes this difficulty. DWI is based on the capacity of fast MRI to detect a signal related to the movement of water molecules between two closely spaced radiofrequency pulses (diffusion). This technique can detect abnormalities caused by ischemia within 3 to 30 minutes of onset, whereas conventional MRI and CT images would still appear normal. Therefore, DWI is helpful in defining the clinically appropriate infarct when multiple subcortical infarcts of various ages are present.

SPECT and PET Imaging

Both SPECT and PET imaging may be useful for identifying brain blood flow or metabolic deficits, but contemporary PET has higher resolution. Combined PET/CT scanners allow for simultaneous function-structure correlations. Fluorodeoxyglucose (FDG)-PET measures glucose uptake in the brain, and patients with Alzheimer's disease show characteristic decreases in temporo-parietal lobe early. FDG-PET findings can help in differential diagnosis of frontotem-poral dementia (FTD) and Alzheimer's disease (Foster et al. 2007). Greater amyloid deposition in cognitively normal older adults is associated with a higher rate of progression to symptomatic Alzheimer's disease (Morris et al. 2009). Antemortem florbetapir F 18 PET imaging has been shown to predict the presence of Aβ in the brain at autopsy with high accuracy (Clark et al. 2011).

Electroencephalography

Electroencephalography (EEG) is most useful in psychiatric evaluation of suspected seizure disorders or sleep disorders. In elderly patients, EEG changes occur in both delirium and dementia, but these changes are not specific to a given diagnosis. In delirium, with the exception of that caused by alcohol or sedative-hypnotic withdrawal, electroencephalograms typically show slowing of the posterior dominant rhythm and increased generalized slow-wave activity (Jacobson and Jerrier 2000). EEG testing may be use-

ful for distinguishing between depression and "quiet" delirium, because no EEG changes are seen in depression, whereas generalized slowing is seen in delirium.

Likewise, EEG changes are seen in dementia, but because of its questionable specificity, EEG has had limited clinical utility in most dementing syndromes. The EEG pattern of periodic sharp-wave complexes is strongly associated with CJD, with a sensitivity of 67% and a specificity of 86% (Steinhoff et al. 1996).

Genetic Testing

Apolipoprotein E Testing

Extensive research has identified mutations on chromosomes 1, 14, and 21 to be linked to rare forms of early-onset familial Alzheimer's disease (Verlinsky et al. 2002). The apolipoprotein E (APOE) gene encodes for an astrocyte-secreted plasma protein that is involved in cholesterol transport. APOE also may play a role in the regeneration of injured nerve tissue.

The presence of the APOE ε4 allele is an established risk factor for Alzheimer's disease (Roses 1997). Additionally, the presence of ε4 alleles increases the specificity of the diagnosis of Alzheimer's disease. Despite these associations, the presence of an ε4 allele, even a homozygous ε4/ε4 genotype, is not diagnostic for Alzheimer's disease because some 30% of Alzheimer's disease subjects are negative for it. APOE testing is not currently recommended to predict dementia risk in asymptomatic individuals. Arguments against routine testing include the lack of an effective treatment to modify the disease course and the lack of evidence that APOE status may influence current supportive treatments.

Ethical and Psychological Concerns in Genetic Testing

The results of genetic testing may have significant psychological, social, and personal repercussions. These possible effects are likely to be of less concern for a patient who already has a dementia diagnosis than for that patient's family members faced with their own risk for inheriting the disease. If a parent with Alzheimer's disease is found to be homozygous for *APOE*E4,* the children, who will have at least one copy of *APOE*E4,* have two to three times the average risk of developing the disease. Unfortunately, this knowledge does not allow offspring to anticipate with certainty whether and when they will develop Alzheimer's disease. Also, no treatment is available to *APOE*E4* carriers to prevent the disease. Financial concerns can include the possibility of losing one's job or insurance. As with other procedures, clinicians must ensure that patients or patients' families understand clearly not only the benefits but also the risks before they proceed with testing.

Future Directions

There is currently great interest in how genomics, proteomics, and metabolomics may improve our understanding of disease in various body systems, including the brain. The costs of whole-genome sequencing are declining rapidly, and many companies are beginning to offer at-home genetic tests. *Proteomics* is the global mapping of proteins, and *metabolomics* refers to the quantification of the complete set of small-molecule metabolites (such as metabolic intermediates, hormones and other signaling molecules, and secondary metabolites) found within a single organism. A subset of metabolomics is *lipidomics,* the study of hundreds of lipid fractions—a technology that has already been applied to map the adverse effects of antipsychotic medications on lipids (Kaddurah-Daouk et al. 2007). Such techniques may help advance our understanding of psychiatric disease mechanisms and aid in tailoring treatment to individual patients.

Key Points

- Laboratory testing is an essential component of the psychiatric evaluation in elderly individuals, who often present with comorbid medical illnesses.

- Laboratory tests are also useful in monitoring medication side effects. New guidelines have been proposed to monitor patients taking atypical antipsychotics.

- Neuroimaging is useful in evaluation of a variety of neuropsychiatric illnesses, including, but not limited to, dementia.

- Genetic testing has great potential in geriatric psychiatry but currently has limited clinical utility. Important ethical issues should be considered when using genetic testing.

References

American Diabetes Association, American Psychiatric Association, American Association of Clinical Endocrinologists, North American Association for the Study of Obesity: Consensus Development Conference on Antipsychotic Drugs and Obesity and Diabetes. Diabetes Care 27:596–601, 2004

Carmel R, Gott PS, Waters CH, et al: The frequently low cobalamin levels in dementia usually signify treatable metabolic, neurologic and electrophysiologic abnormalities. Eur J Haematol 54:245–253, 1995

Clark CM, Schneider JA, Bedell BJ, et al: Use of Florbetapir-PET for imaging beta-amyloid pathology. JAMA 305:275–283, 2011

Cunha UG, Rocha FL, Peixoto JM, et al: Vitamin B_{12} deficiency and dementia. Int Psychogeriatr 7:85–88, 1995

Dagogo-Jack S: Diabetes mellitus and related disorders, in The Washington Manual of Medical Therapeutics. Edited by Ahya SN, Flood K, Paranjothi S. Philadelphia, PA, Lippincott Williams & Wilkins, 2001, p 455

Durga J, van Boxtel MP, Schouten EG, et al: Effect of 3-year folic acid supplementation on cognitive function in older adults in the FACIT trial: a randomised, double blind, controlled trial. Lancet 369:208–216, 2007

Foster NL, Heidebrink JL, Clark CM, et al: FDG-PET improves accuracy in distinguishing frontotemporal dementia and Alzheimer's disease. Brain 130:2616–2635, 2007

Glassman AH, Bigger JT: Antipsychotic drugs: prolonged QTc interval, torsade de pointes, and sudden death. Am J Psychiatry 158:1774–1782, 2001

Graff-Radford NR, Crook JE, Lucas J, et al: Association of low plasma Abeta42/Abeta40 ratios with increased imminent risk for mild cognitive impairment and Alzheimer disease [published erratum in Arch Neurol 64:1246, 2007]. Arch Neurol 64:354–362, 2007

Hsich G, Kenney K, Gibbs CJ, et al: The 14–3–3 brain protein in cerebrospinal fluid as a marker for transmissible spongiform encephalopathies. N Engl J Med 335:924–930, 1996

Jacob S, Spinler SA: Hyponatremia associated with selective serotonin-reuptake inhibitors in older adults. Ann Pharmacother 40:1618–1622, 2006

Jacobson S, Jerrier H: EEG in delirium. Semin Clin Neuropsychiatry 5:86–92, 2000

Kaddurah-Daouk R, McEvoy J, Baillie RA, et al: Metabolomic mapping of atypical antipsychotic effects in schizophrenia. Mol Psychiatry 12:934–945, 2007

Kaplan MM: Clinical perspectives in the diagnosis of thyroid disease. Clin Chem 45:1377–1383, 1999

Klee GG, Hay ID: Biochemical testing of thyroid function. Endocrinol Metab Clin North Am 26:763–775, 1997

Knopman DS, DeKosky ST, Cummings JL, et al: Practice parameter: diagnosis of dementia (an evidence-based review). Report of the Quality Standards Subcommittee of the American Academy of Neurology. Neurology 56:1143–1153, 2001

Mack KA, Ory MG: AIDS and older Americans at the end of the twentieth century. J Acquir Immune Defic Syndr 1 (suppl 2):S68–S75, 2003

Mattsson N, Zetterberg H, Hansson O, et al: CSF biomarkers and incipient Alzheimer disease in patients with mild cognitive impairment. JAMA 302:385–393, 2009

McMahon JA, Green TJ, Skeaff CM, et al: A controlled trial of homocysteine lowering and cognitive performance. N Engl J Med 354:2764–2772, 2006

Meins W, Muller-Thomsen T, Meier-Baumgartner H-P: Subnormal serum vitamin B_{12} and behavioural and psychological symptoms in Alzheimer's disease. Int J Geriatr Psychiatry 15:415–418, 2000

Morris J, Roe C, Grant E, et al: Pittsburgh Compound B imaging and prediction of progression from cognitive normality to symptomatic Alzheimer disease. Arch Neurol 66:1469–1475, 2009

Nickoloff EL, Alderson PO: Radiation exposures to patients from CT: reality, public perception, and policy. AJR Am J Roentgenol 177:285–287, 2001

Nilsson K, Gustafson L, Hultberg B: Improvement of cognitive functions after cobalamin/folate supplementation in elderly patients with dementia and elevated plasma homocysteine. Int J Geriatr Psychiatry 16:609–614, 2001

Robins Wahlin TB, Wahlin A, Winblad B, et al: The influence of serum vitamin B12 and folate status on cognitive functioning in very old age. Biol Psychol 56:247–265, 2001

Roose SP: Considerations for the use of antidepressants in patients with cardiovascular disease. Am Heart J 140:S84–S88, 2000

Roses AD: A model for susceptibility polymorphisms for complex diseases: apolipoprotein E and Alzheimer disease. Neurogenetics 1:3–11, 1997

Selhub J, Bagley LC, Miller J, et al: B vitamins, homocysteine, and neurocognitive function in the elderly. Am J Clin Nutr 71 (suppl):614S–620S, 2000

Stabler SP, Lindenbaum J, Allen RH: Vitamin B$_{12}$ deficiency in the elderly: current dilemmas. Am J Clin Nutr 66:741–749, 1997

Steinhoff BJ, Racker S, Herrendorf G, et al: Accuracy and reliability of periodic sharp wave complexes in Creutzfeldt-Jakob disease. Arch Neurol 53:162–166, 1996

Trannel TJ, Ahmed I, Goebert D: Occurrence of thrombocytopenia in psychiatric patients taking valproate. Am J Psychiatry 158:128–130, 2001

Verlinsky Y, Rechitsky S, Verlinsky O, et al: Preimplantation diagnosis for early onset Alzheimer disease caused by V717L mutation. JAMA 287:1018–1021, 2002

Yaffe K, Weston A, Graff-Radford NR, et al: Association of plasma beta-amyloid level and cognitive reserve with subsequent cognitive decline. JAMA 305:261–266, 2011

Suggested Readings

Knopman DS, DeKosky ST, Cummings JL, et al: Practice parameter: diagnosis of dementia (an evidence-based review). Report of the Quality Standards Subcommittee of the American Academy of Neurology. Neurology 56:1143–1153, 2001

Townsend BA, Petrella JR, Murali Doraiswamy P: The role of neuroimaging in geriatric psychiatry. Curr Opin Psychiatry 15:427–432, 2002

CHAPTER 5

NEUROPSYCHOLOGICAL ASSESSMENT OF DEMENTIA

KATHLEEN A. WELSH-BOHMER, PH.D.
DEBORAH K. ATTIX, PH.D.

Alzheimer's disease (AD) is by far the most common disorder of aging that causes dementia, affecting nearly 5.3 million Americans and more than 30% of those older than 85 (Brookmeyer et al. 2011). Neuropsychological assessment plays a central role in the diagnosis of cognitive disorders in the elderly (for review, see Mayeux et al. 2011), offering a sensitive, reliable, and noninvasive approach to early symptom verification as well as a potentially cost-effective means for managing patients with memory disorders (Welsh-Bohmer et al. 2003). The goals of this chapter are 1) to describe in detail the instances in which neuropsychological assessment can be most useful in geriatric settings, 2) to describe in detail the neuropsychological examination process, and 3) to summarize the neurobehavioral presentations of common disorders in geriatric practices, specifically the profiles of various common dementias, normal aging, and depression.

Neuropsychological Assessment in Geriatric Settings

In geriatric practices, the neuropsychological evaluation finds utility in four common situations, none of which are mutually exclusive. First, it is used to assist in the diagnosis of a cognitive disorder arising from medical, neurological, or psychiatric causes. Second, it is used to establish an objective baseline for evaluating progress and response to treatment. Third, an evaluation is sought to guide clinical care decisions including the determination of functional capacities and competency (for re-view, see Koltai and Welsh-Bohmer 2000). Finally, the neuropsychological evaluation can be used to guide appropriate psychotherapeutic interventions and rehabilitative approaches (for full discussion of topic, see Attix and Welsh-Bohmer 2006).

The actual neuropsychological evaluation process itself can vary in its form across clinical practices. Regardless of approach, standard features are uniformly applied across neuropsychological settings (Lezak et al. 2004). Domains generally assessed include orientation, intelligence, memory, attention/concentration, higher executive functions, language expression and comprehension, visuoperception/spatial abilities, sensorimotor integration, mood, and personality. The tests commonly used in assessing these domains are listed in Table 5–1.

From the battery of tests, a profile of performance can be constructed, examined in reference to normative standards, and then interpreted relative to the established behavioral profiles of known neurobehavioral syndromes. It must be emphasized that the neuropsychological examination is not simply a process of actuarial comparisons to normative tables. Rather, the neuropsychological assessment involves an iterative process, which incorporates multiple sources of information, including patient and informant interviews, to arrive at diagnostic impressions (see Potter and Attix 2006). The psychologist first must determine likely premorbid ability to ascertain the presence of newly acquired weaknesses according to appropriate age- and education–adjusted normative values (Steinberg and Bieliauskas 2005). Consideration is given to any potential confounding influences such as subject anxiety, effort on testing, and motivation. The interpretation of the likely medical and psycho-logical contributions to the cognitive profile requires a thorough appreciation of brain-behavior organization and knowledge of both common and uncommon neurobehavioral syndromes. Before rendering a diagnostic impression, consideration is given to other attendant data such as laboratory findings, neuroimaging results, medical history, and informant report of functional change.

Neuropsychology of Normal Aging

Cognitive change after age 50 is common and reflects biological processes of an aging nervous system (Drachman 2006; Park and Reuter-Lorenz 2009). Compared with young adults, older individuals show selective losses in functions related to speed and efficiency of information processing. Particularly vulnerable are memory retrieval abilities, attentional capacity, executive skills, and divergent thinking (Salthouse 2010). On formal neuropsychological testing, memory measures involving delayed free recall typically show modest declines (Craik 1984), whereas performance on cued memory recall or delayed recognition is typically normal. Beyond memory, older adults also show some decrements compared with their younger counterparts on tests of visuoperceptual, visuospatial, and constructional functions (Salthouse 2010). These modest declines are seen on tests involving visual analysis and integration, such as the Block Design test of the Wechsler Adult Intelligence Scale, 3rd Edition (WAIS-III), and similar tests involving visual integration. Performance on measures of executive control (e.g., Trail Making), language retrieval (verbal fluency), and divided attention (e.g., Digit Span from WAIS-III) also tends to be lower in older groups compared with their younger counterparts (Park and Reuter-Lorenz 2009).

TABLE 5–1. Common neuropsychological tests used in geriatric assessment

Domain	Tests commonly used	References
Orientation/global mental status	Temporal Orientation Test Mini-Mental State Examination Alzheimer's Disease Assessment Scale–Cognitive	Benton et al. 1964 Folstein et al. 1975 Mohs and Cohen 1988
Intellect	Wechsler Adult Intelligence Scale, 3rd Edition (WAIS-III)	Wechsler 1997a
Language	Multilingual Aphasia Examination Category Fluency Boston Naming Test	Benton and Hamsher 1983 Strauss et al. 2006 Kaplan et al. 1978
Memory	Wechsler Memory Scale, 3rd Edition (WMS-III) California Verbal Learning Test, 2nd Edition Selective Reminding Test Consortium to Establish a Registry for Alzheimer's Disease Word List Memory Test Rey Auditory Verbal Learning Test	Wechsler 1997b Delis et al. 1987 Buschke and Fuld 1974 Welsh-Bohmer and Mohs 1997 Ivnik et al. 1992
Attention/ concentration	Subtests from the WMS-III and WAIS-III	Lezak et al. 2004
Executive function	Trail Making Test Symbol Digit Modalities Test Short Category Test Wisconsin Card Sorting Test	Reitan 1958 Smith 1968 Wetzel and Boll 1987 Berg 1948
Visuoperception	Benton Facial Recognition Test Judgment of Line Orientation Test Tests of Constructional Praxis	Benton et al. 1983 Benton et al. 1981 Lezak et al. 2004
Sensorimotor abilities	Grooved Pegboard Finger Oscillation	Strauss et al. 2006 Heaton et al. 1991
Personality and mood	Minnesota Multiphasic Personality Inventory–2 (MMPI-2) Geriatric Depression Scale Beck Depression Inventory–II	Butcher et al. 1989 Yesavage et al. 1983 Beck et al. 1996

Several explanations for age-related cognitive change have been suggested, none of which are mutually exclusive. All basically support a premise of a broad explanatory mechanism for age-related cognitive change rather than unique and specific changes in restricted cognitive domains. Among these are 1) aging-associated decline in the speed of central processing (Finkel et al. 2007) and 2) selective losses in "fluid" cognitive abilities, such as novel problem solving and flexible behavior (Botwinick 1977; Horn 1982), whereas well-rehearsed verbal abilities, so-called crystallized skills, are less susceptible to age-associated change. More contemporary refinements of the latter hypothesis conceptualize normal aging as 3) a selective vulnerability in frontal, dysexecutive processes (Daigneault and Braun 1993). Although this hypothesis is conceptually appealing and capable of explaining many of the observed changes with aging (Coffey et al. 1992; Langley and Madden 2000), some recent work suggests that the deficits may not be localizable to a single brain system (Finkel et al. 2007; Salthouse 2010). Work continues to identify the neurobiological mechanisms of brain senescence and the extent to which these brain changes converge to influence the expression of neurodegenerative diseases (Finch 2009).

Alzheimer's Disease

AD is an age-associated disorder that in its early stages is commonly mistaken for cognitive aging. Unrelentingly progressive, it is the leading cause of functional disability and dementia in the elderly, accounting for approximately 50%–75% of all dementia cases (Breitner et al. 1999; Fratiglioni et al. 1999; Gascon-Bayarri et al. 2007). Vascular dementia accounts for 12%–30% of reported cases (Lobo et al. 2000); dementia with Lewy bodies is seen in 3%–26% of the cases (McKeith et al. 2005; Zaccai et al. 2005); and conditions such as frontotemporal dementia are considered relatively rare in late life, accounting for an additional 3%–5% of the reported cases of dementia in individuals older than 65 (Cairns et al. 2007). Illnesses, such as

hydrocephalus, metabolic disorders, and infectious dementias, are etiologically tied to the remaining cases (Holman et al. 1995; Savolainen et al. 1999). The cognitive profiles of the various dementing disorder subtypes overlap, but unique features to many of them can be of diagnostic utility. These characteristics are summarized in Table 5–2.

The presentation of AD dementia is dominated by a pronounced impairment in recent memory processing, which remains the most affected area of mentation in most cases. On formal neuropsychological testing, the memory problem of AD manifests as a rapid forgetting of new information after very brief delays (Welsh et al. 1991). Patients in the mild prodrome of the illness often show this pronounced memory deficit along with subtle deficits in executive function, language expression, visuoperception, and attention (Bäckman et al. 2005). At this early symptomatic stage, a diagnosis of amnesic mild cognitive impairment (MCI) is often made (for a review, see Petersen and Morris 2005). However, the certainty of a prodromal AD diagnosis is almost ensured if the profile of cognitive disorder includes the classic amnesic disorder of AD and evidence of either functional decline or mild cognitive compromise in other typical domains (language, executive function; Mayeux et al. 2011).

As the disease progresses, other areas of cognition become progressively more involved, reflecting the specific spread of neuropathological involvement (Small et al. 2000). Prototypical changes occur in expressive language, visuospatial function, higher executive control, and semantic knowledge (Locascio et al. 1995; Mickes et al. 2007; Storandt et al. 2006). At these latter stages of the illness, anomia with impaired semantic fluency (e.g., generation of names of animals) is generally seen on examination. Word search and circumlocution tendencies are common in conversational speech, whereas speech comprehension itself is better preserved as are all other fundamental elements of communication (Bayles et al. 1989). Subtle problems in spatial processing can occur early and may be detectable only on formal examination on tests of spatial judgment and visual organization (Rizzo et al. 2000). These visuospatial problems become more prominent in later stages of illness, resulting in dressing apraxia, difficulty in recognizing objects or people, and problems in performing familiar motor acts (Benke 1993). An example of the profound memory loss distinguishing AD and MCI from normal aging appears in Figure 5–1.

Vascular Dementia

The neuropsychological profile of vascular dementia differs in many respects from that of AD, with the largest difference being the absence of the profound memory impairment classic of the latter disorder (Tierney et al. 2001). The presentation of vascular dementia will vary according to the type and extent of the vascular disorder—multiple infarctions, a single strategic stroke, microvascular disease, cerebral hypoperfusion, hemorrhage, or combinations of these etiologies (Cohen et al. 2002). Multi-infarct dementia, arising from multiple large and small vessel strokes, will show a pattern of multifocal impairments on testing that respect the cerebral territories involved by the infarctions (Chui et al. 1992; Roman et al. 1993). In dementia due to diffuse small vessel disease (e.g., Binswanger's disease), the pattern shown on testing reflects the disruption in the dorsolateral prefrontal and subcortical circuitry (Kramer et al. 2002). Memory is involved, but the deficits are often patchy in nature. Patients may show impaired recollection of some recent event but show

surprising recall for other occurrences transpiring over the same time frame.

On formal neuropsychological testing, the pattern on memory testing is one of inefficient acquisition of new information leading to a flattened learning curve over repeating trials (Looi and Sachdev 1999; Padovani et al. 1995). Recall performance can be quite low, similar to that seen in AD and MCI, but generally performance improves dramatically within a recognition format, suggesting a primary difficulty in retrieval rather than in the consolidation of new information (Hayden et al. 2005). Beyond memory, dysexecutive functions are typically involved, leading to slowed sequencing, cognitive inflexibility, and decreased verbal fluency (Kertesz and Clydesdale 1994). Asymmetries on sensory motor function or deficits in coordination are also frequently identified.

Frontotemporal Lobar Dementia

Frontotemporal lobar dementia (FTLD) refers to a heterogeneous group of neurodegenerative conditions that are now recognized as a major non-AD dementia. Typically the onset of disease is in the presenium, distinguishing it from AD, in which the typical period of onset appears to occur later, after age 65. FTLD is also characteristically different from AD, dominated early in its course by changes in behavior, personality, or language as opposed to impairments in memory and other aspects of cognition. The exact prevalence of FTLD in late old age remains inconclusive, but studies suggest that it accounts for approximately 10%–20% of the early-onset dementias (Ratnavalli et al. 2002; Snowden et al. 2002).

The neuropathological features of FTLD are heterogeneous, but uniformly the histo-

TABLE 5–2. Clinical syndromes and associated neuropsychological profiles

Cognitive syndrome	Neuropsychological profile
Normal aging	
Subjective memory complaints	Impaired fluid abilities (novel problem
Annoying but not disabling problems	solving)
Frequent problems with name retrieval	Deficiencies in memory retrieval
Minor difficulties in recalling detailed events	Decreased general speed of processing
	Lowered performance on executive tasks and visuospatial skills/visuomotor speed
Mild cognitive impairment	
Subjective memory complaints	Memory performance 1.5 SD below age-matched peers
Noticeable change in memory as noted by informants	Otherwise intact neurocognitive function
Clinical Dementia Rating score of 0.5	Functional disorder limited to mild interference from the memory difficulty
Problem not disabling	
Alzheimer's disease (AD)	
Insidious onset	Impaired memory consolidation with rapid forgetting
Progressive impairment	
Prominent memory impairment	Diminished executive skills
Disorders in aphasia, apraxia, agnosia	Impaired semantic fluency and naming
	Impaired visuospatial analysis and praxis
Frontotemporal dementia	
Prominent personality/behavior change	Pronounced executive impairments
Disinhibition or apathy	Cognitive inflexibility
Impaired judgment, insight	Impaired sequencing
Normal mental status initially	Perseverative, imitative, utilization behaviors
	Poor use of feedback
	Prone to interference
	Less obvious memory impairments
Lewy body dementia	
Fluctuations in alertness/acute confusional state	Memory impairment of AD but with some partial saving
Visual hallucinations	Pronounced apraxia, visuospatial difficulties
Memory impairment	Rapidly increasing quantifiable deficits in many cases
Parkinsonian signs	
Neuroleptic sensitivity	
Falls resulting from orthostatic hypotension	

TABLE 5–2. Clinical syndromes and associated neuropsychological profiles *(continued)*

Cognitive syndrome	Neuropsychological profile
Vascular dementia	
Variation of symptoms with vascular subtype	Common language/memory retrieval difficulties
Focality on examination	Benefit from structural support/cueing
Abrupt onset	Asymmetric motor speed/dexterity
Stepwise progression in multi-infarct dementia	Executive inefficiencies
Parkinson's disease dementia	
Extrapyramidal motor disturbance	Slowed performance
Gait dysfunction and frequent falls	Retrieval memory deficit
Bradykinesia	Executive deficiencies (slowed sequencing, impaired lexical fluency)
Bradyphrenia	Impaired fine motor speed (asymmetry common)
	Constructional deficits
Huntington's disease	
Early age at onset (midlife)	Slowed performance
Choreiform movements	Memory difficulty in retrieval
Dementia	Benefit from retrieval supports (recognition okay)
Bradyphrenia	Executive compromises
	Poor verbal fluency/preserved naming
Progressive supranuclear palsy	
Extrapyramidal syndrome but no tremor	Mild dysexecutive symptoms: impaired sequencing, fluency, flexibility
Ophthalmic abnormalities (limited downgaze)	Motor slowing
Axial rigidity	Memory weakness characterized as inefficiencies in storage and retrieval
Pseudobulbar palsy	
Frequent falls	
Hydrocephalus	
Memory impairment	Slowed information processing
Gait disturbance	Memory retrieval problems
Incontinence	Benefit from retrieval supports

TABLE 5–2. Clinical syndromes and associated neuropsychological profiles *(continued)*

Cognitive syndrome	Neuropsychological profile
Creutzfeldt-Jakob disease	
Rare	Rapidly evolving dementia
Typically, rapid onset and course	Subtypes include a profile akin to AD or
Dementia with pyramidal and	pronounced complex visuospatial disorder
extrapyramidal signs	(Balint's syndrome)
Transient spikes on electroencephalogram	
Dementia of geriatric depression	
Mood disorder	Impaired performance on tasks involving
Psychomotor slowing	effortful processing
Memory complaints	Impaired attention, concentration,
Cognitive complaints linked temporally	sequencing, cognitive flexibility, and
to the depressive disorder	executive control
	Retrieval memory difficulty
	Memory improvement with cueing/
	recognition
	Behavioral tendencies to abandon tasks,
	poor motivation

logical changes and atrophy are confined to the frontal and anterior temporal cortices. The clinical features of FTLD parallel closely the brain regions affected (Snowden et al. 2002), and three subtypes are now well described (see Hodges 2001). The most common form of FTLD is the behavioral variant, followed by a language variant (Weintraub et al. 1990) and a rare form involving behavioral inertia and mutism (Hodges and Miller 2001). Comparisons of the cognitive profiles of the common behavioral variant of FTLD and AD (Pachana et al. 1996) indicate clear distinctions between the two disorders. AD involves classic rapid forgetting, whereas the behavioral form of FTLD involves impairment in executive function, characterized by slowed information processing, cognitive rigidity, diminished abstract reasoning, poor response inhibition, and impaired planning. At the neurobehavioral level, major changes in personality, general social decorum, and

insight into impairment occur early in the course of FTLD (Rankin et al. 2005). This behavior pattern contrasts with that of AD, in which insight is generally lost later in the dementia (Salmon et al. 2007).

Parkinson's Disease and Lewy Body Dementias

Patients with Parkinson's disease commonly have cognitive complaints, and many go on to develop dementia. Although the cumulative prevalence estimates of Parkinson's disease dementia remain unclear, recent estimates suggest that 10%–30% of patients newly diagnosed with Parkinson's disease develop dementia within 3 years (Williams-Gray et al. 2007). Related to Parkinson's disease dementia is dementia with Lewy bodies, a progressive neurological condition that is heralded by cognitive, behavioral,

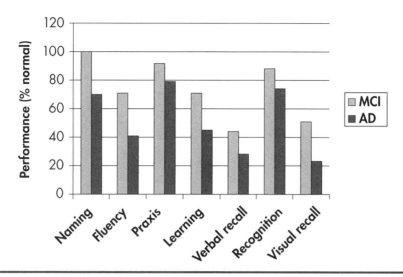

FIGURE 5–1. Profiles of neuropsychological test performance by patients with mild cognitive impairment (MCI) and by patients with moderate Alzheimer's disease (AD).

Bars indicate the performance of patients with MCI (*n*=153) and moderately impaired AD patients (*n*=277) on the subtests of the Consortium to Establish a Registry for Alzheimer's Disease (CERAD) neuropsychological battery, compared with the performance of nonimpaired elderly control subjects (*n*=158) of similar age, sex, and education. The overall neuropsychological test performance of the AD patients is well below that of both patients with MCI and subjects experiencing normal aging. Patients with MCI performed at normal levels on naming and praxis. Learning and verbal fluency were mildly affected in this group, falling at 71% of normal. Memory was particularly affected in both AD and MCI. Verbal recall on the CERAD Word List Memory test was 45% of normal in the MCI sample and only 28% for the AD patients. Visual memory was 51% of normal in MCI and 23% in AD.

Source. Data derived from the Cache County Study of Memory population sample (unpublished).

and functional impairments, as opposed to extrapyramidal motor symptoms, and is associated with a disorder of α-synuclein metabolism (McKeith et al. 2005; Zaccai et al. 2005). The recent recognition that dementia with Lewy bodies and Parkinson's disease dementia share a common biology has led to their being grouped together and referred to collectively as *Lewy body dementias* (LBDs; Lippa et al. 2007).

On neuropsychological evaluation, the cognitive impairments of LBD can be differentiated from those typically observed in AD (for review, see Tröster and Woods 2007). LBD is characterized by a pattern of mem-

ory retrieval problems and mild dysexecutive disturbances, which early in the course are less dramatic and globally impairing than the cognitive deficits of AD (Hamilton et al. 2004). Visuospatial disturbances are commonly observed early in the course of LBD (Salmon et al. 1996), but expressive language such as naming tends to be better preserved than in AD (Heyman et al. 1999). Despite these differences on neuropsychological testing, making a solid differential diagnosis on the basis of the cognitive profile alone will be difficult (e.g., Testa et al. 2001). A history of fluctuations in ability throughout the day is important to the dementia with Lewy bodies diagnosis (Geser et al. 2005). Behavior differences, including the presence of visual hallucinations early in the course and not associated with treatment, can help distinguish LBD from AD (Aarsland et al. 2001; Cahn-Weiner et al. 2002).

Geriatric Depression and Mood Disorders

Serious mood depression in the elderly can result in disabling cognitive impairment that may be mistaken clinically for a neurodegenerative condition (see Breitner and Welsh 1995). Depression also frequently co-occurs in the context of a range of medical disorders, including AD, stroke, and Parkinson's disease, complicating the diagnosis of these disorders and exacerbating functional loss associated with each (Krishnan 2000; Migliorelli et al. 1995; Reichman and Coyne 1995). Distinguishing between depression and other conditions in the elderly can be challenging, in part, because of the heterogeneity in the presentation of late-life depression, such that the severity of the depressive symptoms is not always concordant with the level of cognitive impairment (Alexopoulus et al. 2002). Despite the heterogeneity, some distinctive neurocognitive and behavior changes are characteristic of a rather large subgroup of patients that present without neurological disease (Lockwood et al. 2002). Neuropsychological evaluation can be particularly useful in the differential diagnosis.

On neuropsychological examination, the profile of late-life depression tends to be one of a dysexecutive syndrome with impairments on tests sensitive to frontal lobe function, including tasks of planning, organization, initiation, sequencing, working memory, and behavioral shifting in response to feedback. Difficulties also can be readily appreciated on tests of selective and sustained attention, verbal fluency, inhibitory control, and set shifting (Boone et al. 1994, 1995; Lockwood et al. 2002). Memory is impaired on both acquisition and recall, leading to a profile characterized by a flattened learning curve and impaired free recall of previously learned information after brief delays (Hart et al. 1987). Recognition memory is better preserved but can be characterized by false-negative tendencies (not recognizing previous target material). The profile of impairment in depression leads to the impression of generalized cognitive inefficiency and suppression of performance. Behaviorally, the depressed patients show apathy, a tendency to abandon tasks, and psychomotor retardation.

Importantly, even with treatment, not all of the cognitive impairments associated with geriatric depression remit. In the older patient, this may be a result of the co-occurrence of another disease process, such as AD or vascular dementia. Although far from conclusive, some studies report that depression in the elderly exerts a discernible additional effect on cognition and functional independence and may be a risk factor for later cognitive decline (Steffens et al. 2006). Neuropsychological evaluation of the elderly patient can provide clinically useful information about the nature of the cognitive failures, differential diagnostic information, and a baseline for future comparisons. The information is useful in diagnosis and management, regardless of whether all of the cognitive change detected is reversible.

Conclusion

The neuropsychological evaluation provides a useful and cost-effective management approach for diagnosis and management of memory complaints in the growing geriatric population. The neuropsychological evaluation is particularly useful in diagnostically complicated cases, such as in early AD detection or in geriatric depression. It also is useful in medical management, providing information about patient capacities and deficits that is important for intervention approaches and for guiding future decision making with respect to competency and safety.

Key Points

- The neuropsychological presentation of Alzheimer's disease (AD) is characterized by a pronounced deficit in the consolidation of new information from short-term, immediate memory to a more permanent store. Thus, the deficit early on in the disorder is a problem of rapid forgetting of newly learned information.

- The profile of normal cognitive aging is characterized by modest declines on executive function tests, in large measure because of inefficiencies in multitask processing and declines in perceptual motor speed.

- The neuropsychological deficits associated with Parkinson's disease dementia are clinically very similar to those of dementia with Lewy bodies. However, the neuropsychological profiles of these conditions can be distinguished from AD dementia. Visuospatial deficits are common early in the Parkinson's disease dementia and dementia with Lewy bodies conditions, and the memory disorders are less severe than those of AD.

- Frontotemporal lobar dementia is characterized by profound functional and behavioral changes. The neurocognitive deficits associated with the disorder, particularly in the early stages, may be difficult to discern with mental status instruments. Neuropsychological testing targeting executive functions can tease out the impairments in behavioral regulation, disinhibition, perseveration, judgment, and abstraction.

- Geriatric depression can cause significant impairments in the efficiency of cognitive processing, leading to selective problems in sustained attention, concentration, and memory. It is a risk factor for cognitive decline to dementia. When co-occurring with progressive neurological disorders, such as AD or vascular dementia, depression can lead to excess disability and an overall reduction in the quality of life that might otherwise be achieved.

References

Aarsland D, Cummings JL, Larsen JP: Neuropsychiatric differences between Parkinson's disease with dementia and Alzheimer's disease. Int J Geriatr Psychiatry 16:184–191, 2001

Alexopoulos GS, Kiosses DN, Klimstra S, et al: Clinical presentation of the "depression-executive dysfunction syndrome" of late life. Am J Geriatr Psychiatry 10:98–106, 2002

Attix DK, Welsh-Bohmer KA: Geriatric Neuropsychology: Assessment and Intervention. Edited by Attix DK, Welsh-Bohmer KA. New York, Guilford, 2006

Bäckman L, Jones S, Berger A, et al: Cognitive impairment in preclinical Alzheimer's disease: a meta-analysis. Neuropsychology 19:520–531, 2005

Bayles KA, Boone DR, Tomoeda CK, et al: Differentiating Alzheimer's patients from the normal elderly and stroke patients with aphasia. J Speech Hear Disord 54:74–87, 1989

Beck AT, Steer RA, Brown GK: Beck Depression Inventory, II. San Antonio, TX, Psychological Corporation, 1996

Benke T: Two forms of apraxia in Alzheimer's disease. Cortex 29:715–725, 1993

Benton AL, Hamsher K: Multilingual Aphasia Examination. Iowa City, IA, AJA Associates, 1983

Benton AL, Van Allen MW, Fogel ML: Temporal orientation in cerebral disease. J Nerv Ment Dis 139:110–119, 1964

Benton AL, Eslinger PJ, Damasio AR: Normative observations on neuropsychological test performance in old age. J Clin Neuropsychol 3:33–42, 1981

Benton AL, Hamsher K, Varney NR, et al: Contributions to Neuropsychological Assessment. New York, Oxford University Press, 1983

Berg EA: A simple objective technique for measuring flexibility in thinking. J Gen Psychol 39:15–22, 1948

Boone KB, Lesser I, Miller B, et al: Cognitive functioning in a mildly to moderately depressed geriatric sample: relationship to chronological age. J Neuropsychiatry Clin Neurosci 6:267–272, 1994

Boone KB, Lesser I, Miller B, et al: Cognitive functioning in older depressed outpatients: relationship of presence and severity of depression on neuropsychological test scores. Neuropsychology 9:390–398, 1995

Botwinick J: Intellectual abilities, in The Handbook of the Psychology of Aging. Edited by Birren JE, Schaie KW. New York, Van Nostrand Reinhold, 1977, pp 508–605

Breitner JCS, Welsh KA: An approach to diagnosis and management of memory loss and other cognitive syndromes of aging. Psychiatr Serv 46:29–35, 1995

Breitner JC, Wyse BW, Anthony JC, et al: APOE-epsilon4 count predicts age when prevalence of AD increases, then declines: the Cache County Study. Neurology 53:321–331, 1999

Brookmeyer R, Evans DA, Hebert LE, et al: National estimates of the prevalence of Alzheimer's disease in the United States. Alzheimers Dement 7:61–73, 2011

Buschke H, Fuld PA: Evaluation of storage, retention and retrieval in disordered memory and learning. Neurology 11:1019–1025, 1974

Butcher JN, Dahlstrom WG, Graham JR, et al: Manual for the Restandardized Minnesota Multiphasic Personality Inventory: MMPI2. Minneapolis, University of Minnesota Press, 1989

Cahn-Weiner DA, Grace J, Ott BR, et al: Cognitive and behavioral features discriminate between Alzheimer's and Parkinson's disease. Neuropsychiatry Neuropsychol Behav Neurol 15:79–87, 2002

Cairns NJ, Bigio EH, Mackenzie IR, et al: Neuropathologic diagnostic and nosologic criteria for frontotemporal lobar degeneration: consensus of the Consortium for Frontotemporal Lobar Degeneration. Acta Neuropathol 114:5–22, 2007

Chui HC, Victoroff JI, Margolin D, et al: Criteria for the diagnosis of ischemic vascular dementia proposed by the State of California Alzheimer's Disease Diagnostic and Treatment Centers. Neurology 42(3 pt 1):473–480, 1992

Coffey CE, Wilkinson WE, Parashos IA, et al: Quantitative cerebral anatomy of the aging human brain: a cross-sectional study using magnetic resonance imaging. Neurology 43:527–536, 1992

Cohen RA, Paul RH, Ott BR, et al: The relationship of subcortical MRI hyperintensities and brain volume to cognitive function in vascular dementia. J Int Neuropsychol Soc 8:743–752, 2002

Craik FIM: Age differences in remembering, in Neuropsychology of Memory. Edited by Squire L, Butters N. New York, Guilford, 1984, pp 3–12

Daigneault S, Braun CM: Working memory and the Self-Ordered Pointing Task: further evidence of early prefrontal decline in normal aging. J Clin Exp Neuropsychol 15:881–895, 1993

Delis DC, Kramer JH, Kaplan E, et al: California Verbal Learning Tests: Adult Version. San Antonio, TX, Psychological Corporation, 1987

Drachman DA: Aging of the brain, entropy, and Alzheimer disease. Neurology 67:1340–1352, 2006

Finch CE: The neurobiology of middle-age has arrived. Neurobiol Aging 30:515–520; discussion 530–533, 2009

Finkel D, Reynolds CA, McArdle JJ, et al: Age changes in processing speed as a leading indicator of cognitive aging. Psychol Aging 22:558–568, 2007

Folstein MF, Folstein SE, McHugh PR: "Minimental state": a practical method for grading the cognitive state of patients for the clinician. J Psychiatr Res 12:189–198, 1975

Fratiglioni L, De Ronchi D, Aguero-Torres H: Worldwide prevalence and incidence of dementia. Drugs Aging 15:365–375, 1999

Gascon-Bayarri J, Rene R, Del Barrio JL, et al: Prevalence of dementia subtypes in El Prat de Llobregat, Catalonia, Spain: the PRATICON study. Neuroepidemiology 28:224–234, 2007

Geser F, Wenning GK, Poewe W, et al: How to diagnose dementia with Lewy bodies: state of the art. Mov Disord 20:S11–S20, 2005

Hamilton JM, Salmon DP, Galasko D, et al: A comparison of episodic memory deficits in neuropathologically confirmed dementia with Lewy bodies and Alzheimer's disease. J Int Neuropsychol Soc 10:689–697, 2004

Hart RP, Kwentus JA, Taylor JR, et al: Rate of forgetting in dementia and depression. J Consult Clin Psychol 55:101–105, 1987

Hayden KM, Warren LH, Pieper CF, et al: Identification of VaD and AD prodromes: the Cache County Study. Alzheimers Dement 1:19–29, 2005

Heaton RK, Grant I, Matthews CG: Comprehensive Norms for an Expanded Halstead-Reitan Battery: Demographic Corrections, Research Findings and Clinical Applications. Odessa, FL, Psychological Assessment Resources, 1991

Heyman A, Fillenbaum GG, Gearing M, et al: Comparison of Lewy body variant of Alzheimer's disease with pure Alzheimer's disease: Consortium to Establish a Registry for Alzheimer's Disease, Part XIX. Neurology 52:1839–1844, 1999

Hodges JR: Frontotemporal dementia (Picks disease): clinical features and assessment. Neurology 56:S6–S10, 2001

Hodges JR, Miller B: The classification, genetics and neuropathology of frontotemporal dementia: introduction to the special topic papers: Part I. Neurocase 7(1):31–35, 2001

Holman RC, Khan AS, Kent J, et al: Epidemiology of Creutzfeldt-Jakob disease in the United States 1979–1990: analysis of national mortality data. Neuroepidemiology 14:174–181, 1995

Horn J: The theory of fluid and crystallized intelligence in relation to concepts of cognitive psychology and aging in adulthood, in Aging and Cognitive Processes. Edited by Craik F, Trehub S. New York, Plenum, 1982, pp 237–278

Ivnik RJ, Malec JF, Smith GE, et al: Mayo's older Americans normative studies: updated AVLT norms for ages 56–97. Clin Neuropsychol 6:83–104, 1992

Kaplan EF, Goodglass H, Weintraub S: The Boston Naming Test, 2nd Edition. Philadelphia, PA, Lea & Febiger, 1978

Kertesz A, Clydesdale S: Neuropsychological deficits in vascular dementia vs Alzheimer's disease: frontal lobe deficits prominent in vascular dementia. Arch Neurol 51:1226–1231, 1994

Koltai DC, Welsh-Bohmer KA: Geriatric neuropsychological assessment, in Clinician's Guide to Neuropsychological Assessment, 2nd Edition. Edited by Vanderploeg RD. Mahwah, NJ, Lawrence Erlbaum, 2000, pp 383–415

Kramer JH, Reed BR, Mungas D, et al: Executive dysfunction in subcortical ischaemic vascular disease. J Neurol Neurosurg Psychiatry 72:217–220, 2002

Krishnan KR: Depression as a contributing factor in cerebrovascular disease. Am Heart J 140:70–76, 2000

Langley LK, Madden DJ: Functional neuroimaging of memory: implications for cognitive aging. Microsc Res Tech 51:75–84, 2000

Lezak MD, Howieson DB, Loring DW: Neuropsychological Assessment, 4th Edition. New York, Oxford University Press, 2004

Lippa CF, Duda JE, Grossman M, et al: DLB and PDD boundary issues: diagnosis, treatment, molecular pathology, and biomarkers. Neurology 68:812–819, 2007

Lobo A, Launer LJ, Fratiglioni L, et al: Prevalence of dementia and major subtypes in Europe: a collaborative study of population-based cohorts. Neurologic Diseases in the Elderly Research Group. Neurology 54 (suppl 5):S4–S9, 2000

Locascio JJ, Growdon JH, Corkin S: Cognitive test performance in detecting, staging, and tracking Alzheimer's disease. Arch Neurol 52:1087–1099, 1995

Lockwood KA, Alexopoulos GS, van Gorp WG: Executive dysfunction in geriatric depression. Am J Psychiatry 159:1119–1126, 2002

Looi J, Sachdev PS: Differentiation of vascular dementia from AD on neuropsychological tests. Neurology 53:670–678, 1999

Mayeux R, Reitz C, Brickman AM, et al: Operationalizing diagnostic criteria for Alzheimer's disease and other age-related cognitive impairment—part 1. Alzheimers Dement 7:15–34, 2011

McKeith IG, Dickson DW, Lowe J, et al: Diagnosis and management of dementia with Lewy bodies: third report of the DLB Consortium. Neurology 65:1863–1872, 2005

Mickes L, Wixted JT, Fennema-Notestine C, et al: Progressive impairment on neuropsychological tasks in a longitudinal study of preclinical Alzheimer's disease. Neuropsychology 21:696–705, 2007

Migliorelli R, Teson A, Sabe L, et al: Prevalence and correlates of dysthymia and major depression among patients with Alzheimer's disease. Am J Psychiatry 152:37–44, 1995

Mohs RC, Cohen L: Alzheimer's Disease Assessment Scale (ADAS). Psychopharmacol Bull 24:627–628, 1988

Pachana NA, Boone KB, Miller BL, et al: Comparison of neuropsychological functioning in Alzheimer's disease and frontotemporal dementia. J Int Neuropsychol Soc 2:505–510, 1996

Padovani A, Di Piero V, Bragoni M, et al: Patterns of neuropsychological impairment in mild dementia: a comparison between Alzheimer's disease and multi-infarct dementia. Acta Neurol Scand 92:433–442, 1995

Park DC, Reuter-Lorenz P: The adaptive brain: aging and neurocognitive scaffolding. Annu Rev Psychol 60:173–196, 2009

Petersen RC, Morris JC: Mild cognitive impairment as a clinical entity and treatment target. Arch Neurol 62:1160–1163, 2005

Potter GG, Attix DK: An integrated model for geriatric neuropsychological assessment, in Geriatric Neuropsychology: Assessment and Intervention. Edited by Attix DK, Welsh-Bohmer KA. New York, Guilford, 2006, pp 5–26

Rankin KP, Baldwin E, Pace-Savitsky C, et al: Self awareness and personality change in dementia. J Neurol Neurosurg Psychiatry 76:632–639, 2005

Ratnavalli E, Brayne C, Dawson K, et al: The prevalence of frontotemporal dementia. Neurology 58:1615–1621, 2002

Reichman WE, Coyne AC: Depressive symptoms in Alzheimer's disease and multi-infarct dementia. J Geriatr Psychiatry Neurol 8:96–99, 1995

Reitan RM: Validity of the Trail Making Test as an indicator of organic brain damage. Percept Mot Skills 8:271–276, 1958

Rizzo M, Anderson SW, Dawson J, et al: Vision and cognition in Alzheimer's disease. Neuropsychologia 38:1157–1169, 2000

Roman GC, Tatemichi TK, Erkinjuntti T, et al: Vascular dementia: diagnostic criteria for research studies. Report of the NINDS-AIREN International Workshop. Neurology 43:250–260, 1993

Salmon DP, Galasko D, Hansen LA, et al: Neuropsychological deficits associated with diffuse Lewy body disease. Brain Cogn 31:148–165, 1996

Salmon E, Perani D, Collette F, et al: A comparison of unawareness in frontotemporal dementia and Alzheimer's disease. J Neurol Neurosurg Psychiatry 79:176–179, 2007

Salthouse TA: Selective review of cognitive aging. J Int Neuropsychol Soc 16:754–760, 2010

Savolainen S, Palijarvi L, Vapalahti M: Prevalence of Alzheimer's disease in patients investigated for presumed normal pressure hydrocephalus: a clinical and neuropathological study. Acta Neurochir (Wien) 141:849–853, 1999

Small GW, Ercoli LM, Silverman DHS, et al: Cerebral metabolic and cognitive decline in persons at genetic risk for Alzheimer's disease. Proc Natl Acad Sci U S A 97:6037–6042, 2000

Smith A: The Symbol Digit Modalities Test: a neuropsychologic test for economic screening of learning and other cerebral disorders. Learning Disorders 3:83–91, 1968

Snowden JS, Neary D, Mann DM: Frontotemporal dementia. Br J Psychiatry 180:140–143, 2002

Steffens DC, Otey E, Alexopoulos GS, et al: Perspectives on depression, mild cognitive impairment, and cognitive decline. Arch Gen Psychiatry 63:130–138, 2006

Steinberg B, Bieliauskas L: Introduction to the special edition: IQ-based MOANS norms for multiple neuropsychological instruments. Clin Neuropsychol 19:277–279, 2005

Storandt M, Grant EA, Miller JP, et al: Longitudinal course and neuropathologic outcomes in original vs revised MCI and in pre-MCI. Neurology 67:467–473, 2006

Strauss E, Sherman EM, Spreen O: A Compendium of Neuropsychological Tests: Administration, Norms, and Commentary, 3rd Edition. New York, Oxford University Press, 2006

Testa D, Monza D, Ferrarini M, et al: Comparison of natural histories of progressive supranuclear palsy and multiple system atrophy. Neurol Sci 22:247–251, 2001

Tierney MC, Black SE, Szalai JP, et al: Recognition memory and verbal fluency differentiate probable Alzheimer disease from subcortical ischemic vascular dementia. Arch Neurol 58:1654–1659, 2001

Tröster AI, Woods SP: Neuropsychological aspects, in Handbook of Parkinson's Disease, 4th Edition. Edited by Pahwa R, Lyons KE. New York, Informa, 2007, pp 109–131

Wechsler D: Wechsler Intelligence Scale III Manual. San Antonio, TX, Psychological Corporation, 1997a

Wechsler D: Wechsler Memory Scale III Manual. San Antonio, TX, Psychological Corporation, 1997b

Weintraub S, Rubin NP, Mesulam MM: Primary progressive aphasia: longitudinal course, profile and language features. Arch Neurol 47:1329–1335, 1990

Welsh KA, Butters N, Hughes JP, et al: Detection of abnormal memory decline in mild Alzheimer's disease using CERAD neuropsychological measures. Arch Neurol 48:278–281, 1991

Welsh-Bohmer KA, Mohs RC: Neuropsychological assessment of Alzheimer's disease. Neurology 49:S11–S13, 1997

Welsh-Bohmer KA, Koltai DC, Mason DJ: The clinical utility of neuropsychological evaluation of patients with known or suspected dementia, in Demonstrating Utility and Cost Effectiveness in Clinical Neuropsychology. Edited by Prigatano G, Pliskin N. Philadelphia, PA, Psychology Press–Taylor & Francis Group, 2003, pp 177–200

Wetzel L, Boll TJ: Short Category Test, Booklet Format. Los Angeles, CA, Western Psychological Services, 1987

Williams-Gray CH, Foltynie T, Brayne CEG, et al: Evolution of cognitive dysfunction in an incident Parkinson's disease cohort. Brain 130 (pt 7):1787–1798, 2007

Yesavage J, Brink TL, Rose TL, et al: Development and validation of a geriatric depression scale: a preliminary report. J Psychiatr Res 17:37–49, 1983

Zaccai J, McCracken C, Brayne C: A systematic review of prevalence and incidence studies of dementia with Lewy bodies. Age Ageing 34:561–566, 2005

Suggested Readings

Attix DK, Welsh-Bohmer KA: Geriatric Neuropsychology: Assessment and Intervention. Edited by Attix DK, Welsh-Bohmer KA. New York, Guilford, 2006

Brayne C: The elephant in the room—healthy brains in later life, epidemiology and public health. Nat Rev Neurosci 8:233–239, 2007

Strauss E, Sherman EM, Spreen O: A Compendium of Neuropsychological Tests: Administration, Norms, and Commentary, 3rd Edition. New York, Oxford University Press, 2006

Tröster AI, Woods SP: Neuropsychological aspects, in Handbook of Parkinson's Disease, 4th Edition. Edited by Pahwa R, Lyons KE. New York, Informa, 2007, pp 109–131

PART III

Presentation of Psychiatric Disorders in Late Life

CHAPTER 6

DELIRIUM

LI-WEN HUANG, A.B.
SHARON K. INOUYE, M.D., M.P.H.

Delirium, defined as an acute change in attention and overall cognitive function, is a common, morbid, yet potentially preventable medical problem for older persons. Patients age 65 years and older account for almost half (49%) of all days of hospital care, and although delirium is the most frequent complication affecting this population, it often goes unrecognized (Inouye 2006; U.S. Department of Health and Human Services 2004). Delirium is independently associated with an increased risk of mortality, institutionalization, long-term cognitive decline and dementia, and functional decline (Inouye 2006; MacLullich et al. 2009; Witlox et al. 2010). It is a costly condition, leading to increased costs per hospital stay of at least $2,500 per patient, which translates to $6.9 billion (values in U.S. dollars in 2004) in annual excess Medicare hospital expenditures directly related to delirium and its complications (Inouye 2006). Total health care costs related to delirium are estimated at $38 billion to $152 billion annually (Leslie et al. 2008).

Definition and Assessment Tools

The DSM-IV-TR (American Psychiatric Association 2000) diagnostic criteria for delirium are generally accepted as the diagnostic standard (see Table 6–1). The Confusion Assessment Method (CAM; Inouye et al. 1990) provides a simple yet highly sensitive and specific diagnostic algorithm that has become widely used for the identification of delirium (see Table 6–2). The CAM also has been adapted for use in the intensive care unit (CAM-ICU; Ely et al. 2001) and nursing home (Minimum Data Set Version 3.0; Centers for Medicare and Medicaid Services 2010). Other instruments used to detect delirium include the Delirium Rating Scale—Revised–98 (DRS-R-98; Trzepacz et al. 2001) and the Delirium Symptom Interview (Albert et al. 1992). Both the DRS-R-98 and the Memorial Delirium Assessment Scale (MDAS; Breitbart et al. 1997) are used to rate delirium severity.

Epidemiology

Delirium is often the only sign of an acute and serious medical condition affecting a patient, and it most commonly occurs in frail older persons with an underlying disease process. Occurrence estimates suggest that delirium affects 11%–42% of hospitalized older adults (Siddiqi et al. 2006). Delirium occurs in up to 30% of older patients presenting to the emergency department and in up to 60% of those in nursing home or post–acute care settings (Inouye 2006). It is present in 2%–73% of older patients postoperatively, depending on the type of surgery performed (Sieber 2009). Incidence rates increase to 70%–87% of older patients in intensive care units and in palliative care settings (Inouye 2006).

Clinical Features

Acute onset, fluctuating course, and alteration in attention are the core features of delirium. It is important to establish a patient's level of baseline cognitive function and the course of cognitive change from a reliable informant. Cognitive changes that occur abruptly over a period of days are usually indicative of delirium, whereas changes that progress gradually over a period of months to years are usually indicative of dementia. The cognitive evaluation for delirium should examine for evidence of global cognitive changes, impairment in attention, disorganized thought process, and altered level of consciousness. Other clinical features commonly associated with delirium are psychomotor agitation, paranoid delusions, sleep-wake cycle disruption, emotional lability, and perceptual disturbances or hallucinations.

Clinically, delirium typically presents in one of four psychomotor behavioral subtypes: normal, hypoactive, hyperactive, or mixed (Yang et al. 2009). The hypoactive form, more common in older patients, is characterized by lethargy and reduced psychomotor functioning, which is often misattributed to depression or fatigue. Although the hypoactive form of delirium is associated with a poorer prognosis, it is often unrecognized or misdiagnosed by clinicians and caregivers (Yang et al. 2009). The hyperactive form of delirium, characterized by agitation, increased vigilance, and often hallucinations, rarely goes unnoticed. The mixed form of delirium, in which patients fluctuate between the hypoactive and the hyperactive forms, creates a challenge in distinguishing symptoms of delirium from symptoms of other psychotic or mood disorders.

Pathophysiology

The fundamental pathophysiological mechanisms of delirium remain unclear. Historically, delirium was thought to result from a functional rather than a structural lesion. Several studies of cerebral blood flow that used positron emission tomography (PET) or single-photon emission computed tomography

---

TABLE 6–1. DSM-IV-TR diagnostic criteria for delirium due to a general medical condition

A. Disturbance of consciousness (i.e., reduced clarity of awareness of the environment) with reduced ability to focus, sustain, or shift attention.

B. A change in cognition (such as memory deficit, disorientation, language disturbance) or the development of a perceptual disturbance that is not better accounted for by a preexisting, established, or evolving dementia.

C. The disturbance develops over a short period of time (usually hours to days) and tends to fluctuate during the course of the day.

D. There is evidence from the history, physical examination, or laboratory findings that the disturbance is caused by the direct physiological consequences of a general medical condition.

Source. Reprinted from American Psychiatric Association: *Diagnostic and Statistical Manual of Mental Disorders,* 4th Edition, Text Revision. Washington, DC, American Psychiatric Association, 2000. Copyright American Psychiatric Association, 2000. Used with permission.

TABLE 6–2. Confusion Assessment Method (CAM) diagnostic algorithm

Feature 1. **Acute onset and fluctuating course**

This feature is usually obtained from a reliable reporter, such as a family member, caregiver, or nurse, and is shown by positive responses to these questions: Is there evidence of an acute change in mental status from the patient's baseline? Did the (abnormal) behavior fluctuate during the day, that is, tend to come and go, or did it increase and decrease in severity?

Feature 2. **Inattention**

This feature is shown by a positive response to this question: Did the patient have difficulty focusing attention, for example, being easily distractible, or have difficulty keeping track of what was being said?

Feature 3. **Disorganized thinking**

This feature is shown by a positive response to this question: Was the patient's thinking disorganized or incoherent, such as rambling or irrelevant conversation, unclear or illogical flow of ideas, or unpredictable switching from subject to subject?

Feature 4. **Altered level of consciousness**

This feature is shown by any answer other than "alert" to this question: Overall, how would you rate this patient's level of consciousness (alert [normal], vigilant [hyperalert], lethargic [drowsy, easily aroused], stupor [difficult to arouse], or coma [unarousable])?

Note. The CAM ratings should be completed following brief cognitive assessment of the patient, for example, with the Mini-Mental State Examination. The diagnosis of delirium by CAM requires the presence of features 1 and 2 and of either 3 or 4.

Source. Adapted from Inouye SK, Vandyck CH, Alessi CA, et al.: "Clarifying Confusion: The Confusion Assessment Method—A New Method for Detection of Delirium." *Annals of Internal Medicine* 113:941–948, 1990. Used with permission.

(SPECT) have found that delirium is associated with patterns of localized hypoperfusion. However, other neuroimaging studies that used either computed tomography (CT) or magnetic resonance imaging (MRI) have detected structural abnormalities, such as cortical atrophy, in the brains of patients with delirium (Fong et al. 2009b). Results from neuropsychological testing also suggest that delirium is related to disruptions in higher cortical function, especially frontal lobe functioning (Rudolph et al. 2006). Currently, delirium is viewed as the final common pathway of many different pathogenic mechanisms, including imbalances in neurotransmission, inflammation, and chronic stress.

The most frequently considered mechanism of delirium is cholinergic dysfunction. Acetylcholine plays a key role in mediating consciousness and attentional processes. Evidence for the cholinergic mechanism includes findings that anticholinergic drugs can induce delirium and that serum anticholinergic activity is increased in patients with delirium (Marcantonio et al. 2006). Also, cholinesterase inhibitors have been found to reduce symptoms of delirium (Gleason 2003). An excess of dopaminergic neurotransmission, which regulates the release of acetylcholine, also has been linked with delirium (Trzepacz and van der Mast 2002). Elevated serotonin is another proposed mechanism of delirium (Marcantonio et al. 2006). Other neurotransmitters, including norepinephrine, glutamate, and melatonin, have been implicated in the development of delirium, possibly because of their interactions with cholinergic and dopaminergic pathways; however, support for their involvement is less substantiated (Inouye 2006).

Chronic stress induced by severe illness, trauma, or surgery involves sympathetic

and immune system activation that may lead to delirium. This activation may include increased activity of the hypothalamic-pituitary-adrenal axis with hypercortisolism, release of cerebral cytokines that alter neurotransmitter systems, alterations in the thyroid axis, and modification of blood-brain barrier permeability.

Risk Factors

Delirium usually has multifactorial causes. Although it can be caused by a single factor, delirium more typically develops as a result of the interrelation between patient vulnerability and noxious insults or precipitating factors (Inouye and Charpentier 1996). Clinicians must recognize that addressing a single noxious insult or factor may not improve delirium; instead, appropriate management of delirium requires that *all* predisposing and precipitating factors be considered and addressed.

Existing cognitive impairment and dementia are the leading risk factors for the development of delirium (Trzepacz and van der Mast 2002). Various medical illnesses also serve as predisposing factors for delirium (see Table 6–3; Inouye 2006), including neurological disorders; systemic or non-neurological infections; metabolic alterations; and cardiac, pulmonary, endocrine, renal, and neoplastic conditions. Other predisposing factors include advanced age, number and severity of comorbid conditions, functional impairment, male gender, dehydration, vision or hearing impairments, history of alcohol abuse or dependence, and malnutrition (see Table 6–3; Inouye 2006). Several predictive risk models that identify predisposing factors for delirium in different medical populations have been developed and validated (Boyle 2006; Hamann et al.

TABLE 6–3. Predisposing and precipitating factors for delirium

Predisposing factors

Demographic characteristics
  Age 65 years or older
  Male gender

Coexisting medical conditions
  Severe illness
  Multiple coexisting conditions
  Chronic renal or hepatic disease
  History of stroke
  Infection with HIV
  Metabolic derangements
  Neurological disease
  Terminal illness
  Fracture or trauma

Cognitive status
  Dementia
  Cognitive impairment
  History of delirium
  Depression

Decreased oral intake
  Dehydration
  Malnutrition

Drugs
  Treatment with psychoactive drugs
  Treatment with many drugs
  Alcohol abuse

Functional status
  Functional dependence
  Immobility
  Low level of activity
  History of falls

Sensory impairment
  Visual impairment
  Hearing impairment

Precipitating factors

Drugs
  Sedative-hypnotics
  Narcotics
  Anticholinergic drugs
  Treatment with multiple drugs
  Alcohol or drug withdrawal

Environment
  Admission to intensive care unit
  Use of physical restraints
  Use of bladder catheter
  Use of multiple procedures
  Pain
  Emotional stress

Primary neurological disease
  Stroke, particularly nondominant
  hemispheric
  Intracranial bleeding
  Meningitis or encephalitis

Intercurrent illnesses
  Infections
  Iatrogenic complications
  Severe acute illness
  Hypoxia
  Shock
  Fever or hypothermia
  Anemia
  Dehydration
  Poor nutritional status
  Low serum albumin level
  Metabolic derangements (e.g., electrolytes)

Sensory impairment
  Visual impairment
  Hearing impairment

Surgery
  Orthopedic surgery
  Cardiac surgery
  Prolonged cardiopulmonary bypass
  Noncardiac surgery

Source.   Adapted from Inouye SK: "Current Concepts: Delirium in Older Persons." *New England Journal of Medicine* 354:1157–1165, 2006. Used with permission.

2005; Inouye et al. 1993, 2007), improving the identification of high-risk patients.

Precipitating factors for delirium include medications, immobilization, use of indwelling bladder catheters, use of physical restraints, dehydration, malnutrition, iatrogenic events, medical illnesses, organ insufficiency or failure (particularly renal or hepatic), infections, electrolyte or metabolic derangement, alcohol or drug intoxication or withdrawal, environmental influences, and psychosocial factors (see Table 6–3) (Inouye 2006). Occult infection is a particularly important treatable contributor because older patients may not present with leukocytosis or the typical febrile response. A model of precipitating factors for the development of delirium in hospitalized older patients has been developed and validated (Inouye and Charpentier 1996).

The role of medications in the development of delirium deserves special attention (see Table 6–4; Alagiakrishnan and Wiens 2004; Clegg and Young 2011). Medications contribute to delirium in more than 40% of cases (Inouye and Charpentier 1996). The medications most strongly associated with delirium include sedative-hypnotics such as benzodiazepines, narcotics such as opioids, and histamine H_1 receptor antagonists. Drugs with anticholinergic effects (including antimuscarinics, tricyclic antidepressants, and antiparkinsonian agents), histamine H_2 receptor antagonists, steroids, and nonsteroidal anti-inflammatory drugs also have been associated with delirium (Alagiakrishnan and Wiens 2004; Clegg and Young 2011).

Previous studies suggested that overuse of psychoactive drugs and poor management of medications commonly occur in hospitalized older patients (Bates et al. 1995; Lindley et al. 1992). Given the role of medications in

contributing to the development of delirium, the clinician must conduct a complete review of all prescription and over-the-counter medications being taken by the patient. Medications with known psychoactive effects should be minimized or discontinued whenever possible. In older adults, medications may cause adverse effects even when given at the recommended dosages and with serum drug levels that are within the "therapeutic range."

Diagnosis and Differential Diagnosis

The diagnosis of delirium is based on clinical observation and relies on a thorough cognitive assessment, a detailed history from a reliable informant, and a comprehensive physical and neurological examination. The goal of a thorough history is to establish that a change has occurred from the patient's baseline cognitive functioning. Delirium goes unrecognized by clinicians in up to 70% of patients (Rockwood et al. 1994); therefore, careful clinical assessment is imperative. To facilitate early diagnosis and treatment of delirium, clinicians must identify all of the condition's multifactorial contributors. Guidelines established by the National Institute for Health and Clinical Excellence (2010) outline approaches to diagnosis and management of delirium in the older population.

The clinician's most important and difficult task is to differentiate delirium from dementia. Traditionally, delirium has been conceptualized as a brief and transient condition; however, many studies have shown that delirium symptoms may persist for months to years (Marcantonio et al. 2003; McCusker et al. 2003). Nearly two-thirds

---

TABLE 6–4. Medications associated with delirium

Sedative-hypnotics

    Benzodiazepines (especially long-acting agents such as chlordiazepoxide, diazepam, flurazepam)

    Barbiturates (phenobarbital)

Analgesics

    Opioids (especially meperidine)

    Nonsteroidal anti-inflammatory drugs

Psychoactive medications

    Tricyclic antidepressants (amitriptyline, imipramine, doxepin)

    Antipsychotics (chlorpromazine, haloperidol, thioridazine)

    Antiparkinsonian agents (trihexyphenidyl, benztropine, levodopa)

Cardiovascular medications

    Digitalis glycosides (digoxin)

    Antiarrhythmics (quinidine, procainamide, lidocaine, disopyramide)

    Antihypertensives (β-blockers, methyldopa)

Gastrointestinal medications

    Histamine H_2 receptor antagonists (cimetidine, ranitidine, famotidine)

    Antiemetics (scopolamine, metoclopramide)

    Antidiarrheals (diphenoxylate/atropine, loperamide)

Other

    Incontinence medications (oxybutynin, hyoscyamine)

    Histamine H_1 receptor antagonists (especially first-generation, such as diphenhydramine, hydroxyzine)

    Steroids (prednisone)

    Alternative medicines (atropa belladonna, jimson weed, henbane, mandrake)

---

of cases of delirium occur in patients with dementia (Inouye 2006). Patients with dementia who develop a superimposed delirium experience a more rapid progression of cognitive dysfunction and have a worse long-term prognosis (Fick and Foreman 2000; Fong et al. 2009a). The key diagnostic feature that aids in distinguishing these two conditions is pattern of onset: the acute onset of delirium contrasts with the more gradual progression of dementia. Changes in attention and level of consciousness also point to delirium. However, establishing

the occurrence of those changes can be difficult in the face of missing baseline cognitive assessment data or preexisting cognitive deficits. If the differentiation cannot be made with certainty, then given the life-threatening nature of delirium, the patient should be assumed to have—and should receive treatment for—delirium until proven otherwise.

Other important diagnoses that must be differentiated from delirium include psychiatric conditions such as depression, mania, and nonorganic psychotic disorders including schizophrenia. Differentiating among diagnoses is critical because delirium carries a more serious prognosis without proper evaluation and management. Treatment for certain conditions, such as depression or mood disorders, may involve the use of drugs with anticholinergic activity, which could exacerbate an unrecognized case of delirium. Thus, given the seriousness of delirium and the possibility that certain medical treatments may worsen symptoms, it is best for the clinician to assume that delirium is present until further diagnostic information is available.

No specific laboratory tests currently exist for the definitive identification of delirium. The laboratory evaluation for delirium is intended to identify contributing factors that need to be addressed, and the approach should be guided by astute clinical judgment and tailored to the individual situation. Laboratory tests that should be considered include complete blood count, electrolytes, kidney and liver function, oxygen saturation, and glucose levels. Evaluation of occult infection can be obtained through blood cultures, urinalysis, and urine culture. Other laboratory tests, such as thyroid function, arterial blood gas, vitamin B_{12} level, cortisol level, drug levels, toxicology screen, and ammonia levels, are also helpful in identifying factors that contribute to delirium.

Brain imaging is indicated in cases of head trauma or injury, evaluation of new focal neurological symptoms, evaluation for suspected encephalitis, or development of fever of unknown origin. Electroencephalography serves a limited role in the diagnosis of delirium and is most useful for detecting an occult seizure disorder. Overall, the routine use of neuroimaging in delirium is not recommended because the overall diagnostic yield is low, and the findings change the management of patients in fewer than 10% of cases (Hirano et al. 2006).

Prevention and Management

Prevention

Primary prevention is the most effective strategy to decrease delirium and its complications. The Hospital Elder Life Program (HELP; www.hospitalelderlifeprogram.org) uses a targeted risk factor reduction approach for prevention of delirium (Inouye et al. 1999, 2000). HELP is a hospital-wide program that is cost-effective and contributes to an overall improvement in quality of geriatric care in the hospital setting. Other controlled trials have reported the effectiveness of a combination of staff education and individually tailored treatments to reduce delirium incidence, duration, or severity (Milisen et al. 2005; Naughton et al. 2005). Another study confirmed effectiveness of proactive geriatric consultation in reducing delirium risk following hip fracture (Marcantonio et al. 2001). Overall, these trials suggest that 40% of cases of delirium may be preventable and that prevention strategies should begin as soon as possible after hospital admission.

Studies also have explored the potential of pharmacological prevention of delirium, but the results of trials with haloperidol or risperidone have been inconclusive (Campbell et al. 2009). Cholinesterase inhibitors have not been found to be effective for prevention.

Management

In general, nonpharmacological approaches should be implemented as the first-line treatment of delirium. Nonpharmacological treatment approaches include reorientation, behavioral interventions, increased supervision, correcting sensory deficits, and minimizing use of physical restraints (Inouye et al. 2007). Strategies that increase the patient's mobility, self-care, and independence should be promoted. Other environmental interventions include limiting room and staff changes, providing a quiet patient care setting with low-level lighting at night, and implementing a nonpharmacological sleep protocol (McDowell et al. 1998), allowing for an uninterrupted period for sleep.

Pharmacological management of delirium (see Table 6–5; Campbell et al. 2009) should be used only in patients who have severe agitation that interferes with the application of medical treatments (e.g., intubation) or in patients who pose a danger to themselves, other patients, or staff members. The lowest dose of medication should be prescribed for the shortest amount of time possible, because drugs used to manage delirium can also lead to an increase in acute confusion. The goal of pharmacological management of delirium should be an alert and manageable patient, not one who is lethargic and sedated. No randomized controlled trials to date have compared pharmacological treatments for delirium with placebo in hospitalized patients (Campbell et al. 2009).

If required, haloperidol remains the first line of pharmacological treatment for delirium. Haloperidol is the most widely used agent, with documented efficacy for decreasing delirium symptoms and duration compared with placebo and lorazepam (Breitbart et al. 1996). Although haloperidol can be administered orally, intramuscularly, or intravenously, the oral route appears to be the most optimal because of favorable pharmacokinetics and minimal risk of serious adverse effects. Intravenous administration of haloperidol results in rapid onset of action but should be avoided because of the short duration of effect and potential life-threatening adverse effects. The average geriatric patient naive to antipsychotic treatment should require a total loading dose not exceeding 3 mg of haloperidol. Subsequently, a maintenance dose consisting of one-half of the loading dose should be administered over the next 24-hour period, with doses tapered over the next several days. Vital signs should be monitored before each additional dose. Potential side effects include hypotension, QT interval prolongation and torsades de pointes, sedation, extrapyramidal side effects, acute dystonias, and anticholinergic effects. Atypical antipsychotics may have a lower rate of extrapyramidal side effects but appear to be less efficacious overall for delirium treatment (Lonergan et al. 2007). Benzodiazepines are not recommended for treating non–alcohol-related delirium because they typically lead to oversedation, exacerbation of confusion, and prolonged delirium (Breitbart et al. 1996; Lonergan et al. 2009). However, benzodiazepines remain the treatment of choice for alcohol or sedative-hypnotic drug withdrawal. For older patients, lorazepam is the preferred benzodiazepine because of its shorter half-life, lack of active metabolites, and availability in parenteral form.

TABLE 6–5. Pharmacological management of delirium

Class and drug	Geriatric dosing	Indication and efficacy	Adverse effects
First-generation antipsychotic			
Haloperidol	Oral: 0.25–0.50 mg twice daily, with additional doses every 4 h as needed for severe agitation (peak effect, 4–6 h)	First-line agent	Extrapyramidal symptoms, especially if dose is >3 mg/day
	Intramuscular: 0.25–0.50 mg; observe after 30–60 min and repeat as needed for severe agitation (peak effect, 20–40 min)	Effectiveness shown in randomized controlled trials	Prolonged corrected QT interval and risk for torsades
	Total dose not to exceed 3 mg/day	Avoid intravenous use because of short duration of action	Avoid in patients with withdrawal syndrome, hepatic insufficiency, and neuroleptic malignant syndrome
Second-generation (atypical) antipsychotics			
Risperidone	0.5 mg twice daily	Tested mostly in small nonrandomized studies	Extrapyramidal effects equivalent to or slightly less than those with haloperidol
		Efficacy ≤low-dose haloperidol	
Olanzapine	2.5–5.0 mg once daily	Treatment advantage over haloperidol only for possibly fewer extrapyramidal effects	Prolonged corrected QT interval and risk for torsades
Quetiapine	25 mg twice daily	Tested mostly in small nonrandomized studies	Associated with increased mortality rate among older patients with dementia
		Efficacy comparable to haloperidol, with possibly fewer side effects	

TABLE 6–5. Pharmacological management of delirium *(continued)*

Class and drug	Geriatric dosing	Indication and efficacy	Adverse effects
Benzodiazepine			
Lorazepam	Oral: 0.5–1.0 mg, with additional doses every 4 h as needed Sublingual route can be used if necessary Intravenous use of lorazepam should be reserved for emergencies only	Second-line agent Reserve for use in patients undergoing sedative and alcohol withdrawal, those with Parkinson's disease, and those with neuroleptic malignant syndrome	Paradoxical excitation, respiratory depression, oversedation Associated with prolongation and worsening of delirium symptoms in randomized clinical trial
Antidepressant			
Trazodone	25–150 mg orally at bedtime	Tested only in uncontrolled studies	Oversedation

Key Points

- Delirium is a common problem for older persons that may be preventable.

- Delirium is the most frequent complication of hospitalization affecting older persons and often goes unrecognized.

- Patients with delirium have a worse prognosis than patients without delirium and an increased risk of developing long-term cognitive and functional decline.

- It is important to establish a patient's level of baseline cognitive functioning and course of cognitive change when evaluating for delirium.

- The Confusion Assessment Method provides a simple diagnostic algorithm and has become widely used for identification of delirium.

- Although delirium can be caused by a single factor, it is usually multifactorial.

- Existing cognitive impairment and/or dementia are the leading risk factors for development of delirium.

- Nonpharmacological approaches should be implemented as the first line of treatment for delirium.

- Pharmacological management of delirium should be used only in patients with severe agitation.

- The effectiveness of comprehensive geriatric assessment and management has been validated in several large randomized studies, and the geriatrician has a valuable and essential role in the evaluation and treatment of this population.

References

Alagiakrishnan K, Wiens CA: An approach to drug induced delirium in the elderly. Postgrad Med J 80:388–393, 2004

Albert MS, Levkoff SE, Reilly C, et al: The Delirium Symptom Interview: an interview for the detection of delirium symptoms in hospitalized patients. J Geriatr Psychiatry Neurol 5:14–21, 1992

American Psychiatric Association: Diagnostic and Statistical Manual of Mental Disorders, 4th Edition, Text Revision. Washington, DC, American Psychiatric Association, 2000

Bates DW, Cullen DJ, Laird N, et al: Incidence of adverse drug events and potential adverse drug events: implications for prevention. ADE Prevention Study Group. JAMA 274:29–34, 1995

Boyle DA: Delirium in older adults with cancer: implications for practice and research. Oncol Nurs Forum 33:61–78, 2006

Breitbart W, Marotta R, Platt MM, et al: A double-blind trial of haloperidol, chlorpromazine, and lorazepam in the treatment of delirium in hospitalized AIDS patients. Am J Psychiatry 153:231–237, 1996

Breitbart W, Rosenfeld B, Roth A, et al: The Memorial Delirium Assessment Scale. J Pain Symptom Manage 13:128–137, 1997

Campbell N, Boustani MA, Ayub A, et al: Pharmacological management of delirium in hospitalized adults—a systematic evidence review. J Gen Intern Med 24:848–853, 2009

Centers for Medicare and Medicaid Services: MDS 3.0 for Nursing Homes and Swing Bed Providers. Available at: http://www.cms.hhs.gov/NursingHomeQualityInits/25_NHQIMDS30.asp. Accessed December 8, 2010.

Clegg A, Young JB: Which medications to avoid in people at risk of delirium: a systematic review. Age Ageing 40:23–29, 2011

Ely EW, Margolin R, Francis J, et al: Evaluation of delirium in critically ill patients: validation of the Confusion Assessment Method for the Intensive Care Unit (CAM-ICU). Crit Care Med 29:1370–1379, 2001

Fick D, Foreman M: Consequences of not recognizing delirium superimposed on dementia in hospitalized elderly individuals. J Gerontol Nurs 26:30–40, 2000

Fong TG, Jones RN, Shi P, et al: Delirium accelerates cognitive decline in Alzheimer disease. Neurology 72:1570–1575, 2009a

Fong TG, Tulebaev SR, Inouye SK: Delirium in elderly adults: diagnosis, prevention and treatment. Nat Rev Neurol 5:210–220, 2009b

Gleason OC: Donepezil for postoperative delirium. Psychosomatics 44:437–438, 2003

Hamann J, Bickel H, Schwaibold H, et al: Postoperative acute confusional state in typical urologic population: incidence, risk factors, and strategies for prevention. Urology 65:449–453, 2005

Hirano LA, Bogardus ST, Saluja S, et al: Clinical yield of computed tomography brain scans in older general medical patients. J Am Geriatr Soc 54:587–592, 2006

Inouye SK: Current concepts: delirium in older persons. N Engl J Med 354:1157–1165, 2006

Inouye SK, Charpentier PA: Precipitating factors for delirium in hospitalized elderly persons: predictive model and interrelationship with baseline vulnerability. JAMA 275:852–857, 1996

Inouye SK, Vandyck CH, Alessi CA, et al: Clarifying confusion: the Confusion Assessment Method—a new method for detection of delirium. Ann Intern Med 113:941–948, 1990

Inouye SK, Viscoli CM, Horwitz RI, et al: A predictive model for delirium in hospitalized elderly medical patients based on admission characteristics. Ann Intern Med 119:474–481, 1993

Inouye SK, Bogardus ST, Charpentier PA, et al: A multicomponent intervention to prevent delirium in hospitalized older patients. N Engl J Med 340:669–676, 1999

Inouye SK, Bogardus ST, Baker DI, et al: The Hospital Elder Life Program: a model of care to prevent cognitive and functional decline in hospitalized older patients. J Am Geriatr Soc 48:1697–1706, 2000

Inouye SK, Zhang Y, Jones RN, et al: Risk factors for delirium at discharge: development and validation of a predictive model. Arch Intern Med 167:1406–1413, 2007

Leslie DL, Marcantonio ER, Zhang Y, et al: One-year health care costs associated with delirium in the elderly population. Arch Intern Med 168:27–32, 2008

Lindley CM, Tully MP, Paramsothy V, et al: Inappropriate medication is a major cause of adverse drug reactions in elderly patients. Age Ageing 21:294–300, 1992

Lonergan E, Britton AM, Luxenberg J, et al: Antipsychotics for delirium. Cochrane Database of Systematic Reviews 2007, Issue 2. Art. No.: CD005594.

Lonergan E, Luxenberg J, Areosa Sastre A: Benzodiazepines for delirium. Cochrane Database of Systematic Reviews, 2009, Issue 4. Art. No.: CD006379.

MacLullich AM, Beaglehole A, Hall RJ, et al: Delirium and long-term cognitive impairment. Int Rev Psychiatry 21:30–42, 2009

Marcantonio ER, Flacker JM, Wright RJ, et al: Reducing delirium after hip fracture: a randomized trial. J Am Geriatr Soc 49:516–522, 2001

Marcantonio ER, Simon S, Bergmann M, et al: Delirium symptoms in post-acute care: prevalent, persistent, and associated with poor functional recovery. J Am Geriatr Soc 51:4–9, 2003

Marcantonio ER, Rudolph JL, Culley D, et al: Serum biomarkers for delirium. J Gerontol A Biol Sci Med Sci 61:1281–1286, 2006

McCusker J, Cole M, Dendukuri N, et al: The course of delirium in older medical inpatients: a prospective study. J Gen Intern Med 18:696–704, 2003

McDowell JA, Mion LC, Lydon TJ, et al: A nonpharmacologic sleep protocol for hospitalized older patients. J Am Geriatr Soc 46:700–705, 1998

Milisen K, Lemiengre J, Braes T, et al: Multicomponent intervention strategies for managing delirium in hospitalized older people: systematic review. J Adv Nurs 52:79–90, 2005

National Institute for Health and Clinical Excellence: Delirium: diagnosis, prevention and management (NICE Clinical Guideline 103). July 2010. Available at: http://guidance. nice.org.uk/CG103. Accessed December 8, 2010.

Naughton BJ, Saltzman S, Ramadan F, et al: A multifactorial intervention to reduce prevalence of delirium and shorten hospital length of stay. J Am Geriatr Soc 53:18–23, 2005

Rockwood K, Cosway S, Stolee P, et al: Increasing the recognition of delirium in elderly patients. J Am Geriatr Soc 42:252–256, 1994

Rudolph JL, Jones RN, Grande LJ, et al: Impaired executive function is associated with delirium after coronary artery bypass graft surgery. J Am Geriatr Soc 54:937–941, 2006

Siddiqi N, House AO, Holmes JD: Occurrence and outcome of delirium in medical in-patients: a systematic literature review. Age Ageing 35:350–364, 2006

Sieber FE: Postoperative delirium in the elderly surgical patient. Anesthesiol Clin 27:451–464, 2009

Trzepacz PT, van der Mast R: The neuropathophysiology of delirium, in Delirium in Old Age. Edited by Lindesay J, Rockwood K, MacDonald AJ. New York, Oxford University Press, 2002, pp 51–90

Trzepacz PT, Mittal D, Torres R, et al: Validation of the Delirium Rating Scale—Revised–98: comparison with the Delirium Rating Scale and the Cognitive Test for Delirium. J Neuropsychiatry Clin Neurosci 13:229–242, 2001

U.S. Department of Health and Human Services: 2004 CMS statistics. Washington, DC, Centers for Medicare and Medicaid Services, 2004

Witlox J, Eurelings LS, de Jonghe JF, et al: Delirium in elderly patients and the risk of postdischarge mortality, institutionalization, and dementia: a meta-analysis. JAMA 304:443–451, 2010

Yang FM, Marcantonio ER, Inouye SK, et al: Phenomenological subtypes of delirium in older persons: patterns, prevalence, and prognosis. Psychosomatics 50:248–254, 2009

CHAPTER 7

DEMENTIA AND MILDER COGNITIVE SYNDROMES

CONSTANTINE G. LYKETSOS, M.D., M.H.S.

Dementia is a clinical syndrome that can be caused by a range of diseases or injuries to the brain. Although it can affect young people, it is most commonly seen in older individuals because dementia prevalence increases with age. In the United States, as many as 15 million new cases of dementia are expected in the next several decades (Hebert et al. 2003). Given that dementia is a chronic disease, with estimates of its duration ranging from 3–4 years in community settings (Graham et al. 1997) to 10–12 years in clinical settings (Rabins et al. 2006), it poses a unique public health problem with serious effects on its victims, their families, and society at large. In the United States alone, it is estimated that by 2050, the annual cost of dementia will be close to $400 billion in direct and indirect expenses (Murman 2001; Murman et al. 2007).

In this chapter, I discuss definitions, clinical presentation, evaluation, and differential diagnosis of dementia and related cognitive disorders; describe specific dementia syndromes according to their etiology; and discuss how to approach treatment. For an in-depth discussion of the clinical management of dementia, the reader is referred to *Practical Dementia Care* by Rabins et al. (2006).

Definitions

Table 7–1 provides definitions related to dementia espoused by the American Association for Geriatric Psychiatry (Lyketsos et al. 2006).

Although these definitions are important to the clinical world, one should recognize that uncertainty remains about linking cognitive syndrome to brain pathology. For example, in community settings, most patients with dementia have mixed brain

---

TABLE 7–1. Definitions related to dementia

Cognitive impairment not dementia (CIND): A clinical syndrome consisting of a measurable or evident decline in memory or other cognitive abilities, with little effect on day-to-day functioning; does not meet criteria for dementia.

Mild cognitive impairment (MCI): A clinical subsyndrome of CIND, most likely the prodrome to Alzheimer's dementia. Can be amnestic (having memory deficits) or nonamnestic.

Dementia: A clinical syndrome not entirely due to delirium, consisting of global cognitive decline, with several areas of cognition affected, and significant effect on day-to-day functioning.

Alzheimer's dementia: A dementia syndrome that has gradual onset and slow progression and is best explained as caused by Alzheimer's disease.

Alzheimer's disease: A brain disease characterized by plaques, tangles, and neuronal loss.

Source. Adapted from Lyketsos CG, Colenda CC, Beck C, et al: "Position Statement of the American Association for Geriatric Psychiatry Regarding Principles of Care for Patients With Dementia Resulting From Alzheimer Disease." *American Journal of Geriatric Psychiatry* 14:561–572, 2006. Used with permission.

---

pathologies including Alzheimer's disease, micro infarcts, lacunar infarcts, and Lewy bodies (Neuropathology Group, Medical Research Council Cognitive Function and Aging Study 2001; White and Launer 2006).

Clinical Presentation, Evaluation, and Differential Diagnosis

Clinical Presentation of the Dementia Syndrome

Dementia is defined entirely on clinical grounds. Table 7–2 lists the four critical elements of the definition. Dementia is a condition that affects *cognition*. For the dementia syndrome to be present, *several* areas of cognition must be affected (*global*). To differentiate dementia from mental retardation, the cognitive symptoms must represent a cognitive *decline* for the individual. The decline

must be significant, typically sufficient to affect the person's daily functioning. Finally, because delirium can cause the full range of cognitive symptoms associated with dementia, it is critical that the cognitive syndrome be present in the *absence of delirium*. This broad definition has been operationalized in several diagnostic systems, with the criteria of DSM-IV-TR (American Psychiatric Association 2000) being the most commonly used.

Although dementia is defined around cognitive disturbances, individuals with dementia have a wider range of impairments. These include functional, neuropsychiatric (behavioral), and neurological impairments. In the functional realm, patients with dementia have problems in their social and interpersonal functioning and in their ability to live independently. Patients with milder dementia have difficulties with instrumental abilities, whereas patients with more severe dementia develop impairments in their basic abilities of daily living.

TABLE 7–2. Four key elements of the dementia syndrome

---

1. Global
2. Cognitive
3. Decline
4. Absence of delirium

Dementia also has been associated with several neuropsychiatric symptoms, such as apathy, depression, agitation, psychosis, and disinhibited behaviors. Over the course of a progressive dementia, essentially all patients develop one or more of these symptoms (Steinberg et al. 2008).

Finally, patients with dementia develop a range of neurological findings. Most common are gait disorders, especially unstable, ataxic, or labored gait. Other neurological symptoms include incontinence, focal findings, seizures, and, less commonly, cranial nerve findings.

Clinical Presentation of Milder Cognitive Syndromes

Large numbers of older people have cognitive impairments that are troubling to them or family members but not sufficiently severe or broad to meet criteria for dementia. The prevalence of these impairments might be as high as 18% after age 65 (Lopez et al. 2003). Most patients who develop progressive dementia do so in stages and typically go through a prodromal period of cognitive impairment, most often with memory symptoms, that is characteristic of the specific cause of the dementia. Thus, for example, it appears that mild cognitive impairment (MCI) is a prodrome to Alzheimer's disease because many patients who meet MCI criteria have Alzheimer's disease pathology. The term *vascular cognitive impairment* (Ha-

chinski 2007) refers to nondementia disturbances associated with brain vascular disease, likely the prodrome of vascular dementia. Whereas the prodrome of Alzheimer's disease, MCI, appears to have primarily cortical features, the prodrome of vascular dementia, vascular cognitive impairment, typically affects executive functions (Hayden et al. 2006).

Conducting an Evaluation

In this section, I highlight critical aspects of the evaluation. A thorough discussion of the evaluation of the patient with suspected dementia, including reasons for doing an evaluation, the setting for the evaluation, and ways to communicate the diagnosis to the patient, can be found in *Practical Dementia Care* (Rabins et al. 2006).

History Taking

The patient's medical history is critical to a good dementia evaluation. The inclusion of an informant is critical. Informants must be people who know the patient well, such as spouses, children, friends, neighbors, or other family members. Because informants themselves can be influenced by their own mental states, it is often useful to have additional informants to confirm or disconfirm discrepancies between the history and the evaluation of the patient. Dating the onset of cognitive symptoms is critical. It is important to spend a lot of time trying to determine when the patient was last well as opposed to when the first symptom started. Informants may minimize early symptoms by attributing them to "normal aging." The history should survey for cognitive symptoms; functional losses in social, interpersonal, and daily functioning; the full range of neuropsychiatric symptoms; and neurological deficits.

Cognitive Assessment

Conducting a cognitive assessment is the central aspect of the dementia evaluation. Many specialists tend to use the Mini-Mental State Examination (MMSE; Folstein et al. 1975) as their primary tool. The MMSE is inefficient in evaluating milder cognitive symptoms or mild dementia. The Modified Mini-Mental State provides a broader assessment (Teng and Chui 1987) and has many advantages. For closer assessments of executive functioning, clinicians should consider incorporating the Clock Drawing test (van der Burg et al. 2004), the Frontal Assessment Battery (Dubois et al. 2000), and the Mental Alternation Test (Jones et al. 1993).

Differential Diagnosis and Diagnostic Testing

The establishment of a careful differential diagnosis is a key aspect of the dementia evaluation. The first step is to develop a differential diagnosis of the syndrome. Figure 7–1 provides a useful flowchart for this purpose.

Neuropsychological testing is often useful in differentiating dementia from milder cognitive syndromes or normal aging, especially in investigating profiles of cognitive impairment that suggest specific etiologies. However, neuropsychological testing is not needed in every case. When conducted, neuropsychological testing should be requested with specific questions in mind.

Further workup using laboratory studies is needed in most cases. Blood tests and brain imaging are typically used in all cases. The American Academy of Neurology (Knopman et al. 2001) recommends thyroid studies, liver tests, metabolic panel, complete blood count, and vitamin B_{12} and folate levels. Additional tests, such as heavy metal screen, syphilis serology, toxicology, electrocardiogram, and chest X ray, should be considered to determine possible underlying causes. Computed tomography (CT) of the head is usually adequate, but some believe it is important to perform magnetic resonance imaging (MRI), especially when brain vascular disease may be involved. Functional brain imaging with positron emission tomography (fluorodeoxyglucose [^{18}FDG]-PET) has come into broader use (Kulasingam et al. 2003). This is most useful in the differential diagnosis of dementia caused by Alzheimer's disease or by frontotemporal degeneration (FTD).

More than 100 different disease processes have been associated with dementia (Rabins et al. 2006). Most can be assessed adequately with the approach discussed in this section. In the past, reference was made to treatable and nontreatable dementias. This differentiation is no longer useful, for two reasons. First, reversibility of a "treatable dementia" depends on the severity of the brain damage that has occurred, not its cause. Second, the implication that Alzheimer's disease, vascular dementia, and other dementias are not treatable is also incorrect. Although these cases tend to be progressive, the application of available treatments makes a big difference to patients, caregivers, and families.

Specific Dementias

Dementia Due to Alzheimer's Disease

Alzheimer's dementia is the most common form of dementia. Depending on the population series, 50%–70% of individuals with dementia are diagnosed clinically as having dementia due to Alzheimer's disease

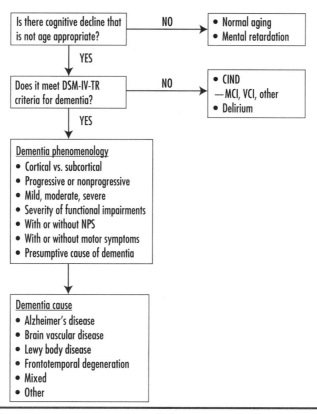

FIGURE 7–1. Flowchart in the diagnosis of dementia.

CIND = cognitive impairment not dementia; MCI = mild cognitive impairment; NPS = neuro-psychiatric symptoms; VCI = vascular cognitive impairment.

(McKhann et al. 1984; Ranginwala et al. 2008).

The prevalence of Alzheimer's dementia is closely tied to age, which is the primary risk factor. Other risk factors include traumatic brain injury, reduced reserve capacity of the brain, limited educational or occupational attainment, brain vascular disease, hyperlipidemia, hypertension, atherosclerosis, coronary heart disease, atrial fibrillation, smoking, obesity, and diabetes.

A major risk factor is genetic (Blennow et al. 2006). Alzheimer's disease is a heterogeneous genetic disorder with familial and polygenic forms. Several mutations have been associated with the familial conditions; all involve mutations in genes associated with the amyloid precursor protein on chromosome 21 and also include the presenilin 1 and 2 genes (on chromosomes 14 and 1, respectively). Most cases of Alzheimer's disease are polygenic. Several genes, most unknown, likely increase risk but do not absolutely determine the occurrence of the disease. The most well-known gene is the *APOE* gene, whose ε4 allele is a risk factor for Alzheimer's dementia.

Neuropsychiatric symptoms are nearly universal. Affective, psychotic, and sleep symptoms relapse and remit through the course of Alzheimer's dementia and are very troubling for patients and caregivers (Steinberg et al. 2008). Apathy, in contrast, appears to be a steadily accumulating symptom in that many but not all patients gradually develop persistent and pervasive apathy (Onyike et al. 2007; Steinberg et al. 2008).

The brain changes seen in Alzheimer's dementia are well known. Even in early disease, atrophy in the hippocampus occurs bilaterally, which progresses throughout the brain. In early stages, brain imaging using ^{18}FDG-PET typically shows bitemporoparietal hypoperfusion.

Pathologically, the characteristic lesions of Alzheimer's disease include senile or neuritic plaques and neurofibrillary tangles, with associated loss of neurons in several neurotransmitter systems: cholinergic, serotonergic, and dopaminergic. These changes typically occur early in the disease and affect both the nuclei and the cortical projections of neurons. The current hypothesis about etiopathogenesis suggests a cascade (Blennow et al. 2006). Genetic and environmental risk factors interact to increase the production or to decrease the clearance of amyloid derived from the amyloid precursor protein (APP). APP may be processed through cleavage by β-secretase preferentially over α-secretase, leading to the formation of a form of amyloid beta ($A\beta_{1-42}$). The latter is prone to dimerization, oligomerization, and deposition in the extracellular space. The deposition of this toxic form of $A\beta$ accumulates close to the synaptic cleft and is thought to lead over time to synaptic disconnection, the loss of neurotransmitter systems, and the emergence of symptoms. A range of downstream factors have been implicated in the disease cascade, including activation of microglia that might injure neurons through several mechanisms (Rosenberg 2005). Other downstream factors involved in the progression include glutamatergic toxicity, lipid peroxidation products, and the loss of trophic factor.

Dementia Due to Brain Vascular Disease (Vascular Dementia)

Vascular dementia is a controversial nosological entity. It is difficult to differentiate on clinical grounds those patients who have Alzheimer's dementia from those who have vascular dementia (Groves et al. 2000). Further complicating the differentiation, recent evidence suggests that cerebrovascular risk factors and diseases influence the progression of Alzheimer's dementia (Mielke et al. 2007) and the emergence of Alzheimer's pathology in the brain (Beach et al. 2007; Roher et al. 2006). Most patients with vascular dementia who come to autopsy have mixed pathology, often with significant Alzheimer's disease pathology (Jellinger and Attems 2006).

Vascular dementia, therefore, is best understood as a heterogeneous group of dementias. On one end of the spectrum are pure genetic forms, such as 1) cerebral autosomal dominant arteriopathy with subcortical infarcts and leukoencephalopathy and 2) mitochondrial encephalopathy with lactic acidosis and strokelike episodes. At the other end are patients who develop dementia after multiple strokes in which significant portions of the brain are damaged. Between those two end points are patients with mixtures of pathologies and clinical presentations that affect one another (e.g., smaller strokes or chronic subcortical hypoxia might both damage brain tissue and lead to the onset and progression of Alzheimer's pathology).

In addition to genetic conditions such as those mentioned in the previous paragraph, genes that predispose to cerebrovascular disorders are risk factors for vascular dementia (Meschia et al. 2005; Schneider et al. 2007). The following are some of the risk factors for cerebrovascular disease that are also risk factors for vascular dementia: disease of the large and small vessels of the brain, diabetes, hypertension, and atrial fibrillation and other cardiac disease.

The clinical presentation of vascular dementia is variable. Typically, it presents in fits and spurts, often with acute or subacute onset after a cerebrovascular event. A mix of symptoms usually presents, often including apathy, depression, and motor symptoms. Of patients with vascular dementia or Alzheimer's dementia who have similar MMSE scores, those with vascular dementia are usually more functionally impaired. Gait disorders, parkinsonism, and incontinence are early features.

The diagnosis of vascular dementia is based on a typical clinical history and associated physical examination findings. The diagnosis requires brain imaging that shows completed infarcts or lacunas in brain areas associated with the cognitive changes. A temporal relationship between the brain vascular disease and the cognitive changes should be demonstrable, but this might be difficult. Radiological findings of white matter change alone, with no evidence of completed strokes or associated examination findings (e.g., motor focality or gait disorder), are not supportive of a diagnosis of vascular dementia. White matter changes, as evident on MRI, are common in older people who are cognitively normal (Longstreth 1998; Longstreth et al. 2005). The diagnosis becomes more complex when patients with established Alzheimer's dementia develop strokes; many such patients also meet criteria for a diagnosis of vascular dementia.

Dementias Due to Lewy Body Disease

A recent consensus panel (Lippa et al. 2007) has proposed the term *Lewy body disorders* as an umbrella term for Parkinson's disease (PD), Parkinson's disease dementia (PDD), and dementia with Lewy bodies (DLB). This proposal appropriately recognizes the existence of a spectrum of dementias associated with Lewy body deposition in the brain whose shared pathology involves impairments in alpha synuclein metabolism. The hypothesis is that these three conditions, which can also be termed *synucleinopathies,* represent brain diseases in which abnormal synuclein metabolism leads to dementia. The sequence of events involved is poorly known. One of the complicating factors in determining a diagnosis is that many patients with Lewy body pathologies have coexisting pathologies, in particular Alzheimer's and vascular pathology. Additionally, the clinical presentations of PDD and DLB can be similar, with motor parkinsonism, gait imbalance, visual hallucinations, and dementia being the unifying clinical features. The discussion that follows focuses on each of these conditions separately.

Parkinson's Disease Dementia

With the advent of the use of L-dopa to help control Parkinson's motor symptoms, it has become apparent that some of the most common and impairing symptoms of PD are in the cognitive realm. Patients with PD typically show impairments in executive functioning. They also have memory impairments, affecting working memory and the organization of explicit memory. In early to mid-stage PD, 16%–20% of patients develop dementia, with as many as 80% in later PD. In early stages, a further 15%–30% of patients have milder cognitive symptoms. *PDD* refers to patients who have had PD for many years and then develop dementia most likely caused by the PD itself. PDD can be quite impairing of daily functioning and adversely affects caregivers (Mehta 2005). PDD has become a therapeutic target, leading to the U.S. Food and Drug Administration's (FDA's) approval of the cholinesterase inhibitor rivastigmine for treatment of PDD.

Dementia With Lewy Bodies

The Consortium on Dementia With Lewy Bodies continues to systematically update diagnostic and management recommendations for DLB. The most recent DLB diagnostic criteria (McKeith et al. 2005) present central, core, suggestive, and supportive features. The central feature is a progressive dementia with primary persistent memory impairment and deficits in attention and executive and visuospatial abilities. Core features, at least one of which is necessary for the diagnosis of DLB, include fluctuating cognition with pronounced variations in attention and alertness, visual hallucinations, or spontaneous parkinsonism. Suggestive features include REM (rapid eye movement) sleep behavior disorder, severe neuroleptic sensitivity, and low dopamine transporter uptake in the basal ganglia demonstrated on PET or single-photon emission computed tomography (SPECT) imaging. The long list of supportive features includes falls and syncope, unexplained loss of consciousness, autonomic dysfunction, nonvisual hallucinations, delusions, depression, and brain imaging or electroencephalographic findings consistent with the diagnosis.

If dementia and parkinsonism coexist, the differential diagnosis is sorted out by examining the relative course of the cognitive and motor symptoms. The emergence of dementia after many years of motor symptoms supports a diagnosis of PDD. In contrast, the early presence of dementia in a patient with motor parkinsonism supports a

diagnosis of DLB. Note that many patients with Alzheimer's dementia develop a DLB picture, which is reflected in the neuropathology, and many DLB patients have concurrent Alzheimer's dementia pathology. It is difficult to clinically distinguish Alzheimer's dementia patients with and without DLB pathology (Lopez et al. 2000).

Although the progression of DLB tends to be similar overall to that of Alzheimer's dementia, the course of DLB is more variable. Because many patients have a more fulminant course, some experts believe that DLB has a worse prognosis than Alzheimer's dementia (McKeith et al. 2003, 2004). DLB is associated with considerable suffering for patients, particularly because of the very common, persistent, and hard-to-treat neuropsychiatric symptoms, especially hallucinations, delusions, and affective symptomatology (Ballard et al. 1999; McKeith and Cummings 2005). Patients also tend to become affected early with balance, sleep, and motor disorders and to become confined in their mobility.

Dementia Due to Frontotemporal Degeneration

FTD is in many ways the paradigmatic non-Alzheimer's dementia and has recently become a major focus of interest because in individuals younger than 65 years, FTD is the second most common form of dementia (Neary et al. 2005). Previously referred to as *Pick's disease,* FTD is heterogeneous both clinically and pathologically (Kertesz 2005; Neary et al. 2005). The clinical syndrome typically begins with changes in behavior, affect, and personality, which result in disinhibition, hyperorality, social inappropriateness, apathy, and related symptoms of loss of executive control. Cognitive changes leading to difficulties in attention, memory, set shifting, and organization occur early in the disease (Kertesz et al. 2005). The phenotype, however, is variable because many patients develop progressive expressive aphasia, whereas others develop semantic dementia early on (Shinagawa et al. 2006). As the condition progresses, disinhibited behaviors and apathy—often at the same time—worsen, leading to admixtures of productive-type and deficit-type loss of executive control.

Pathologically, FTD is characterized by knife-edge lobar atrophy, typically in the anterior temporal and posterior inferior areas of the frontal lobes. Microscopically, neurons appear enlarged and vacuolar, with extensive gliosis. Revised consensus neuropathological criteria reflect the diversity of pathological pictures (Cairns et al. 2007a). Most of these conditions appear to be tauopathies and include the pathologies of FTD with Pick bodies, corticobasal degeneration, progressive supranuclear palsy, hippocampal sclerosis, and other less common pathologies. TDP-43 proteinopathy appears to be the most frequent histological finding in FTD. FTD is familial in a considerable number of patients; mutations in the tau, progranulin, and ubiquitin genes have been associated with the condition. Familial TDP-43 proteinopathy is associated with defects in multiple genes and several neuropathological types (Cairns et al. 2007b).

FTD is almost invariably progressive, especially if language symptoms occur early on. In clinical settings, the time from an FTD diagnosis to death is on the order of 3–5 years, shorter than the periods associated with Alzheimer's dementia (Chow et al. 2006). Also, compared with Alzheimer's dementia, FTD is a greater burden to care-givers, given the disinhibited behaviors that are hard to treat and require aggressive supervision to manage.

Treatment

Treatment for Milder Cognitive Syndromes

Given the increased public awareness of dementia, memory clinics and primary care physicians anecdotally report that patients are presenting with increasingly milder cognitive symptoms to request diagnosis and treatment. At present, little empirical knowledge exists about how to manage these patients clinically; most experts recommend continued observation, the use of nonpharmacological therapies such as exercise and mental activity, and possibly cognitive rehabilitation. The results of at least one randomized trial suggest that the cholinesterase inhibitor donepezil may delay progression to dementia, especially in patients who are *APOE*E4* carriers (Petersen et al. 2005), but this has not been replicated or supported by other trials (Rosenberg et al. 2006). Initiation of pharmacological therapy is reserved for cases for which there is strong evidence of likely benefit—for example, when the patient appears to be about to transition to Alzheimer's dementia. For more a detailed approach to this issue, see Rosenberg et al. (2006).

The Four Pillars of Dementia Care

Dementia care has four basic elements or pillars (Lyketsos et al. 2006). The first relates to management of key aspects of the disease with the goal of reversing its effects or delaying its progression in the brain. Although few disease therapies exist at present, several therapies are being developed for different types of dementia targeted at underlying pathophysiological mechanisms. The second pillar relates to the management of symptoms, whether they are cognitive, neuropsychiatric, or functional. The final pillars involve supportive care to patients and caregivers in ways that are systematic and evidence based. Evidence from randomized trials now indicates that the "package" of dementia care as currently conceived provides significant benefits to patients and caregivers by reducing symptoms, improving disability and quality of life, and reducing caregiver effects (Callahan et al. 2006; Drentea et al. 2006; Mittelman et al. 2006).

Disease Therapies: Alzheimer's Dementia

Estrogen, anti-inflammatory agents, and ginkgo biloba are not effective treatments for Alzheimer's dementia. High doses of the antioxidant vitamin E were found, in one large randomized controlled trial, to delay progression of Alzheimer's dementia, lengthening the time before onset of the next phase (Sano et al. 1997). Given safety concerns about dosing, the American Association for Geriatric Psychiatry recommended that vitamin E be considered for Alzheimer's dementia but that doses higher than 400 IU/day should be avoided.

Probably the most effective therapy for Alzheimer's disease is management of associated vascular risk factors—blood pressure in particular—and treatment with the glutamatergic antagonist memantine. Reduction of blood pressure, weight loss, exercise, management of diabetes, and a healthy diet all probably constitute effective therapy for Alzheimer's disease. For patients with moderate or more severe Alzheimer's dementia, memantine titrated to 10 mg twice daily has very small but measurable effects, especially in patients with more severe disease.

Therapies for Cognitive Symptoms

The cholinesterase inhibitors donepezil, rivastigmine, and galantamine are all approved by the FDA or otherwise available in the United States for treatment of the cognitive symptoms of Alzheimer's dementia. Most of these medications have been approved for the treatment of mild to moderate Alzheimer's dementia; donepezil has been approved for the treatment of severe Alzheimer's dementia. They are available in a variety of formulations as pills, delayed-release pills, and patch form (rivastigmine only). Although clinical trials have suggested that these medications may be of value in treating vascular dementia, none of them has been approved by the FDA for that purpose. The results of one study suggested that donepezil is associated with increased mortality in vascular dementia relative to placebo. Rivastigmine has been approved for the treatment of PDD and also has been found in randomized trials to be effective in DLB.

Currently, most experts recommend, and the data support, initiation of one of these medications titrated to the highest approved and tolerated dose and assessment of response over 6–12 months (Rabins et al. 2006). There is debate, however, about whether patients should continue a cholinesterase inhibitor for a longer time. In primary care settings in the United States, most patients who start a prescription do not continue it for more than a few months.

Nevertheless, many experts recommend continuation of therapy once it is started because discontinuation studies suggest that patients may get worse when a cholinesterase inhibitor is stopped. However, other experts point out that some patients do well after a discontinuation trial and that many benefit from switching to another agent when they do not respond to an earlier one (Tariot et al. 2006).

Therapies for Neuropsychiatric Symptoms

Neuropsychiatric symptoms are nearly universal over the course of dementia. They have severe adverse effects for patients and caregivers and are a frequent target of treatment. Nevertheless, uncertainty about how to manage these symptoms continues. Detailed discussion of the evaluation and management of neuropsychiatric symptoms in dementia is beyond the scope of this chapter (see Rabins et al. 2006 for an in-depth discussion); however, a few principles are articulated here.

A useful approach to the management of neuropsychiatric symptoms uses a mnemonic of four D's: define, decode, devise, and determine. *Define* refers to an evaluation phase in which the patient, caregivers, and other relevant informants (e.g., charts and professional caregivers in long-term care facilities and hospitals) provide the history, which is used to describe in detail the phenomenology of the patient's disturbance. Then, the patient undergoes an examination, which sometimes involves laboratory studies. This information is used to decide what type of disturbance is present: delirium, mood disorder, psychotic disorder, sleep disturbance, apathy, executive dysfunction, and so on (Lyketsos 2007).

Subsequently, the clinician, working as part of a team, seeks contributing factors to the disorder; this is the *decode* phase. Contributing causes to neuropsychiatric symptoms are listed in Table 7–3. In general, most disturbances are multifactorial; therefore, it is best to address several factors at once. The *devise* phase, which derives from the decoding process, consists of pharmacological, behavioral, environmental, and educational approaches that target the causes identified and are often delivered through the patient's caregiver. For example, a patient's urinary tract infection or constipation might be treated while teaching the caregiver how not to rush the patient during toileting.

Occasionally, management with psychotropics is needed, especially if nonpharmacological approaches have failed. Although extensive effort has been put into the development of nonpharmacological approaches, little controlled evidence suggests that they work, and they are often hard to implement in real-world settings, especially in primary and institutional care (Livingston et al. 2005). The interventions with the best evidence to support their use are outlined in Table 7–4. Finally, the *determine* phase refers to setting reasonable goals for assessing the effect of the intervention and readjusting the plan if the intervention is not successful.

If medication treatments are indicated, it is important to follow an approach similar to the one outlined in Table 7–5. Several different classes of medications have been studied, but for some of them, safety concerns exist and efficacy remains uncertain. The use of antipsychotics, especially the atypical antipsychotics, is controversial because their efficacy is modest (Schneider et al. 2005, 2006), and they have been associated with a higher risk of cerebrovascular or cardiovascular conditions and mortality in patients with dementia specifically (Schneider et al. 2005). Both conventional and atypical antipsychotics carry this risk in dementia, whereas other psychotropics, such as antidepressants and anticonvulsants, do not (Kales et al. 2007). Although these antipsychotics are not contraindicated in dementia, the risk-benefit threshold has recently been raised, and they should be used with caution (Rabins and Lyketsos 2005). Evidence is limited regarding the efficacy of cholinesterase inhibitors and memantine for behavior. In general, although these medications may delay the emergence of neuropsychiatric symptoms or treat very mild symptoms, they should not be considered first-line agents in managing acute neuropsychiatric symptoms of moderate or greater severity until better evidence of their efficacy emerges (Weintraub and Katz 2005). Similarly, evidence suggests that the selective serotonin reuptake inhibitor citalopram (Pollock et al. 2002) has efficacy for the treatment of agitation in patients with Alzheimer's dementia. Putting this information together, a widely used algorithm for use of medications to treat neuropsychiatric symptoms in dementia has been published (Sink et al. 2005).

Supportive Care for Patients

The provision of systematic supportive care to patients with dementia is critical. This care is typically tailored to individual patients and is implemented in collaboration with caregivers and other team members. Table 7–6 lists areas that should be addressed in every case (Lyketsos et al. 2006). In addition, when appropriate, patients should be educated as much as possible about their condition and their prognosis.

Supportive Care for Caregivers

Because caregivers are greatly affected by dementia and are the lifeline of the patient, they should be involved intimately in the development and implementation of any dementia care program. Table 7–7 lists key intervention areas involving caregivers (Lyketsos et al. 2006; Rabins et al. 2006; Selwood et al. 2007).

TABLE 7–3. Contributing causes of neuropsychiatric symptoms

Biological stress or delirium that accompanies a recurrent or new medical condition (e.g., constipation, urinary or upper respiratory infection, pain, poor dentition, headaches, hunger, thirst)

Identifiable psychiatric syndrome that is either recurrent or associated with the dementia

Aspects of the cognitive disturbance itself (catastrophic reaction due to inability to express oneself vocally)

Environmental stressor (e.g., too much noise, not enough heat)

Unmet needs (e.g., hunger, thirst, feeling lonely)

Unsophisticated or intrusive caregiving (e.g., poor communication, being rushed)

Medication side effects, whether from new medications or previously prescribed medications

TABLE 7–4. Evidence-based nonpharmacological treatments for neuropsychiatric symptoms

Cognitive stimulation and behavioral management techniques centered on patient behavior or caregiver behavior are effective treatments whose benefits last for months.

Music therapy and controlled multisensory stimulation (Snoezelen) are useful during the treatment session but have no longer-term effects.

Specific education for caregiving staff about managing neuropsychiatric symptoms is very beneficial, but other educational interventions are not.

Changing the visual environment (e.g., painting doors to disguise them) is promising, but more research is needed.

TABLE 7–5. Guidelines for use of medications to treat neuropsychiatric symptoms

Differentiate which disturbance is present; they are not all the same.

Consider possible contributing causes and the need for medical workup.

Implement nonpharmacological interventions.

Decide whether to treat with medications.

Use medications cautiously, with defined targets and close monitoring.

Be mindful that select *isolated* disturbances are unlikely to respond to medications.

Have in place a backup plan and a plan to deal with after-hours crisis.

TABLE 7–6. Supportive care for patients

Comfort and emotional support

Safety in regard to driving, living alone, medications, falls

Proper approach and communication

A safe, predictable place to live with support for independent activities of daily living and activities of daily living

Structure, activity, and stimulation in day-to-day life

Planning and assistance with decision making

Aggressive management of medical comorbidity

Good nursing care in advanced stages

TABLE 7–7. Supportive care for the caregiver

Comfort and emotional support

Education about dementia and caregiving

Instruction in the skills of caregiving

Support with problem solving

Availability of an expert clinician, especially for crisis intervention

Respite from caregiving

Attention to general and mental health

Maintenance of social network

Key Points

- Dementia is a clinical syndrome that can be accurately diagnosed and differentiated from cognitive impairment not dementia and mild cognitive impairment.

- The evaluation and differential diagnosis of dementia, and of milder cognitive syndromes, involves an initial focus on defining the phenomenology of the syndrome and its associated features, followed by a workup for a putative cause.

- The concept of treatable and nontreatable dementias is no longer relevant; all dementias are treatable albeit not necessarily curable.

- The four pillars of dementia treatment are disease treatment, symptom treatments, supportive care for the patient, and supportive care for the caregiver. All of these areas must be addressed in contemporary dementia care.

- Nonpharmacological interventions, in the context of carefully orchestrated dementia care, can be as effective as currently available medications (and in some cases more effective).

References

American Psychiatric Association: Diagnostic and Statistical Manual of Mental Disorders, 4th Edition, Text Revision. Washington, DC, American Psychiatric Association, 2000

Ballard C, Holmes C, McKeith I, et al: Psychiatric morbidity in dementia with Lewy bodies: a prospective clinical and neuropathological comparative study with Alzheimer's disease. Am J Psychiatry 156:1039–1045, 1999

Beach TG, Wilson JR, Sue LI, et al: Circle of Willis atherosclerosis: association with Alzheimer's disease, neuritic plaques and neurofibrillary tangles. Acta Neuropathol 113:13–21, 2007

Blennow K, de Leon MJ, Zetterberg H: Alzheimer's disease. Lancet 368:387–403, 2006

Cairns NJ, Bigio EH, Mackenzie IR, et al: Neuropathologic diagnostic and nosologic criteria for frontotemporal lobar degeneration: consensus of the Consortium for Frontotemporal Lobar Degeneration. Acta Neuropathol 114:5–22, 2007a

Cairns NJ, Neumann M, Bigio EH, et al: TDP-43 in familial and sporadic frontotemporal lobar degeneration with ubiquitin inclusions. Am J Pathol 171:227–240, 2007b

Callahan CM, Boustani MA, Unverzagt FW, et al: Effectiveness of collaborative care for older adults with Alzheimer disease in primary care: a randomized controlled trial. JAMA 295:2148–2157, 2006

Chow TW, Hynan LS, Lipton AM: MMSE scores decline at a greater rate in frontotemporal degeneration than in AD. Dement Geriatr Cogn Disord 22:194–199, 2006

Drentea P, Clay OJ, Roth DL, et al: Predictors of improvement in social support: five-year effects of a structured intervention for caregivers of spouses with Alzheimer's disease. Soc Sci Med 63:957–967, 2006

Dubois B, Slachevsky A, Litvan I, et al: The FAB: a frontal assessment battery at bedside. Neurology 55:1621–1626, 2000

Folstein MF, Folstein SE, McHugh PR: "Mini-Mental State": a practical method for grading the cognitive state of patients for the clinician. J Psychiatr Res 12:189–198, 1975

Graham JE, Rockwood K, Beattie BL, et al: Prevalence and severity of cognitive impairment with and without dementia in an elderly population. Lancet 349:1793–1796, 1997

Groves WC, Brandt J, Steinberg M, et al: Vascular dementia and Alzheimer's disease: is there a difference? A comparison of symptoms by disease duration. J Neuropsychiatry Clin Neurosci 12:305–315, 2000

Hachinski V: The 2005 Thomas Willis lecture: stroke and vascular cognitive impairment: a transdisciplinary, translational and transactional approach. Stroke 38:1396, 2007

Hayden KM, Zandi PP, Lyketsos CG, et al: Vascular risk factors for incident Alzheimer disease and vascular dementia: the Cache County study. Alzheimer Dis Assoc Disord 20:93–100, 2006

Hebert LE, Scherr PA, Bienias JL, et al: Alzheimer disease in the U.S. population: prevalence estimates using the 2000 census. Arch Neurol 60:1119–1122, 2003

Jellinger KA, Attems J: Prevalence and impact of cerebrovascular pathology in Alzheimer's disease and parkinsonism. Acta Neurol Scand 114:38–46, 2006

Jones BN, Teng EL, Folstein MF, et al: A new bedside test of cognition for patients with HIV infection. Ann Intern Med 119:1001–1004, 1993

Kales HC, Valenstein M, Kim HM, et al: Mortality risk in patients with dementia treated with antipsychotics versus other psychiatric medications. Am J Psychiatry 164:1568–1576, 2007

Kertesz A: Frontotemporal dementia: one disease, or many? Probably one, possibly two. Alzheimer Dis Assoc Disord 19 (suppl 1):S19–S24, 2005

Kertesz A, McMonagle P, Blair M, et al: The evolution and pathology of frontotemporal dementia. Brain 128 (pt 9):1996–2005, 2005

Knopman DS, DeKosky ST, Cummings JL, et al: Practice parameter: diagnosis of dementia (an evidence-based review): report of the Quality Standards Subcommittee of the American Academy of Neurology. Neurology 56:1143–1153, 2001

Kulasingam SL, Samsa GP, Zarin DA, et al: When should functional neuroimaging techniques be used in the diagnosis and management of Alzheimer's dementia? A decision analysis. Value 6:542–550, 2003

Lippa CF, Duda JE, Grossman M, et al: DLB and PDD boundary issues: diagnosis, treatment, molecular pathology, and biomarkers. Neurology 68:812–819, 2007

Livingston G, Johnston K, Katona C, et al, for the Old Age Task Force of the World Federation of Biological Psychiatry: Systematic review of psychological approaches to the management of neuropsychiatric symptoms of dementia. Am J Psychiatry 162:1996–2021, 2005

Longstreth WT Jr, for the Cardiovascular Health Study Collaborative Research Group: Brain abnormalities in the elderly: frequency and predictors in the United States (the Cardiovascular Health Study). J Neural Transm 53(suppl):9–16, 1998

Longstreth WT Jr, Arnold AM, Beauchamp NJ Jr, et al: Incidence, manifestations, and predictors of worsening white matter on serial cranial magnetic resonance imaging in the elderly: the Cardiovascular Health Study. Stroke 36:56–61, 2005

Lopez OL, Wisniewski S, Hamilton RL, et al: Predictors of progression in patients with AD and Lewy bodies. Neurology 54:1774–1779, 2000

Lopez OL, Jagust WJ, DeKosky ST, et al: Prevalence and classification of mild cognitive impairment in the Cardiovascular Health Study Cognition Study, part 1. Arch Neurol 60:1385–1389, 2003

Lyketsos CG: Neuropsychiatric symptoms (behavioral and psychological symptoms of dementia) and the development of dementia treatments. Int Psychogeriatr 19:409–420, 2007

Lyketsos CG, Colenda CC, Beck C, et al: Position statement of the American Association for Geriatric Psychiatry regarding principles of care for patients with dementia resulting from Alzheimer disease. Am J Geriatr Psychiatry 14:561–572, 2006

McKeith I, Cummings J: Behavioural changes and psychological symptoms in dementia disorders. Lancet Neurol 4:735–742, 2005

McKeith IG, Burn DJ, Ballard CG, et al: Dementia with Lewy bodies. Semin Clin Neuropsychiatry 8:46–57, 2003

McKeith I, Mintzer J, Aarsland D, et al: Dementia with Lewy bodies. Lancet Neurol 3:19–28, 2004

McKeith IG, Dickson DW, Lowe J, et al: Diagnosis and management of dementia with Lewy bodies: third report of the DLB consortium. Neurology 65:1863–1872, 2005

McKhann G, Drachman D, Folstein M, et al: Clinical diagnosis of Alzheimer's disease: report of the NINCDS-ADRDA Work Group under the auspices of Department of Health and Human Services Task Force on Alzheimer's Disease. Neurology 34:939–944, 1984

Mehta KK: Stress among family caregivers of older persons in Singapore. J Cross Cult Gerontol 20:319–334, 2005

Meschia JF, Brott TG, Brown RD Jr: Genetics of cerebrovascular disorders. Mayo Clin Proc 80:122–132, 2005

Mielke MM, Rosenberg PB, Tschanz J, et al: Vascular factors predict rate of progression in Alzheimer disease. Neurology 69:1850–1858, 2007

Mittelman MS, Haley WE, Clay OJ, et al: Improving caregiver well-being delays nursing home placement of patients with Alzheimer disease. Neurology 67:1592–1599, 2006

Murman DL: The costs of caring: medical costs of Alzheimer's disease and the managed care environment. J Geriatr Psychiatry Neurol 14:168–178, 2001

Murman DL, Von Eye A, Sherwood PR, et al: Evaluated need, costs of care, and payer perspective in degenerative dementia patients cared for in the United States. Alzheimer Dis Assoc Disord 21:39–48, 2007

Neary D, Snowden J, Mann D: Frontotemporal dementia. Lancet Neurol 4:771–780, 2005

Neuropathology Group, Medical Research Council Cognitive Function and Aging Study: Pathological correlates of late-onset dementia in a multicentre, community-based population in England and Wales. Lancet 357:169–175, 2001

Onyike CU, Sheppard JM, Tschanz JT, et al: Epidemiology of apathy in older adults: the Cache County study. Am J Geriatr Psychiatry 15:365–375, 2007

Petersen RC, Thomas RG, Grundman M, et al: Vitamin E and donepezil for the treatment of mild cognitive impairment. N Engl J Med 352:2379–2388, 2005

Pollock BG, Mulsant BH, Rosen J, et al: Comparison of citalopram, perphenazine, and placebo for the acute treatment of psychosis and behavioral disturbances in hospitalized, demented patients. Am J Psychiatry 159:460–465, 2002

Rabins PV, Lyketsos CG: Antipsychotic drugs in dementia: what should be made of the risks? JAMA 294:1963–1965, 2005

Rabins PV, Lyketsos CG, Steele CD: Practical Dementia Care, 2nd Edition. New York, Oxford University Press, 2006

Ranginwala NA, Hynan LS, Weiner MF, et al: Clinical criteria for the diagnosis of Alzheimer disease: still good after all these years. Am J Geriatr Psychiatry 16:384–388, 2008

Roher AE, Kokjohn TA, Beach TG: An association with great implications: vascular pathology and Alzheimer disease. Alzheimer Dis Assoc Disord 20:73–75, 2006

Rosenberg PB: Clinical aspects of inflammation in Alzheimer's disease. Int Rev Psychiatry 17:503–514, 2005

Rosenberg PB, Johnston D, Lyketsos CG: A clinical approach to mild cognitive impairment. Am J Psychiatry 163:1884–1890, 2006

Sano M, Ernesto C, Thomas RG, et al: A controlled trial of selegiline, alpha-tocopherol, or both as treatment for Alzheimer's disease: the Alzheimer's Disease Cooperative Study. N Engl J Med 336:1216–1222, 1997

Schneider JA, Arvanitakis Z, Bang W, et al: Mixed brain pathologies account for most dementia cases in community-dwelling older persons. Neurology 69:2197–2204, 2007

Schneider LS, Dagerman KS, Insel P: Risk of death with atypical antipsychotic drug treatment for dementia: meta-analysis of randomized placebo-controlled trials. JAMA 294:1934–1943, 2005

Schneider LS, Tariot PN, Dagerman KS, et al: Effectiveness of atypical antipsychotic drugs in patients with Alzheimer's disease. N Engl J Med 355:1525–1538, 2006

Selwood A, Johnston K, Katona C, et al: Systematic review of the effect of psychological interventions on family caregivers of people with dementia. J Affect Disord 101:75–89, 2007

Shinagawa S, Ikeda M, Fukuhara R, et al: Initial symptoms in frontotemporal dementia and semantic dementia compared with Alzheimer's disease. Dement Geriatr Cogn Disord 21:74–80, 2006

Sink KM, Holden KF, Yaffe K: Pharmacological treatment of neuropsychiatric symptoms of dementia: a review of the evidence. JAMA 293:596–608, 2005

Steinberg M, Shao H, Zandi P, et al: Point and 5-year period prevalence of neuropsychiatric symptoms in dementia: the Cache County study. Int J Geriatr Psychiatry 23:170–177, 2008

Tariot P, Cummings J, Ismael S, et al: New paradigms in the treatment of Alzheimer's disease. J Clin Psychiatry 67:2002–2013, 2006

Teng EL, Chui HC: The Modified Mini-Mental State (3MS) examination. J Clin Psychiatry 48:314–318, 1987

van der Burg M, Bouwen A, Stessens J, et al: Scoring Clock Tests for dementia screening: a comparison of two scoring methods. Int J Geriatr Psychiatry 19:685–689, 2004

Weintraub D, Katz IR: Pharmacologic interventions for psychosis and agitation in neurodegenerative diseases: evidence about efficacy and safety. Psychiatr Clin North Am 28:941–983, ix–x, 2005

White L, Launer L: Relevance of cardiovascular risk factors and ischemic cerebrovascular disease to the pathogenesis of Alzheimer disease: a review of accrued findings from the Honolulu-Asia Aging Study. Alzheimer Dis Assoc Disord 20 (suppl 2):S79–S83, 2006

Suggested Readings

Blennow K, de Leon MJ, Zetterberg H: Alzheimer's disease. Lancet 368:387–403, 2006

Ferri CP, Prince M, Brayne C, et al: Global prevalence of dementia: a Delphi consensus study. Lancet 366:2112–2117, 2005

Lyketsos CG: Lessons from neuropsychiatry. J Neuropsychiatry Clin Neurosci 18:445–449, 2006

Metzler-Baddeley C: A review of cognitive impairments in dementia with Lewy bodies relative to Alzheimer's disease and Parkinson's disease with dementia. Cortex 43:583–600, 2007

Neary D, Snowden J, Mann D: Frontotemporal dementia. Lancet Neurol 4:771–780, 2005

Rosenberg PB, Johnston D, Lyketsos CG: A clinical approach to mild cognitive impairment. Am J Psychiatry 163:1884–1890, 2006

White L, Launer L: Relevance of cardiovascular risk factors and ischemic cerebrovascular disease to the pathogenesis of Alzheimer disease: a review of accrued findings from the Honolulu-Asia Aging Study. Alzheimer Dis Assoc Disord 20 (suppl 2):S79–S83, 2006

CHAPTER 8

MOOD DISORDERS

DAVID C. STEFFENS, M.D., M.H.S.
DAN G. BLAZER, M.D., PH.D.

Clinical entities listed under the mood disorders in DSM-IV-TR (American Psychiatric Association 2000) relevant to depression in elderly patients include 1) bipolar disorder, 2) major depressive disorder (with or without psychotic features), 3) dysthymic disorder, and 4) minor or subsyndromal depression (found in Appendix B of DSM-IV-TR). Depressive symptoms are also present in other DSM-IV-TR disorders, such as bereavement, adjustment disorder with depressed mood, and mood disorder due to a general medical condition (see Table 8–1).

Manic episodes in later life also may present with a mixture of manic, dysphoric, and cognitive symptoms, with euphoria being less common (Post 1978). When mania is associated with significant changes in cognitive function—so-called manic delirium—it may be difficult to distinguish from organic conditions or schizophrenia (Shulman 1986).

TABLE 8–1. Subtypes of depression in later life

Bipolar disorder

Major depression, single episode or recurrent

Psychotic depression

Dysthymic disorder

Minor or subsyndromal depression

Bereavement

Adjustment disorder with depressed mood

Depression associated with medical illness

Epidemiology

In a community survey of more than 1,300 older adults living in urban and rural communities, 27% reported depressive symptoms; of these, 19% had mild dysphoria only (Blazer et al. 1987). Persons with symptomatic depression—that is, subjects with more severe depressive symptoms—made up 4% of the population. These individuals were primarily experiencing stressors, such as physical illness and stressful life events. Only 2% had a dysthymic disorder, and 0.8% were experiencing a current major depressive episode. No cases of current manic episode were identified. Finally, 1.2% had a mixed depression and anxiety syndrome. These data suggest that the traditional DSM-IV-TR depression categories do not apply to most depressed older adults in the community. Subsequent surveys confirmed the lower frequency of major depression in the community (Kessler et al. 2005), but a more recent, population-representative study of 851 older community-dwelling adults reported a combined prevalence of major and minor depression of 11.2% (Steffens et al. 2009). White and Hispanic older adults had nearly three times the prevalence of depression found in African American older adults.

In hospital and long-term care settings, the frequency of major depression among older adults is much higher than in community settings. Up to 21% of hospitalized elders meet criteria for a major depressive episode, and an additional 20%–25% have a minor depression (Koenig et al. 1988). Rates of major depression among elderly nursing home patients are even higher, exceeding 25% in some studies (Parmelee et al. 1989).

The Epidemiologic Catchment Area surveys identified bipolar disorder in 9.7% of nursing home patients, which suggests that nursing homes may have become a dumping ground for such patients (Weissman et al. 1991). In clinical settings, about 10%–25% of geriatric patients with mood disorder have bipolar disorder, and 3%–10% of all older psychiatric patients have this disorder (Wylie et al. 1999; Young and Kler-

man 1992). About 5% of all individuals admitted as geropsychiatry inpatients present with mania (Yassa et al. 1988).

Clinical Course

Episodes of depression across the life cycle, especially episodes of more severe major depression, almost always remit or at least partially remit. Nevertheless, depression is a chronic and recurrent illness. Data from a community study from the Netherlands illustrate this chronicity. Among subjects with clinically significant depressive symptoms, 23% improved, 44% experienced an unfavorable but fluctuating course, and 33% experienced a severe and chronic course. In a second group of subjects with less severe depression, 25% experienced a chronic course. Overall, 35% of those subjects with a diagnosis of major depression and 52% of the subjects with a diagnosis of dysthymic disorder experienced a chronic course (Beekman et al. 2002).

Studies that have focused on older adults in clinical settings have found similar chronicity (Alexopoulos et al. 1996; Baldwin and Jolley 1986; Murphy 1983; Post 1962). The prognosis from clinical studies of depressed older adults with uncomplicated late-life depression, however, is similar to that found among younger adults if the older adult is not plagued with comorbid medical illness, functional impairment, or cognitive impairment (Keller et al. 1982a, 1982b). Comorbid depression is associated with a less favorable prognosis. For example, when major depression is comorbid with dysthymic disorder, the prognosis is poor. Factors predicting partial remission were similar to those predicting no remission, and poor social support and functional limitations increased the risk for poor outcome in these subjects (Hybels et al. 2005).

Cognitive impairment is often associated with depressive symptoms. When the depression improves, the cognitive impairment often improves as well. Nevertheless, comorbid depression and cognitive impairment are a risk for the later emergence of Alzheimer's disease (Alexopoulos et al. 1993). Therefore, early depressive symptoms associated with mild cognitive impairment may represent a preclinical sign and should be considered a risk for impending Alzheimer's disease or vascular dementia (Li et al. 2001). Depression can further complicate Alzheimer's disease over time by increasing disability and physical aggression, thereby contributing to depression among caregivers (Gonzalez-Salvador et al. 1999). Depressive symptoms in patients with Alzheimer's disease resolve spontaneously at a greater frequency without requiring intensive therapy (such as medication therapy) than among older adults experiencing depression and vascular dementia, in which depressive symptoms tend to be persistent and refractory to drug treatment (Li et al. 2001).

Depression and medical problems are frequently comorbid, and the causal pathway may be bidirectional (Blazer and Hybels 2005). Depression, for example, is a frequent and important contributing cause of weight loss in late life (Morley and Kraenzle 1994). Frailty, leading to profound weight loss, can contribute to clinically important depressive symptoms (Fried 1994). Many chronic medical illnesses are associated with depression, including cardiovascular disease, diabetes, osteoporosis, and hip fracture (Blazer et al. 2002b; Lenze et al. 2007; Lyles 2001; Williams et al. 2002).

Perhaps the best-established association between depression and physical problems is the association between depression and functional impairment (Blazer et al. 1991; Bruce 2001). For example, in one study, older adults who were depressed were 67% more likely to experience impairment in activities of daily living and 73% more likely to experience mobility restrictions 6 years following initial evaluation than were those not depressed (Penninx et al. 1999). Disability, in turn, can increase the risk for depressive symptoms (Kennedy et al. 1990; Roberts et al. 1997). Functional decline, however, is not inevitable when the older adult becomes depressed. For example, the instrumental support provided to older adults, such as help in tasks necessary for daily living, can be protective against the worsening of performance on instrumental abilities, which buffers against the onset of depression (Hays et al. 2001).

Most clinicians and clinical investigators report that more than 70% of elderly patients with major depression who receive antidepressant medication (at an adequate dose for a sufficient time) recover from the index episode of depression if the depression is uncomplicated by comorbid factors. Reynolds et al. (1992) reported that treatment of depression in physically healthy elders with combined interpersonal psychotherapy and nortriptyline was associated with response rates nearing 80%. In a long-term outcome study of treatment-resistant depression in older adults, 47% of patients were clinically improved 15 months after treatment with an antidepressant or electroconvulsive therapy (ECT); at 4-year follow-up, the percentage had increased to 71% (Stoudemire et al. 1993). Once an older patient has experienced one or more moderate to severe episodes of major depression, he or she may need to continue antidepressant therapy permanently to minimize the risk of relapse (Reynolds et al. 2006).

Persons with a dysthymic disorder (depressive neurosis) experience a more chronic clinical course than do persons with major depression. By DSM-IV-TR definition, an individual's depressive symptoms must last at least 2 years for a dysthymic disorder diagnosis to be made. An undetermined percentage (as high as 4%–8%) of community-dwelling (and possibly institutionalized) elders experience moderately severe depressive symptoms for more than 2 years, although they report intermittent periods, lasting longer than a few days, of relative freedom from depressive symptoms. Among older patients with major depression, those with comorbid dysthymia had a less favorable trajectory of recovery over 3 years (Hybels et al. 2008).

Factors associated with improved outcome in late-life depression include a history of recovery from previous episodes, a family history of depression, female gender, extroverted personality, current or recent employment, absence of substance abuse, no history of major psychiatric disorder, less severe depressive symptomatology, and absence of major life events and serious medical illness (Baldwin and Jolley 1986; Cole et al. 1999; Post 1972). The results of several studies suggested a relation between social support during an index episode and outcome in psychological distress and depression. In one study involving 493 community respondents, Holahan and Moos (1981) found that decreases in social support of family and in work environments were related to increases in psychological maladjustment over a 1-year follow-up period.

An association between depression and mortality has held in many studies, despite the addition of potentially confounding variables. In studies conducted in North Carolina and New York, however, investigators failed to find an association (Blazer et al. 2001; Thomas et al. 1992). One reason for the lack of association in some studies may be the selection of specific control variables, especially chronic disease and functional impairment.

For example, in a study of the North Carolina Established Populations for Epidemiologic Study of the Elderly cohort, the unadjusted relative odds of mortality among depressed subjects at baseline was 1.98 (Blazer et al. 2001). These odds moved toward unity when other risk factors, such as chronic disease, were controlled and when health habits, cognitive impairment, functional impairment, and social support were added to the model. The effect of depression on mortality may vary by sex (Hybels et al. 2002; Takeshita et al. 2002; Whooley and Browner 1998).

The outcome of bipolar disorder in elderly patients remains virtually unknown. In a long-term follow-up study involving 500 patients in Iowa, Winokur (1975) found that bipolar disorder tended to occur in clusters over time and speculated that early-onset bipolar illness may "burn itself out" in time. Shulman and Post (1980) studied elderly patients with bipolar disorder and found that only 8% had their first episode of mania before age 40. In a review of records of a small number of untreated patients with severe and prolonged bipolar disorder, Cutler and Post (1982) found a tendency toward more rapid recurrences late in the illness, with decreasing periods of remission. In other words, if bipolar disorder re-emerges in the later years, the episodes of mania—or mania mixed with depression—may once again cluster, just as the disorder typically clusters at earlier periods of life. Most clinicians who have worked with patients with bipolar disorder in late life recognize the tendency of these disorders to recur frequently for a time, only to remit for an extended period. Ambelas (1987) emphasized a relation between life events and onset of mania, noting that stressful events were more likely to precede early-onset mania than late-onset mania.

Controversy exists over whether age at onset of first manic episode affects response to treatment. Glasser and Rabins (1984) described no significant age-related differences in presentation or treatment response. Young and Falk (1989) reported that late-onset mania was associated with lower activity level, lower sexual drive, and less-disturbed thought processes; however, they also found that older age was associated with longer hospitalization, greater residual psychopathology, and poorer response to pharmacotherapy. Eastham et al. (1998) suggested that elderly patients with bipolar disorder often require lithium doses that are 25%–50% lower than those used in younger patients. Data on the use of valproic acid in elderly patients with this disorder are limited but encouraging. Almost no information is available on the use of carbamazepine or other drugs in late-life bipolar disorder. ECT has been reported to be well tolerated and effective in the treatment of these patients (Eastham et al. 1998).

Etiology[1]

Biological Origins

Genetics

The etiology of late-life mood disorders is undoubtedly multifactorial (see Table 8–2). Twin and family studies, along with studies focusing on molecular genetics, provide strong evidence for a heritable contribution to the etiology of major depression and bipolar disorder (Gatz et al. 1992). Evidence that these genetic factors weigh heavily in the etiology of bipolar disorders in late life is virtually nonexistent, although the biological nature of this disorder would suggest some genetic contribution. Evidence from studies of unipolar depression in late life suggests that the genetic contribution is weaker in late-life depression than in depression at earlier stages of the life cycle. In a study of elderly twins in Sweden, genetic influences accounted for 16% of the variance in total depression scores on the Center for Epidemiologic Studies Depression Scale (CES-D) and 19% of the somatic symptoms. In contrast, genetic influences minimally contributed to the variance of symptoms of depressed mood and positive affect (Gatz et al. 1992).

Hypothesized genetic markers for late-life depression usually have not stood the test of well-controlled studies, yet some studies present intriguing possibilities. Many candidate genes, such as genes encoding enzymes for serotonin synthesis, the norepinephrine transporter, have been hypothesized and explored in animal studies, but they await further testing in older adults with depression (Smith et al. 2007). Some pharmacological studies with depressed elders have shown associations between speed of response and antidepressant side effects with the serotonin transporter promoter polymorphism (Pollock 2000). Polymorphisms in genes coding for the brain-derived neurotrophic factor (Taylor et al. 2007) and for the enzymes methylene tetrahydrofolate reductase (Hickie et al. 2001) and tryptophan hydroxylase-2 (Zhang et al. 2005) have been associated with geriatric depression. Despite many studies of the ε4 allele of the apolipoprotein E gene, no association was found in a community sample between the ε4 allele and depressive symptoms (Blazer et al. 2002a).

---

[1] The discussion on etiology is abstracted, with permission, from Blazer DG, Hybels CF: "Origins of Depression in Later Life." *Psychological Medicine* 35:1241–1252, 2005.

TABLE 8–2. Origins of late-life depression

Biological risks

Genetics (e.g., abnormalities in the serotonin transporter gene)

Female sex

Neurotransmitter dysfunction (e.g., underactivity of serotonergic neurotransmission)

Endocrine changes (e.g., long-standing elevated blood levels of cortisol)

Vascular changes (e.g., vascular depression secondary to subcortical vascular changes)

Medical illness (e.g., cardiovascular disease)

Other psychiatric disorders (e.g., long-standing anxiety disorder)

Psychological risks

Personality attributes (e.g., hopelessness and ambivalence)

Neuroticism

Cognitive distortions (e.g., feelings of abandonment when left alone for short periods)

Social origins

Stressful life events (e.g., the death of a close friend or a change of residence)

Chronic stress or strain (e.g., residence in an unsafe neighborhood)

Low socioeconomic status

Neurotransmitter Dysfunction

Decreased activity of serotonergic neurotransmission has been the focus of much research on the pathophysiology of depression in younger adults. Dysfunctions in the transmission of norepinephrine and dopamine also have been implicated. Serotonin activity, specifically serotonin type 2A (5-HT_{2A}) receptor binding, decreases dramatically in a variety of brain regions through midlife, yet less decrease occurs from midlife to late life. 5-HT_{2A} receptors in nondepressed subjects decreased markedly from young adulthood to midlife (70% from the levels at age 20 years through the fifth decade) and then leveled off as age advanced (Sheline et al. 2002). Activity of these receptors, however, may vary with age.

Endocrine Changes

Hypersecretion of corticotropin-releasing factor (CRF) has been associated with depression for many years across the life cycle. CRF is thought to mediate sleep and appetite disturbances, reduced libido, and psychomotor changes (Arborelius et al. 1999) and is diminished with normal aging (Gottfries 1990). Aging is associated with an increased responsiveness of dehydroepiandrosterone sulfate to CRF (Luisi et al. 1998).

Serum testosterone levels decline with aging (Liverman and Blazer 2004) and have been found to be even lower in elderly men with dysthymic disorder than in men without depressive symptoms (Seidman et al. 2002). The efficacy of testosterone treatment for major depression in men, however, has not been established (Liverman and Blazer 2004). In women, improvement of mood has resulted from hormone replacement (Sherwin and Gelfand 1985).

Endocrine dysregulation over time has been associated with anatomical changes related to late-life depressive symptoms, suggesting a vicious cycle downward to chronic and moderately severe depressive symptoms. Depressive symptoms have been hypothesized to cause atrophy of the hippocampus (Sapolsky 1996, 2001; Sheline et al. 1996; Steffens et al. 2002). Stress that accumulates over the life cycle may lead to a sustained increase in secretion of cortisol, leading to loss of preexisting hippocampal neurons (Sapolsky 1996). This loss may be prevented in part by use of antidepressant medications (Czéh et al. 2001).

Vascular Depression

Vascular risk factors have been known to be associated with depressive symptoms for many years (Post 1962). Because major depression is a frequent outcome of stroke (Robinson and Price 1982) and hypertension (Rabkin et al. 1983), investigators have proposed a vascular-based depression affecting elderly individuals (Coffey et al. 1990; Krishnan et al. 1988; Kumar et al. 2002; Olin et al. 2002; Post 1962). In a study of 139 depressed older adults, 54% met neuroimaging criteria for subcortical ischemic vascular depression. Older age was most strongly associated with the increased prevalence of subcortical changes; also associated were lassitude, a history of hypertension, and poorer outcome (Krishnan et al. 2004; Taylor et al. 2003). Vascular depression is associated with white matter hyperintensities (Guttmann et al. 1998; Krishnan et al. 1997). These lesions probably contribute to the disruption of neural circuits associated with depression (Taylor et al. 2003).

The clinical symptoms and signs associated with these vascular impairments resemble impairments found in frontal lobe syndromes. Magnetic resonance imaging (MRI) studies of depressed patients have detected structural abnormalities in areas related to limbic-cortical-striatal-pallidal-thalamic-cortical pathways (George et al. 1994), including the frontal lobes (Krishnan et al. 1993), caudate (Krishnan et al. 1992), and putamen (Husain et al. 1991; Sheline 2003). In MRI studies of mood disorders, structures that make up this tract show volume loss or structural abnormalities (Sheline 2003).

These studies linking cerebrovascular disease and late-life depression have led investigators to examine genes associated with vascular risk and development of depression. For example, polymorphisms in the angiotensin II type 1 receptor gene have been associated with depression outcome (Kondo et al. 2007) and with change in vascular brain lesions (Taylor et al. 2010).

Medical and Psychiatric Comorbidity

Myocardial infarction and other heart conditions often lead to late-life depression (Sullivan et al. 1997), as do diabetes (Blazer et al. 2002b), hip fracture (Magaziner et al. 1990), and stroke (Robinson and Price 1982). In a survey of community-dwelling Mexican Americans, depressive symptoms were found to be associated with diabetes, arthritis, urinary incontinence, bowel incontinence, kidney disease, and ulcers (Black et al. 1998). Poor functional status secondary to physical illness and dementing disorders are the most important causes of depressive symptoms in older adults (Bruce 2001; Hays et al. 1997). Depressive symptoms are consistently associated with health status in cross-sectional studies of older adults (Kraaij et al. 2002); however, the association is not always clear-cut (Fiske et al. 2003).

Psychological Origins

Psychological factors, such as personality attributes, neuroticism, cognitive distortions, and emotional control, may contribute to the onset of late-life depression yet are not specific to the origins of depression in older adults. Therefore, we briefly address examples of recent studies.

In a study comparing older patients with and without personality disorder, Morse and Lynch (2004) found that those with a personality disorder were four times more likely to continue with or experience a reemergence of depressive symptoms. Specific personality traits were not correlated with clinical features of depression, such as age at onset and number of previous episodes. Nevertheless, some of the traits were associated with depressive symptoms such as hopelessness. Basic personality attributes often underlie the origin and expression of depressive symptoms in older adults.

Cognitive distortions (Beck 1987) are among the most extensively studied psychological origins of depression across the life cycle. Depressed individuals may overreact to life events or misinterpret these events and exaggerate their adverse outcome. For example, in a study of the experience and effect of adverse life events, older patients with major depression reported more adverse life events in the recent past and a greater negative effect of these events (particularly for interpersonal conflicts) than did comparison groups of elderly patients with dysthymia and healthy control subjects (Devanand et al. 2002). It is not clear whether the reported effect reflects an increased vulnerability to events or a bias in reporting because of current depressed mood.

Beekman et al. (1995), in the Longitudinal Aging Study Amsterdam, found that major and minor depression, as well as the persistence and emergence of depressive symptoms over 3 years, were predicted by external locus of control (Beekman et al. 2001). Higher levels of mastery—that is, a perception of being able to accomplish tasks and having control over one's life—have been shown to have a direct association with fewer depressive symptoms in older adults and to buffer the adverse effect of disability on depression (Jang et al. 2002). Self-efficacy may have a direct effect and also may work indirectly through its effect on social support to prevent depressive symptoms, as was indicated in a sample of older adults followed up for 1 year (Holahan and Holahan 1987).

Social Origins

In addition to having biological and psychological origins, late-life depression derives from social origins, including stressful life events, bereavement, chronic stress or strain, low socioeconomic status, and impaired social support. The relative contribution of these factors appears to vary across the life cycle.

Murphy (1982) found a strong association between both severe life events (e.g., bereavement, life-threatening illness of someone else, major personal illness) and social difficulties (e.g., difficulties in health of someone close to subject, housing issues, marital and family relationships) and the onset of late-life depression. Elders lacking a confidant were especially vulnerable to the effects of life stress. Social support may therefore buffer the effect of a stressful event. The association, however, may not be straightforward. On the basis of a meta-analysis of 25 studies of the relation between negative life events and depression in late life, Kraaij et al. (2002) reported that the total number of life events and the total number of daily hassles were strongly associated with depressive symptoms, as would be expected. In contrast, sudden unexpected events were not related to depression.

Compared with younger adults, older adults are at greater risk for depressive symptoms secondary to stressful life events. However, at least three factors modify this risk. First, ongoing problems may have a smaller effect on the risk for depression in older adults than in younger adults (Bruce 2002). For example, in one study, the onset of depressive symptoms was not associated with baseline psychosocial stressors but was associated with factors that changed over time (Kennedy et al. 1990). Second, stressful events that are predictable or "on-time" events often cause less depression in older adults than in younger adults. For example, death of a spouse is a severe and at times catastrophic event leading to depression. For young or middle-aged adults, this event is unexpected, and the adjustment is especially difficult. Older adults, in contrast, recognize that death of a spouse is frequent (by observing their peers) and have actually rehearsed the event, such as by considering what they might do if a spouse dies. Third, many events that can lead to depression, such as divorce and difficulties with the law, are more frequent early in life than in late life. In one study, significant difficulty with the law (something more serious than a traffic violation) was reported during the preceding year by 9% of younger adults but by fewer than 1% of older adults (Hughes et al. 1988). Bereavement is a common cause of depressive symptoms in late life (Clayton 1990; de Beurs et al. 2001; Prigerson et al. 1994). In a study of 1,810 community-dwelling older adults, onset of clinically significant depressive symptoms over a 3-year follow-up was predicted by the death of a partner or other relatives (Prigerson et al. 1994). Although some studies have found

bereavement to predict depressive symptoms, other studies have not (Prince et al. 1998).

Lower socioeconomic status has been associated with depression across the life cycle. Both the frequency of depressive symptoms and their persistence over 2–4 years were associated with socioeconomic disadvantage in a sample of community-dwelling adults age 50 years or older who originally met criteria for major depression (Mojtabai and Olfson 2004). In another study, although the level of education did not predict emergence of depressive symptoms over 1 year, emergence of depression over a 3-year period was predicted by lower level of education (Beekman et al. 2001).

Perceived social support has proved to be a most consistent predictor of late-life depressive symptoms (Bruce 2002). Investigators from Hong Kong, in a community study, found that depressive symptoms were associated with impaired social support (including network size, network composition, social contact frequency, satisfaction with social support, and instrumental-emotional support) (Chi and Chou 2001). Findings from another longitudinal study substantiated that poor social support predicted depressive symptoms at follow-up after 3–6 years (Henderson et al. 1997). The clinician must not assume that older adults in general experience a deficit in social support. Social support is perceived to be adequate in older adults, even among clinical samples (Blazer 1982). Old social networks thin out, but new ones emerge for many people. Most older people believe that they have enough contact with both family and friends and assess the relationships that they have with their social networks as positive (Cornoni-Huntley et al. 1990). Even so, when the social network is depleted suddenly, either through loss of someone close to the older adult (such as a spouse or child) or through a change in the quality of the relationship (such as a dispute within the family), impaired social support may emerge as a most important contributor to late-life depression.

Diagnosis of Late-Life Mood Disorders

Clinical entities listed under the mood disorders in DSM-IV-TR that are relevant to depression in elderly patients are listed in Table 8–1, presented earlier in this chapter. Depressive symptoms are likewise present in other DSM-IV-TR disorders, such as bereavement and mood disorder due to a general medical condition (Blazer 2002, 2003). The major mood disorders in older adults include the following:

- *Bipolar disorder,* characterized by inflated self-esteem or grandiosity, decreased need for sleep, more talkativeness than usual, flight of ideas, distractibility, psychomotor agitation, and excessive involvement in pleasurable activities (such as unrestricted buying episodes).
- *Major depressive disorder,* for which a diagnosis is made when the older adult has one or both of two core symptoms (depressed mood and lack of interest), as well as four or more of the following symptoms for at least 2 weeks: feelings of worthlessness or inappropriate guilt, diminished ability to concentrate or make decisions, fatigue, psychomotor agitation or retardation, insomnia or hypersomnia, significant decrease or increase in appetite, and recurrent thoughts of death or suicidal ideation.
- *Major depressive episode with psychotic features,* which deserves special attention, because patients with onset after age 60

have a higher risk of psychotic depression and may include somatic, nihilistic, or guilty delusions.
- *Dysthymic disorder,* with fewer criteria symptoms than major depressive disorder, but with symptoms that must last 2 years or more.
- *Adjustment disorder with depressed mood,* reserved for those individuals who show a maladaptive mood reaction to an identifiable stressor.
- *Depression associated with a medical illness,* because depressive disorders have been associated with a variety of physical illnesses, including cardiovascular disease (Glassman and Shapiro 1998; Musselman et al. 1998), endocrine disturbances (Blazer et al. 2002b), Parkinson's disease (Zesiewicz et al. 1999), stroke (Robinson and Price 1982), and cancer (Spiegel 1996).

Diagnostic Workup of the Depressed Older Adult

At its core, the diagnosis of a mood disorder in older adults is made on the basis of a history, augmented with a physical examination and fine-tuned by laboratory studies (Blazer 2003) (see Table 8–3). No biological markers or tests are available to confirm the diagnosis of depression, yet some tests may assist in identifying subtypes of depression; for example, MRI scans for subcortical white matter hyperintensities to confirm the presence of vascular depression (Krishnan et al. 1988) and polysomnography for unexplained sleep disturbances. Of special importance in evaluating the depressed elder are the following: the duration of the current depressive episode; the history of previous episodes; the history of drug and alcohol abuse; the response to previous therapeutic interventions for the depressive illness; a family history of depression, suicide, and/or alcohol abuse; and the severity of the depressive symptoms. Establishing some indication of the risk of suicide is essential, for suicidal risk may determine where the patient is treated.

Screening for depression with standardized scales such as the Geriatric Depression Scale (GDS; Yesavage et al. 1983) and the CES-D (Radloff 1977) is helpful. In primary care settings, the clinical effectiveness of screening is mixed. One reason is that clinical trials typically exclude the type of patients who are most likely to present to the busy internist, such as the patient with comorbid depression and medical illness. Assessment of cognitive status is critical to the evaluation of depressed older patients. Use of a screening scale such as the Mini-Mental State Examination (MMSE; Folstein et al. 1975) or the Montreal Cognitive Assessment (Nasreddine et al. 2005) is a good adjunct to the diagnostic workup.

The physical examination must include a thorough neurological examination to determine whether soft neurological signs (e.g., frontal release signs) or laterality is present. Weight loss and psychomotor retardation in the depressed older adult may lead to peroneal nerve palsy, documented by electromyography and nerve conduction studies (Massey and Bullock 1978). Because the older adult is less occupied with physical activities and therefore tends to be sedentary, the peroneal nerve is subject to chronic trauma.

TABLE 8–3. Diagnostic workup of late-life depression

Routine studies

Screening (especially in a primary care setting, use standard symptom checklists such as the Geriatric Depression Scale [Yesavage et al. 1983] or the Center for Epidemiologic Studies Depression Scale [Radloff 1977])

Thorough history and assessment, including present and past history of depressive episodes, family history, medication history, and assessment of psychological functioning and of social stressors; medical history, including assessment of nutritional status, current medications, past and current medical history, and functional status

Screening for cognitive impairment with an instrument such as the Mini-Mental State Examination (Folstein et al. 1975)

Physical examination

Laboratory tests, such as chemistry screen and electrocardiogram if antidepressants are prescribed (previous medical records may provide these data)

Elective studies

Magnetic resonance imaging to establish the diagnosis of vascular depression

Blood screens for evidence of vitamin deficiency such as a deficiency of B_{12} or folate

Polysomnography when sleep abnormalities persist and cannot be explained

Screen for thyroid dysfunction (triiodothyronine, thyroxine, radioactive iodine uptake, thyrotropin levels)

The laboratory workup of the depressed older adult is important. It should include a thyroid panel (triiodothyronine, thyroxine, and radioactive iodine uptake) and determination of thyrotropin levels. A blood screen enables the clinician to detect the presence of anemia. However, at least one study has shown that red blood cell enlargement and abnormalities are not good predictors of deficits in vitamin B_{12} or folate (Mischoulon et al. 2000). Because both depressive and cognitive symptoms can result from deficits in vitamin B_{12} or folate, it is important to obtain levels of these vitamins.

Treatment

Treatment of depression in late life is four-pronged, involving psychotherapy, pharmacotherapy, ECT, and family therapy. These four approaches are discussed in this section.

Psychotherapy

Cognitive-behavioral therapy is the only psychotherapy that was designed specifically to treat depression (Beck 1987). Even the more recently developed technique of interpersonal therapy is primarily a cognitive-behavioral orientation to improving interpersonal relationships (Klerman et al. 1984). The advantage of using cognitive-behavioral therapy in treating the older adult is that the therapy is directive and time limited, usually involving between 10 and 25 sessions. Cognitive-behavioral therapy has been found to be effective in elderly patients with depression (Gallagher and Thompson 1982; Steuer et al. 1984) and in patients with chronic medical illnesses such as type 2 diabetes (Lustman et al. 1998), heart disease (Kohn et al. 2000), and irritable bowel syndrome (Boyce et al. 2000). It may be particularly

useful in patients who show only a partial response to antidepressant pharmacotherapy (Scott et al. 2000). Problem-solving therapy, another cognitively based approach, also has been shown to be an effective treatment for depression in older individuals, particularly those in primary care settings (Arean et al. 2008).

Results of empirical studies suggest that compared with control subjects, elders who engage in psychotherapy experience incremental improvement. Not only does the percentage of elders who respond to these treatments compare favorably with the percentage of younger subjects who respond, but the degree of improvement appears equal to that obtained with medications, especially for individuals with milder forms of depression. Drug therapy is not appropriate for some elders, and cognitive therapy, behavioral therapy, and brief dynamic psychotherapy are viable alternatives. In addition, evidence has emerged that suggests that the long-term benefit of cognitive-behavioral therapy may be greater than that of pharmacotherapy, especially if the medications are discontinued during the first year of treatment (Reynolds et al. 1999).

Older adults who have minor depression or adjustment disorders, or who experience dysphoria because of losses of various types, often require less intensive forms of psychotherapy. Active listening and simple support may be sufficient to help distressed elders cope with their situation. Because religion is an important factor in the lives of many older adults, referral to a pastoral counselor may be particularly helpful and acceptable (Koenig et al. 2004).

Pharmacotherapy

The use of selective serotonin reuptake inhibitors (SSRIs) has been growing in elderly patients (with or without medical illness). Citalopram (Nyth and Gottfries 1990), escitalopram (Gorwood et al. 2007), fluoxetine (Heiligenstein et al. 1995), paroxetine (Bump et al. 2001), and sertraline (Cohn et al. 1990) have been shown to be effective in geriatric depression. SSRIs also have proved effective in depressed older adults who have had a stroke (Cole et al. 2001) or who have vascular disease in general (Krishnan et al. 2001) or Alzheimer's disease (Lyketsos et al. 2000). These agents have become the drugs of first choice for treating mild to moderate forms of depression. Important advantages of the use of these drugs in treating elderly patients are the lack of anticholinergic, orthostatic, and cardiac side effects; lack of sedation; and safety in overdose. Nevertheless, for a significant number of older individuals, these newer antidepressants cause other unacceptable effects, including excessive activation and disturbance of sleep, tremor, headache, significant gastrointestinal side effects, hyponatremia, and weight loss.

Other agents that affect both the serotonergic and the noradrenergic systems are often considered the best second-line therapy if the patient's response to an SSRI is not adequate. Duloxetine (Raskin et al. 2008) and venlafaxine (Staab and Evans 2000) have been shown to be effective in geriatric depression.

Tricyclic antidepressants (TCAs) are the agents of choice for some patients with more severe forms of major depression who can tolerate the side effects and who do not respond to the medications mentioned earlier. Medications that are effective yet relatively free of side effects (especially cardiovascular effects) are preferred. In recent years, nortriptyline and desipramine have become the more popular medications for treating endogenous or melancholic major depression in older adults. However, doxepin remains a favorite among many practitioners. It is recommended that all elderly patients have an electrocardiogram (ECG) before initiation of treatment and again after therapeutic blood levels have been achieved. If the ECG reveals a second-degree (or higher) block, a bifascicular bundle branch block, a left bundle branch block, or a QTc interval greater than 480 ms, treatment with TCAs should not be initiated or should be stopped in patients already taking these medications.

Antidepressant doses administered to persons in late life should be case specific but are generally lower than those given to persons in midlife (see Table 8–4). Starting therapeutic daily doses of antidepressants are as follows: citalopram, 10–40 mg; fluoxetine, 5–20 mg; paroxetine, 10–30 mg; sertraline, 12.5–50 mg; mirtazapine, 7.5–30 mg; and venlafaxine, 37.5–200 mg (in divided doses). Bupropion therapy should be initiated at 75 mg twice daily, with an increase to 150 mg twice daily (not to exceed 150 mg in a single dose). With regard to tricyclics, 25 mg of desipramine orally twice a day or 25–50 mg of nortriptyline orally at bedtime is frequently adequate for relieving depressive symptoms. Plasma levels of tricyclic medications can be helpful in determining dosing: desipramine plasma levels greater than 125 ng/mL and nortriptyline plasma levels between 50 and 150 ng/mL have been found to be therapeutic.

Trazodone and bupropion (Steffens et al. 2001; Weihs et al. 2000) are alternatives in patients who cannot tolerate TCAs or one of the newer antidepressants. Trazodone has advantages over TCAs in that it is virtually free of anticholinergic effects, and it has advantages over the newer antidepressants in that it

TABLE 8–4. Pharmacological treatment of late-life depression

Medication	Dosage
Selective serotonin reuptake inhibitors	
Citalopram	10–40 mg daily
Escitalopram	10–20 mg daily
Fluoxetine	5–20 mg daily
Paroxetine	10–30 mg daily
Sertraline	12.5–50 mg daily
Serotonin-norepinephrine reuptake inhibitors	
Desvenlafaxine	50–100 mg daily
Duloxetine	40–60 mg daily
Mirtazapine	7.5–30 mg daily
Venlafaxine	37.5–200 mg tid
Tricyclic antidepressants	
Desipramine	25 mg bid
Doxepin	100 mg daily
Nortriptyline	25–50 mg daily
Other agents	
Bupropion	75–150 mg bid
Trazodone	300 mg daily

Note.   bid=twice a day; tid=three times a day.

has strong sedative effects. Nevertheless, the drug is not without side effects, including excessive daytime sedation, priapism (occasionally), and significant orthostatic hypotension. The therapeutic daily dose of trazodone is 300 mg or more, an amount that many older patients cannot tolerate because of sedation. Bupropion can be effective in treating depression in the elderly but generally is used once other medications have proved ineffective. Agitation is the most common side effect that troubles older adults.

Monoamine oxidase inhibitors (MAOIs) are another alternative to TCAs and the newer antidepressants. However, if MAOIs are being considered because of intolerance of side effects of other antidepressants, older adults usually do not tolerate MAOIs any better. If treatment with an MAOI is to follow treatment with an SSRI, a minimum of 1–2 weeks (following fluoxetine, 2–4 weeks) must elapse after discontinuation of SSRI therapy before initiation of MAOI therapy to avoid a serotonergic syndrome. If a patient's depression is severe and ECT is contemplated, use of an MAOI also precludes initiation of ECT until 10–14 days after the drug is discontinued. Such a delay may seriously impede clinical management of the suicidal elder.

Some clinicians prescribe low morning doses of stimulant medications, such as 5 mg of methylphenidate, to improve mood in the apathetic older adult. Although the effectiveness of stimulants has not been conclusively established, these agents are generally safe at low doses, and rarely does the clinician encounter an elder with a propensity to abuse stimulants or to become addicted when these drugs are given once daily. Another recent addition to the pharmacological armamentarium is use of adjunctive atypical antipsychotics such as aripiprazole, which has shown effectiveness among depressed patients up to age 67 years (Steffens et al. 2011).

For further details on psychopharmacological treatment in the older adult, see Mulsant and Pollock, Chapter 16, "Psychopharmacology."

Electroconvulsive Therapy

ECT continues to be the most effective form of treatment for individuals with more severe major depressive episodes (O'Conner et al. 2001). The induction of a seizure via

ECT appears to be effective in reversing a major depression. ECT was first established as a treatment in 1938, but it is not used as much today as it was immediately after its development. Despite its effectiveness, ECT is not the first-line treatment of choice for a patient with major depression and should be prescribed only because other therapeutic modalities have been ineffective. ECT has been shown to be effective in selected individuals, primarily those who have major depression with melancholia, and especially those who have major depression with psychotic symptoms associated with agitation or withdrawal. Many older adults with such syndromes either fail to respond to antidepressant medications or experience toxicity (usually postural hypotension) when taking antidepressant agents. The presence of self-destructive behavior, such as a suicide attempt or refusal to eat, increases the necessity for intervening effectively; in such situations, ECT may be the treatment of choice.

The medical workup before ECT includes acquisition of a complete medical history, a physical examination, and consultation with a cardiologist if any cardiac abnormalities are recognized. Knowledge of any family history of psychiatric disorders, suicide, or treatment with ECT is helpful in predicting a patient's response to treatment. Laboratory examination includes a complete blood count, a urinalysis, routine chemistries, chest and spinal X rays (the latter to document previous compression fractures), an ECG, and a computed tomography (CT) scan or MRI (with CT or MRI available, an electroencephalogram and skull X ray are not routinely required). The presence of some abnormalities seen in magnetic resonance images does not militate against the use of ECT, however. For example, a series of older adults with major depression were found to have subcortical arteriosclerotic encephalopathy, as documented by MRI, but promptly improved after undergoing ECT (Coffey et al. 1987).

ECT treatments are generally administered three times per week, and usually 6–12 treatments are necessary for adequate therapeutic response. A clear improvement is often noted after one of the treatments, with the patient reporting a remarkable improvement in mood and functioning. Two or three treatments are generally given after the ECT administration that leads to improvement.

The risks and side effects of ECT in elderly patients are similar to those in the general population. Cardiovascular effects are of greatest concern and include premature ventricular contractions, ventricular arrhythmias, and transient systolic hypertension. Multiple monitoring during treatment decreases the (infrequent) risk that one of these side effects will lead to permanent problems. Confusion and amnesia often result after a treatment, but the duration of this confusional episode is brief. Even with the use of unilateral nondominant treatment, however, some patients have prolonged memory difficulties. Headaches are a common symptom with ECT; they usually respond to nonnarcotic analgesics. Status epilepticus and vertebral compression fractures are some of the rare but more serious adverse effects. Compression fractures are a particular risk in older women because of the high incidence of osteoporosis in the postmenopausal population.

The overall success rate of ECT in patients who have not responded to drug therapy is usually 80% or greater, and no evidence indicates that effectiveness is lower in older adults (Avery and Lubrano 1979). Wesner and Winokur (1989) examined the influence of age on the natural history of major depressive disorder and found that ECT reduced the rate of chronicity when it was used in patients age 40 years or older but, surprisingly, not in those younger than 40 years.

The relapse rate with no prophylactic intervention may exceed 50% in the year after a course of ECT. This relapse rate can be decreased if antidepressants or lithium carbonate is prescribed after the treatment. Maintenance ECT may be necessary for some patients who have a high likelihood of recurrence despite use of prophylactic medication and/or who experience high toxicity and therefore cannot tolerate prophylactic medications. For such patients, weekly or monthly treatments (usually on an outpatient basis) are prescribed, with careful monitoring of response and side effects. Following an effective course of ECT, the combination of continuation ECT and antidepressant drug therapy has been shown to have greater efficacy than use of medications alone (Gagné et al. 2000).

Despite the effectiveness of ECT, few deny that treatment may lead to memory difficulties. In a study by Frith et al. (1983), 70 severely depressed patients were randomly assigned to eight real or sham ECT treatments and were divided according to the degree of recovery from depression afterward. Compared with nondepressed control subjects, the depressed patients were impaired on a wide range of tests of memory and concentration before treatment, but after treatment, performance on most tests improved. Real ECT induced impairments in concentration, short-term memory, and learning but significantly facilitated access to remote memories. At 6-month follow-up, all differences between real and sham ECT groups had disappeared.

Family Therapy

The final component of therapy for the depressed elderly patient is work with the family. Not only may family dysfunction contribute to the depressive symptoms experienced by the older adult, but also family support is critical to a successful outcome in the treatment of depression in the elder. A clinician must attend to 1) those members of the family who will be available to the elder; 2) the frequency and quality of interactions between the older adult and family members, as well as among other family members; 3) the overall family atmosphere; 4) family values regarding psychiatric disorders; 5) family support and tolerance of symptoms (such as expressions of wishing not to live); and 6) stressors encountered by the family other than the depression experienced by the elder (Blazer 2002).

Most depressed elderly individuals do not resist interaction between the clinician and family members. With the patient's permission, the family should be instructed regarding the nature of the depressive disorder and the potential risks associated with depression in late life, especially suicide. Family members can assist the clinician in observing changes in the patient's behavior, such as an increase in discomfort (either physical or emotional), increased withdrawal and decreased verbalization, and preoccupation with medications or weapons. The family can assist by removing possible implements of suicide from places of easy access. The family can also take responsibility for administering medications to an older adult who is unreliable or whose potential for suicide is high.

When the symptoms of depression become so severe that hospitalization is required, family members are valuable in facilitating hospitalization. Without a proper alliance between clinician and family, a family may be resistant to hospitalization and undermine the clinician's attempts to treat the older adult appropriately. It is usually necessary for the clinician to take responsibility for saying that hospitalization is essential—that the situation has reached the point at which the family has no choice. The clinician informs the patient—in the presence of the family—of the necessity of hospitalization, and the family in turn can support the clinician's position. In such a situation, the patient rarely resists hospitalization for long.

Key Points

- Late-life depression overall may not be as frequent as at other stages of the life cycle, yet the frequency is much higher in physically and cognitively impaired older adults than in community-based samples.

- The biopsychosocial model works well in placing the origins of late-life depression in context. Most cases derive from a variety of causes.

- Older adults appear more vulnerable to biological causes of depression, such as depression secondary to vascular lesions in the brain.

- Social causes of depression in older adults do not appear to be more frequent but differ from social causes of depression in young or middle-aged adults.

- Older adults who are cognitively intact may experience a buffering of depression because of a lifetime of cumulative wisdom coupled with a different view of events given their age.

- The diagnostic workup of the depressed older adult is centered on a detailed history, ideally from the patient and family.

- For moderately severe depression, a combination of antidepressant therapy and psychotherapy (e.g., interpersonal therapy) is optimal.

- Electroconvulsive therapy is indicated for more severe and treatment-resistant depressive disorders in late life and is generally well tolerated.

References

Alexopoulos GS, Meyers BS, Young RC, et al: The course of geriatric depression with "reversible dementia": a controlled study. Am J Psychiatry 150:1693–1699, 1993

Alexopoulos GS, Meyers BS, Young RC, et al: Recovery in geriatric depression. Arch Gen Psychiatry 53:305–312, 1996

Ambelas A: Live events and mania. Br J Psychiatry 150:235–240, 1987

American Psychiatric Association: Diagnostic and Statistical Manual of Mental Disorders, 4th Edition, Text Revision. Washington, DC, American Psychiatric Association, 2000

Arborelius L, Owens M, Plotsky P, et al: The role of corticotropin-releasing factor in depression and anxiety disorders. J Endocrinol 160:1–12, 1999

Arean P, Hegel, Vannoy S, et al: Effectiveness of problem-solving therapy for older, primary care patients with depression: results from the IMPACT project. Gerontologist 48:311–323, 2008

Avery D, Lubrano A: Depression treated with imipramine and ECT: the DeCarolis study reconsidered. Am J Psychiatry 136:559–562, 1979

Baldwin RC, Jolley DJ: The prognosis of depression in old age. Br J Psychiatry 149:574–583, 1986

Beck A: Cognitive model of depression. Journal of Cognitive Psychotherapy 1:2–27, 1987

Beekman A, Deeg D, van Tilberg T, et al: Major and minor depression in later life: a study of prevalence and risk factors. J Affect Disord 36:65–75, 1995

Beekman AT, Deeg DJ, Geerlings SW, et al: Emergence and persistence of late life depression: a 3-year follow-up of the Longitudinal Aging Study Amsterdam. J Affect Disord 65:131–138, 2001

Beekman A, Geerlings S, Deeg D, et al: The natural history of late-life depression. Arch Gen Psychiatry 59:605–611, 2002

Black S, Goodwin J, Markides K: The association between chronic diseases and depressive symptomatology in older Mexican Americans. J Gerontol A Biol Sci Med Sci 53:M118–M194, 1998

Blazer DG: Social support and mortality in an elderly community population. Am J Epidemiol 115:684–694, 1982

Blazer DG: Depression in Late Life, 3rd Edition. New York, Springer, 2002

Blazer DG: Depression in late life: review and commentary. J Gerontol A Biol Sci Med Sci 58:249–265, 2003

Blazer DG 2nd, Hybels CF: Origins of depression in later life. Psychol Med 35:1241–1252, 2005

Blazer D, Hughes DC, George LK: The epidemiology of depression in an elderly community population. Gerontologist 27:281–287, 1987

Blazer D, Burchett B, Service C, et al: The association of age and depression among the elderly: an epidemiologic exploration. J Gerontol 46:M210–M215, 1991

Blazer DG, Hybels CF, Pieper CF: The association of depression and mortality in elderly persons: a case for multiple independent pathways. J Gerontol A Biol Sci Med Sci 56A:M505–M509, 2001

Blazer DG, Burchett B, Fillenbaum G: APOE ε4 and low cholesterol as risks for depression in a biracial elderly community sample. Am J Geriatr Psychiatry 10:515–520, 2002a

Blazer DG, Moody-Ayers S, Craft-Morgan J, et al: Depression in diabetes and obesity: racial/ethnic/gender issues in older adults. J Psychosom Res 53:913–916, 2002b

Boyce P, Gilchrist J, Talley NJ, et al: Cognitive-behaviour therapy as a treatment for irritable bowel syndrome: a pilot study. Aust N Z J Psychiatry 34:300–309, 2000

Bruce ML: Depression and disability in late life: directions for future research. Am J Geriatr Psychiatry 9:102–112, 2001

Bruce ML: Psychosocial risk factors for depressive disorders in late life. Biol Psychiatry 52:175–184, 2002

Bump GM, Mulsant BH, Pollock BG, et al: Paroxetine versus nortriptyline in the continuation and maintenance treatment of depression in the elderly. Depress Anxiety 13:38–44, 2001

Chi I, Chou KL: Social support and depression among elderly Chinese people in Hong Kong. Int J Aging Hum Dev 52:231–252, 2001

Clayton PJ: Bereavement and depression. J Clin Psychiatry 51(suppl):34–40, 1990

Coffey CE, Hinkle PE, Weiner RD, et al: Electroconvulsive therapy of depression in patients with white matter hyperintensity. Biol Psychiatry 22:629–636, 1987

Coffey CE, Figiel GS, Djang WT: Subcortical hyperintensity on magnetic resonance imaging: a comparison of normal and depressed elderly subjects. Am J Psychiatry 147:187–189, 1990

Cohn CK, Shrivastava R, Mendels J, et al: Double-blind, multicenter comparison of sertraline and amitriptyline in elderly depressed patients. J Clin Psychiatry 51 (suppl B):28–33, 1990

Cole MG, Bellavance F, Mansour A: Prognosis of depression in elderly community and primary care populations: a systematic review and meta-analysis. Am J Psychiatry 156:1182–1189, 1999

Cole MG, Elie LM, McCusker J, et al: Feasibility and effectiveness of treatments of post-stroke depression in elderly inpatients: systematic review. J Geriatr Psychiatry Neurol 14:37–41, 2001

Cornoni-Huntley J, Blazer D, Lafferty M, et al (eds): Established Populations for Epidemiologic Studies of the Elderly: Resource Data Book, Vol 2. Bethesda, MD, National Institute on Aging, 1990

Cutler NR, Post RM: Life course of illness in untreated manic-depressive patients. Compr Psychiatry 23:101–115, 1982

Czéh B, Michaelis T, Watanabe T, et al: Stress-induced changes in cerebral metabolites, hippocampal volume, and cell proliferation are prevented by antidepressant treatment with tianeptine. Proc Natl Acad Sci U S A 98:12796–12801, 2001

de Beurs E, Beekman A, Geerlings S, et al: On becoming depressed or anxious in late life: similar vulnerability factors but different effects of stressful life events. Br J Psychiatry 179:426–431, 2001

Devanand DP, Kim MK, Paykina N, et al: Adverse life events in elderly patients with major depression or dysthymia and in healthy-control subjects. Am J Geriatr Psychiatry 10:265–274, 2002

Eastham JH, Jeste DV, Young RC: Assessment and treatment of bipolar disorder in the elderly. Drugs Aging 12:205–224, 1998

Fiske A, Gatz M, Pedersen NL: Depressive symptoms and aging: the effects of illness and non-health-related events. J Gerontol B Psychol Sci Soc Sci 58:P320–P328, 2003

Folstein M, Folstein S, McHugh P: "Mini-mental state": a practical method for grading the cognitive state of patients for the clinician. J Psychiatr Res 12:189–198, 1975

Fried L: Frailty, in Principles of Geriatric Medicine and Gerontology, 3rd Edition. Edited by Hazzard W, Bierman E, Blass J, et al. New York, McGraw-Hill, 1994, pp 1149–1156

Frith CD, Stevens M, Johnstone EC, et al: Effects of ECT and depression on various aspects of memory. Br J Psychiatry 142:610–617, 1983

Gagné GG Jr, Furman MJ, Carpenter LL, et al: Efficacy of continuation ECT and antidepressant drugs compared to long-term antidepressants alone in depressed patients. Am J Psychiatry 157:1960–1965, 2000

Gallagher DE, Thompson LW: Treatment of major depressive disorder in older outpatients with brief psychotherapies. Psychotherapy Theory, Research, Practice, Training 19:482–490, 1982

Gatz M, Pedersen N, Plomin R, et al: Importance of shared genes and shared environments for symptoms of depression in older adults. J Abnorm Psychol 101:701–708, 1992

George MS, Ketter TA, Post RM: Prefrontal cortex dysfunction in clinical depression. Depression 2:59–72, 1994

Glasser M, Rabins P: Mania in the elderly. Age Ageing 13:210–213, 1984

Glassman AH, Shapiro PA: Depression and the course of coronary artery disease. Am J Psychiatry 155:4–11, 1998

Gonzalez-Salvador MT, Arango C, Lyketsos CG, et al: The stress and psychological morbidity of the Alzheimer patient caregiver. Int J Geriatr Psychiatry 14:701–710, 1999

Gorwood P, Weiller E, Lemming O, et al: Escitalopram prevents relapse in older adults with major depressive disorder. Am J Geriatr Psychiatry 15:581–593, 2007

Gottfries CG: Neurochemical aspects on aging and diseases with cognitive impairment. J Neurosci Res 27:541–547, 1990

Guttmann CR, Jolesz F, Kikinis R, et al: White matter changes with normal aging. Neurology 50:972–978, 1998

Hays JC, Saunders WB, Flint EP, et al: Social support and depression as risk factors for loss of physical function in late life. Aging Mental Health 3:209–220, 1997

Hays JC, Steffens DC, Flint EP, et al: Does social support buffer functional decline in elderly patients with unipolar depression? Am J Psychiatry 158:1850–1855, 2001

Heiligenstein JH, Ware JE Jr, Beusterien KM, et al: Acute effects of fluoxetine versus placebo on functional health and well-being in late-life depression. Int Psychogeriatr 7 (suppl):125–137, 1995

Henderson AS, Korten AE, Jacomb PA, et al: The course of depression in the elderly: a longitudinal community-based study in Australia. Psychol Med 27:119–129, 1997

Hickie I, Scott E, Naismith S, et al: Late-onset depression: genetic, vascular and clinical contributions. Psychol Med 31:1403–1412, 2001

Holahan CK, Holahan CJ: Self-efficacy, social support, and depression in aging: a longitudinal analysis. J Gerontol 42:65–68, 1987

Holahan CJ, Moos RH: Social support and psychological distress: a longitudinal analysis. J Abnorm Psychol 90:365–370, 1981

Hughes DC, Blazer DG, George LK: Age differences in life events: a multivariate controlled analysis. Int J Aging Hum Dev 127:207–220, 1988

Husain MM, McDonald WM, Doraiswamy PM, et al: A magnetic resonance imaging study of putamen nuclei in major depression. Psychiatry Res 40:95–99, 1991

Hybels CF, Pieper CF, Blazer DG: Sex differences in the relationship between subthreshold depression and mortality in a community sample of older adults. Am J Geriatr Psychiatry 10:283–291, 2002

Hybels CF, Blazer DG, Steffens DC: Predictors of partial remission in older patients treated for major depression: the role of comorbid dysthymia. Am J Geriatr Psychiatry 13:713–721, 2005

Hybels CF, Pieper CF, Blazer DG, et al: The course of depressive symptoms in older adults with comorbid major depression and dysthymia. Am J Geriatr Psychiatry 16:300–309, 2008

Jang Y, Haley WE, Small BJ: The role of mastery and social resources in the associations between disability and depression in later life. Gerontologist 42:807–813, 2002

Keller MB, Shapiro RW, Lavori PW, et al: Recovery in major depressive disorder: analyses with the life table and regression models. Arch Gen Psychiatry 39:905–910, 1982a

Keller MB, Shapiro RW, Lavori PW, et al: Relapse in major depressive disorder: analysis with the life table. Arch Gen Psychiatry 39:911–915, 1982b

Kennedy GJ, Kelman HR, Thomas C: The emergence of depressive symptoms in late life: the importance of declining health and increasing disability. J Community Health 15:93–104, 1990

Kessler RC, Chiu WT, Demler O, et al: Prevalence, severity, and comorbidity of 12-month DSM-IV disorders in the National Comorbidity Survey Replication [published erratum appears in Arch Gen Psychiatry 62:709, 2005]. Arch Gen Psychiatry 62:617–627, 2005

Klerman GL, Weissman MM, Rounsaville BJ, et al: Interpersonal Psychotherapy of Depression. New York, Basic Books, 1984

Koenig HG, Meador KG, Cohen HJ, et al: Depression in elderly hospitalized patients with medical illness. Arch Intern Med 148:1929–1936, 1988

Koenig HG, George LK, Titus P: Religion, spirituality, and health in medically ill hospitalized older patients. J Am Geriatr Soc 52:554–562, 2004

Kohn CS, Petrucci RJ, Baessler C: The effect of psychological intervention on patients' long-term adjustment to the ICD: a prospective study. Pacing Clin Electrophysiol 23:450–456, 2000

Kondo DG, Speer MC, Krishnan KR, et al: Association of AGTR1 with 18-month treatment outcome in late-life depression. Am J Geriatr Psychiatry 15:564–572, 2007

Kraaij V, Arensman E, Spinhoven P: Negative life events and depression in elderly persons: a meta-analysis. J Gerontol B Psychol Sci Soc Sci 57:P87–P94, 2002

Krishnan KR, Goli V, Ellinwood EH, et al: Leukoencephalopathy in patients diagnosed as major depressive [published erratum appears in Biol Psychiatry 25:822, 1989]. Biol Psychiatry 23:519–522, 1988

Krishnan KR, McDonald WM, Escalona PR, et al: Magnetic resonance imaging of the caudate nuclei in depression: preliminary observations. Arch Gen Psychiatry 49:553–557, 1992

Krishnan KR, McDonald WM, Doraiswamy PM, et al: Neuroanatomical substrates of depression in the elderly. Eur Arch Psychiatry Clin Neurosci 243:41–46, 1993

Krishnan KR, Hays JC, Blazer DG: MRI-defined vascular depression. Am J Psychiatry 154:497–501, 1997

Krishnan KR, Doraiswamy PM, Clary CM: Clinical and treatment response characteristics of late-life depression associated with vascular disease: a pooled analysis of two multicenter trials with sertraline. Prog Neuropsychopharmacol Biol Psychiatry 25:347–361, 2001

Krishnan KR, Taylor WD, McQuoid DR, et al: Clinical characteristics of magnetic resonance imaging–defined subcortical ischemic depression. Biol Psychiatry 55:390–397, 2004

Kumar A, Mintz J, Bilker W, et al: Autonomous neurobiological pathways to late-life depressive disorders: clinical and pathophysiological implications. Neuropsychopharmacology 26:229–236, 2002

Lenze EJ, Munin MC, Skidmore ER, et al: Onset of depression in elderly persons after hip fracture: implications for prevention and early intervention of late-life depression. J Am Geriatr Soc 55:81–86, 2007

Li YS, Meyer JS, Thornby J: Longitudinal follow-up of depressive symptoms among normal versus cognitively impaired elderly. Int J Geriatr Psychiatry 16:718–727, 2001

Liverman C, Blazer D (eds): Testosterone and Aging: Clinical Research Directions. Washington, DC, National Academies Press, 2004

Luisi S, Tonetti A, Bernardi F, et al: Effect of acute corticotropin releasing factor on pituitary-adrenocortical responsiveness in elderly women and men. J Endocrinol Invest 21:449–453, 1998

Lustman PJ, Griffith LS, Freedland KE, et al: Cognitive behavior therapy for depression in type 2 diabetes mellitus: a randomized, controlled study. Ann Intern Med 129:613–621, 1998

Lyketsos CG, Sheppard JM, Steele CD, et al: Randomized, placebo-controlled, double-blind, clinical trial of sertraline in the treatment of depression complicating Alzheimer's disease: initial results from the Depression in Alzheimer's Disease Study. Am J Psychiatry 157:1686–1689, 2000

Lyles KW: Osteoporosis and depression: shedding more light upon a complex relationship. J Am Geriatr Soc 49:827–828, 2001

Magaziner J, Simonsick EM, Kashner TM, et al: Predictors of functional recovery one year following hospital discharge for hip fracture: a prospective study. J Gerontol 45:M101–M107, 1990

Massey EW, Bullock R: Peroneal palsy in depression. J Clin Psychiatry 39:287, 291–292, 1978

Mischoulon D, Burger JK, Spillmann MK, et al: Anemia and macrocytosis in the prediction of serum folate and vitamin B12 status, and treatment outcome in major depression. J Psychosom Res 49:183–187, 2000

Mojtabai R, Olfson M: Major depression in community-dwelling middle-aged and older adults: prevalence and 2- and 4-year follow-up symptoms. Psychol Med 34:623–634, 2004

Morley J, Kraenzle D: Causes of weight loss in a community nursing home. J Am Geriatr Soc 42:583–585, 1994

Morse JQ, Lynch TR: A preliminary investigation of self-reported personality disorders in late life: prevalence, predictors of depressive severity, and clinical correlates. Aging Ment Health 8:307–315, 2004

Murphy E: Social origins of depression in old age. Br J Psychiatry 141:135–142, 1982

Murphy E: The prognosis of depression in old age. Br J Psychiatry 142:111–119, 1983

Musselman DL, Evans DL, Nemeroff CB: The relationship of depression to cardiovascular disease: epidemiology, biology, and treatment. Arch Gen Psychiatry 55:580–592, 1998

Nasreddine ZS, Phillips NA, Bédirian V, et al: The Montreal Cognitive Assessment: MoCA, a brief screening tool for cognitive assessment. J Am Geriatr Soc 53:695–699, 2005

Nyth AL, Gottfries CG: The clinical efficacy of citalopram in treatment of emotional disturbances in dementia disorders: a Nordic multicentre study. Br J Psychiatry 157:894–901, 1990

O'Conner M, Knapp R, Husain M, et al: The influence of age on the response of major depression to electroconvulsive therapy: a C.O.R.E. Report. Am J Geriatr Psychiatry 9:382–390, 2001

Olin J, Schneider L, Katz I, et al: Provisional diagnostic criteria for depression of Alzheimer disease. Am J Geriatr Psychiatry 10:125–128, 2002

Parmelee PA, Katz IR, Lawton MP: Depression among institutionalized aged: assessment and prevalence estimation. J Gerontol 44:M22–M29, 1989

Penninx BW, Leveille S, Ferrucci L, et al: Exploring the effect of depression on physical disability: longitudinal evidence from the Established Populations for Epidemiologic Studies of the Elderly. Am J Public Health 89:1346–1352, 1999

Pollock BG: Geriatric psychiatry: psychopharmacology: general principles, in Kaplan and Sadock's Comprehensive Textbook of Psychiatry. Edited by Sadock BJ, Sadock VA. Baltimore, MD, Williams & Wilkins, 2000, pp 3086–3090

Post F: The Significance of Affective Symptoms at Old Age. London, Oxford University Press, 1962

Post F: The management and nature of depressive illnesses in late life: a follow-through study. Br J Psychiatry 121:393–404, 1972

Post F: The functional psychoses, in Geriatric Psychiatry. Edited by Isaacs A, Post F. New York, Wiley, 1978, pp 77–98

Prigerson H, Reynolds CF 3rd, Frank E, et al: Stressful life events, social rhythms, and depressive symptoms among the elderly: an examination of hypothesized causal linkages. Psychiatry Res 51:33–49, 1994

Prince MJ, Harwood RH, Thomas A, et al: A prospective population-based study of the effects of disablement and social milieu on the onset and maintenance of late-life depression: the Gospel Oak Project VII. Psychol Med 28:337–350, 1998

Rabkin JG, Charles E, Kass F: Hypertension and DSM-III depression in psychiatric outpatients. Am J Psychiatry 140:1072–1074, 1983

Radloff LS: The CES-D Scale: a self-report depression scale for research in the general population. Applied Psychological Measurement 1:385–401, 1977

Raskin J, Xu JY, Kajdasz DK: Time to response for duloxetine 60 mg once daily versus placebo in elderly patients with major depressive disorder. Int Psychogeriatr 20:309–327, 2008

Reynolds CF 3rd, Frank E, Perel JM, et al: Combined pharmacotherapy and psychotherapy in the acute and continuation treatment of elderly patients with recurrent major depression: a preliminary report. Am J Psychiatry 149:1687–1692, 1992

Reynolds CF 3rd, Frank E, Perel JM, et al: Nortriptyline and interpersonal psychotherapy as maintenance therapies for recurrent major depression: a randomized controlled trial in patients older than 59 years. JAMA 281:39–45, 1999

Reynolds CF 3rd, Dew MA, Pollock BG, et al: Maintenance treatment of major depression in old age. N Engl J Med 354:1130–1138, 2006

Roberts RE, Kaplan GA, Shema SJ, et al: Does growing old increase the risk for depression? Am J Psychiatry 154:1384–1390, 1997

Robinson RG, Price TR: Post-stroke depressive disorders: a follow-up study of 103 patients. Stroke 13:635–641, 1982

Sapolsky RM: Why stress is bad for your brain. Science 273:749–750, 1996

Sapolsky RM: Depression, antidepressants, and the shrinking hippocampus. Proc Natl Acad Sci U S A 98:12320–12322, 2001

Scott J, Teasdale JD, Paykel ES, et al: Effects of cognitive therapy on psychological symptoms and social functioning in residual depression. Br J Psychiatry 177:440–446, 2000

Seidman SN, Araujo AB, Roose SP, et al: Low testosterone levels in elderly men with dysthymic disorder. Am J Psychiatry 159:456–459, 2002

Sheline YI: Neuroimaging studies of mood disorder effects on the brain. Biol Psychiatry 54:338–352, 2003

Sheline YI, Wang PW, Gado MH, et al: Hippocampal atrophy in recurrent major depression. Proc Natl Acad Sci U S A 93:3908–3913, 1996

Sheline YI, Mintun MS, Moerlein SM, et al: Greater loss of 5-HT(2A) receptors in midlife than in late life. Am J Psychiatry 159:430–435, 2002

Sherwin B, Gelfand M: Sex steroids and affect in the surgical menopause: a double-blind, cross-over study. Psychoneuroendocrinology 10:325–335, 1985

Shulman KI: Mania in old age, in Affective Disorders in the Elderly. Edited by Murphy E. Edinburgh, Scotland, Churchill Livingstone, 1986, pp 203–216

Shulman K, Post F: Bipolar affective disorder in old age. Br J Psychiatry 136:26–32, 1980

Smith GS, Gunning-Dixon FM, Lotrich FE, et al: Translational research in late-life mood disorders: implications for future intervention and prevention research. Neuropsychopharmacology 32:1857–1875, 2007

Spiegel D: Cancer and depression. Br J Psychiatry 169(suppl):109–116, 1996

Staab JP, Evans DL: Efficacy of venlafaxine in geriatric depression. Depress Anxiety 12 (suppl 1):63–68, 2000

Steffens DC, Doraiswamy PM, McQuoid DR: Bupropion SR in the naturalistic treatment of elderly patients with major depression. Int J Geriatr Psychiatry 16:862–865, 2001

Steffens DC, Payne ME, Greenberg DL, et al: Hippocampal volume and incident dementia in geriatric depression. Am J Geriatr Psychiatry 10:62–71, 2002

Steffens DC, Fisher GG, Langa KM, et al: Prevalence of depression among older Americans: the Aging, Demographics and Memory Study. Int Psychogeriatr 21:878–888, 2009

Steffens DC, Nelson JC, Eudicone JM, et al: Efficacy and safety of adjunctive aripiprazole in major depressive disorder in older patients: a pooled subpopulation analysis. Int J Geriatr Psychiatry 26:564–572, 2011

Steuer JL, Mintz J, Hammen CL, et al: Cognitive-behavioral and psychodynamic group psychotherapy in treatment of geriatric depression. J Consult Clin Psychol 52:180–189, 1984

Stoudemire A, Hill CD, Morris R, et al: Long-term outcome of treatment-resistant depression in older adults. Am J Psychiatry 150:1539–1540, 1993

Sullivan MD, LaCroix AZ, Baum C, et al: Functional status in coronary artery disease: a one year prospective study of the role of anxiety and depression. Am J Med 103:348–356, 1997

Takeshita J, Masaki K, Ahmed I, et al: Are depressive symptoms a risk factor for mortality in elderly Japanese American men? The Honolulu Asia Aging Study. Am J Psychiatry 159:1127–1132, 2002

Taylor WD, Steffens DC, MacFall JR, et al: White matter hyperintensity progression and late-life depression outcomes. Arch Gen Psychiatry 60:1090–1096, 2003

Taylor WD, Zücher S, McQuoid DR, et al: Allelic differences in the brain-derived neurotrophic factor Val66Met polymorphism in late-life depression. Am J Geriatric Psychiatry 15:850–857, 2007

Taylor WD, Steffens DC, Ashley-Koch A, et al: Angiotensin receptor gene polymorphisms and 2-year change in hyperintense lesion volume in men. Mol Psychiatry 15:816–822, 2010

Thomas C, Kelman HR, Kennedy GJ, et al: Depressive symptoms and mortality in elderly persons. J Gerontol 47:S80–S87, 1992

Weihs KL, Settle EC Jr, Batey SR, et al: Bupropion sustained release versus paroxetine for the treatment of depression in the elderly. J Clin Psychiatry 61:196–202, 2000

Weissman MM, Bruce ML, Leaf PJ, et al: Affective disorders, in Psychiatric Disorders in America: The Epidemiologic Catchment Area Study. Edited by Robins LN, Regier DA. New York, Free Press, 1991, pp 53–80

Wesner RB, Winokur G: The influence of age on the natural history of unipolar depression when treated with electroconvulsive therapy. Eur Arch Psychiatry Neurol Sci 238:149–154, 1989

Whooley MA, Browner WS: Association between depressive symptoms and mortality in older women: study of Osteoporotic Fractures Research Group. Arch Intern Med 158:2129–2135, 1998

Williams SA, Kasl SV, Heiat A, et al: Depression and risk of heart failure among the elderly: a prospective community-based study. Psychosom Med 64:6–12, 2002

Winokur G: The Iowa 5000: heterogeneity and course of manic-depressive illness (bipolar). Compr Psychiatry 16:125–131, 1975

Wylie ME, Mulsant BH, Pollock BG, et al: Age of onset in geriatric bipolar disorder: effects on clinical presentation and treatment outcomes in an inpatient sample. Am J Geriatr Psychiatry 7:77–83, 1999

Yassa R, Nair V, Nastase C, et al: Prevalence of bipolar disorder in a psychogeriatric population. J Affect Disord 14:197–201, 1988

Yesavage JA, Brink TL, Rose TL, et al: Development and validation of a geriatric depression screening scale: a preliminary report. J Psychiatr Res 17:37–49, 1983

Young RC, Falk JR: Age, manic psychopathology, and treatment response. Int J Geriatr Psychiatry 4:73–78, 1989

Young RC, Klerman GL: Mania in late life: focus on age at onset. Am J Psychiatry 149:867–876, 1992

Zesiewicz TA, Gold M, Chari G, et al: Current issues in depression in Parkinson's disease. Am J Geriatr Psychiatry 7:110–118, 1999

Zhang X, Gainetdinov RR, Beaulieu JM, et al: Loss-of-function mutation in tryptophan hydroxylase-2 identified in unipolar major depression. Neuron 45:11–16, 2005

Suggested Readings

Alexopoulos G, Meyers B, Young RC, et al: The course of geriatric depression with "reversible dementia": a controlled study. Am J Psychiatry 150:1693–1699, 1993

Blazer DG: Psychiatry and the oldest old. Am J Psychiatry 157:1915–1924, 2000

Blazer DG: Depression in Late Life, 3rd Edition. New York, Springer, 2002

Blazer DG: Depression in late life: review and commentary. J Gerontol A Biol Sci Med Sci 58:249–265, 2003

Blazer DG 2nd, Hybels CF: Origins of depression in later life. Psychol Med 35:1241–1252, 2005

Koenig HG, Meador KG, Cohen HJ, et al: Depression in elderly hospitalized patients with medical illness. Arch Intern Med 148:1929–1936, 1988

Krishnan KR, Goli V, Ellinwood EH, et al: Leukoencephalopathy in patients diagnosed as major depressive [published erratum appears in Biol Psychiatry 25:822, 1989]. Biol Psychiatry 23:519–522, 1988

Reynolds CF 3rd, Dew MA, Pollock BG, et al: Maintenance treatment of major depression in old age. N Engl J Med 354:1130–1138, 2006

Steffens DC, Payne ME, Greenberg DL, et al: Hippocampal volume and incident dementia in geriatric depression. Am J Geriatr Psychiatry 10:62–71, 2002

Taylor WS, Steffens DC, MacFall JR, et al: White matter hyperintensity progression and late-life depression outcomes. Arch Gen Psychiatry 60:1090–1096, 2003

CHAPTER 9

BIPOLAR DISORDER

JOHN L. BEYER, M.D.

Diagnosis

Bipolar disorder is a cycling illness that affects an individual's ability to regulate moods. DSM-IV-TR (American Psychiatric Association 2000) has defined four types of bipolar disorder:

1. **Bipolar disorder, type I**—This diagnosis describes a condition in which a patient has experienced at least one manic episode. A *manic episode* is defined as an alteration in mood that is euphoric, expansive, or irritable; lasts for at least 1 week; and occurs with three other associated symptoms (e.g., decreased need for sleep, increased energy, racing thoughts, pressured speech, increased behaviors that may have high likelihood for bad outcome). It is not necessary for a patient to have experienced a depressive episode to be given the diagnosis of bipolar disorder, although the vast majority have experienced depression, and many report it to be the most common mood problem.
2. **Bipolar disorder, type II**—A diagnosis of bipolar II disorder can be made

when a patient has experienced one or more depressive episodes accompanied by at least one hypomanic episode. A *hypomanic episode* is defined as at least 4 days of altered mood (expansive, euphoric, irritable) occurring with at least three other associated symptoms (see previous point).

3. **Cyclothymia**—*Cyclothymia* is defined as cycling moods that do not fully meet the criteria for either depression or mania.
4. **Bipolar disorder not otherwise specified (NOS)**—*Bipolar disorder NOS* is defined as disorders with bipolar features that do not meet the criteria for specific bipolar disorders.

Epidemiology and Clinical Presentation

Prevalence

Based on four large-scale studies that used very different sampling methods, the prevalence of bipolar disorder in the community generally has been reported to range from 1.0% to 1.4% but only 0.08% to 0.5% in the elderly (Hirschfeld et al. 2003; Klap et al. 2003; Unutzer et al. 1998; Weissman et al. 1988). Interestingly, each of the surveys suggested that the prevalence of bipolar disorder declines with age or in aging cohorts, a finding consistent with other mental illnesses, such as depression and schizophrenia.

Because most of the large-scale prevalence surveys excluded patients who were institutionalized, critics suggested that the prevalence data may underrepresent bipolar disorder because older mentally ill patients are more likely to require institutionalized care. Two surveys of mental illness in nursing home patients found a 3%–10% prevalence of bipolar disorder (Koenig and Blazer 1992; Tariot et al. 1993). Speer (1992) reported that bipolar disorder was present in 17.4% of residential psychiatric programs for older adults. A systematic review of psychiatric inpatient units showed a mean prevalence rate of 8.7%, although Depp and Jeste (2004) suggested that this was likely an underestimation because many inpatient surveys did not include bipolar depressed subjects or reported prevalence only for those with late onset.

Gender

Epidemiological studies in the United States have indicated that men and women are equally affected by bipolar disorder (American Psychiatric Association 2000). Depp and Jeste (2004) pooled 17 studies reporting various samples of late-life bipolar disorder and found that the weighted mean of elderly women with bipolar disorder was 69% (range=45%–89%). However, they noted that this percentage was similar to the gender ratio among older adults in the general population.

Comorbidity

Psychiatric Comorbidity

Psychiatric comorbidity is frequently seen in bipolar patients. Sajatovic et al. (2006) conducted a review of the national Veterans Health Administration database and found that 4.5% of older adults with bipolar disorder had comorbid dementia, 5.4% had posttraumatic stress disorder, and 9.4% had an anxiety disorder. In a study at a state psychiatric hospital, Cassidy et al. (2001) found that nearly 60% of bipolar patients had a history of substance abuse (consistent with the findings of the National Comorbidity Study; Kessler et al. 1997); but in patients older than 60, only 29% had a history of substance abuse. Supporting this finding of lower-than-expected substance abuse in older bipolar patients are two small inpatient studies (Sajatovic et al. 1996), a review of mental health system elderly bipolar outpatients (Depp et al. 2005), and a review of the Veterans Health Administration database (Sajatovic et al. 2006). The reason for this finding is unclear.

Medical Comorbidity

Because of the high association that secondary mania has with late-life bipolar disorder, several studies have assessed the presence of comorbid medical problems. Shulman et al. (1992) compared 50 geriatric patients hospitalized for mania with 50 age-matched patients hospitalized for unipolar depression. They found that the rates of neurological illness in manic patients were significantly higher (36% vs. 8%), suggesting that neurological disease is a risk factor for the development of mania in late life. Depp and Jeste (2004) reviewed eight studies that reported the presence of neurological illness and noted that despite a wide variety in reporting strategies, the sample-weighted prevalence was 23.1%.

Other comorbid medical disorders of note include diabetes. Regenold et al. (2002) reviewed the inpatient charts of 243 older (ages 50–74 years) psychiatric inpatients and found that type 2 diabetes was present in 26% of those with bipolar disorder, a much higher rate than for unipolar depression or schizophrenia.

Mortality and Suicide

Individuals with mental illness at all ages have higher mortality rates, from both natural and unnatural causes, than does the general population (Laursen et al. 2007). Dhingra and Rabins (1991) found that mortality rates among elderly patients with bipolar disorder who had been hospitalized 5–7 years previously were higher than expected compared with population norms. Shulman et al. (1992) found that the mortality rate over a 10- to 15-year follow-up for elderly hospitalized bipolar patients was significantly higher than that for elderly hospitalized unipolar depressed patients (50% vs. 20%).

Despite the high risk of suicide reported with aging and among individuals with bipolar disorder, the risk of suicide in late-life bipolar disorder appears be lower than expected. Tsai et al. (2002) studied suicide rates in Taiwan among patients with bipolar disorder and found that the highest risk was during the first 7–12 years after the onset of the illness and for individuals younger than 35 years. Depp and Jeste (2004) suggested that older, early-onset bipolar patients may constitute a "survivor cohort."

Course

Goodwin and Jamison (1990) reported that depression was the initial episode most often seen in older adults than in younger patients. Shulman and Post (1980) described a group of elderly bipolar patients who had a depressive episode as their index episode and then experienced a long latency period (mean = 15 years) before the onset of mania. They hypothesized that this group may have developed cerebral changes that converted them to mania. Other investigators have described a similar latency period of 10–20 years in a subgroup of patients between their first depressed episode and the onset of mania (Broadhead and Jacoby 1990; Shulman et al. 1992; Snowdon 1991; Stone 1989).

Age at Onset

The mean age at onset for bipolar disorder is in the late teens to early 20s (Weissman et al. 1996). However, some researchers have divided bipolar disorder into early- and late-onset subtypes (Hopkinson 1964; James 1977; Taylor and Abrams 1973). DSM-IV-TR does not make such a distinction, and although some evidence supports this division, differences in opinion exist as to the importance of making such a distinction. Several studies (Baron et al. 1981; Hopkinson 1964; James 1977; Mendlewicz et al. 1972; Post 1968; Snowdon 1991; Stenstedt 1952; Taylor and Abrams 1973) have suggested that patients with an early-onset illness may have an increased prevalence of family members with mood disorders, suggesting a higher genetic loading for early-onset patients and/or a higher incidence of secondary bipolar disorder for late-onset patients, although six other studies did not show any difference (Broadhead and Jacoby 1990; Carlson et al. 1977; Depp et al. 2004; Glasser and Rabins 1984; Hays et al. 1998; Tohen et al. 1994).

The relation between late-onset illness and neurological abnormalities is a much more consistent finding. Although the definition of neurological illness varied, three of the five studies showed significantly higher rates in the late-onset patients (Almeida and Fenner 2002; Tohen et al. 1994; Wylie et al. 1999), whereas the other two studies showed trends toward increased levels of neurological illness (Broadhead and Jacoby 1990; Hays et al. 1998).

Neuroimaging

Volumetric Neuroimaging

Neuroimaging results specific to late-life bipolar disorders are limited, but studies have supported significant volumetric abnormalities consistent with those seen in younger patients. These include smaller caudate (Beyer et al. 2004a) and larger hippocampal (Beyer et al. 2004b) volumes. Young et al. (1999) compared 30 geriatric manic patients with control subjects but did not find any difference in the ventricular-brain ratios. They did note that bipolar subjects had greater cortical sulcal widening, which correlated with age at onset and age at first manic episode. Beyer et al. (2004a) did not find any differences in total brain volume between elderly bipolar subjects and control subjects; however, they did find a volume decrease in late-onset (after age 45 years) compared with early-onset bipolar subjects.

Magnetic Resonance Imaging Hyperintensities

Possibly related to strokes, "hyperintense" signals viewed on T_2-weighted magnetic resonance imaging have been one of the earliest and most consistent neuroimaging findings in bipolar disorder. Hyperintensities represent areas of neuron death, but the mechanism is unclear (Bradley et al. 1984; Braffman et al. 1988; Chimowitz et al. 1992; Fazekas et al. 1993; Fujikawa et al. 1997; George et al. 1986). Fujikawa et al. (1997) called them *silent cerebral ischemia*. Electroencephalographic studies in patients with dementia suggest that white matter hyperintensities may cause functional brain disconnection, prompting some researchers to suggest that hyperintensities may "disconnect" various pathways in mood regulation circuits. Most (Altshuler et al. 1995; Aylward et al. 1994; Botteron et al. 1995; Dupont et al. 1987, 1990, 1995; Figiel et al. 1991; Krabbendam et al. 2000; McDonald et al. 1991, 1999; Swayze et al. 1990), but not all (Brown et al. 1992; Strakowski et al. 1993), studies found increased hyperintensities in bipolar patients. Because of differences in study groups and methodology, a wide range in frequency of T_2 hyperintensities is found in bipolar subjects (5%–62%) and nonbipolar control subjects (0%–42%) (Bearden et al. 2001). Two meta-analyses reported odds ratios of 3.3 (Altshuler et al. 1995) and 3.29 (Videbech 1997), strongly supporting the relation between hyperintensities and bipolar disorder.

Specific studies of bipolar disorder in late life have consistently found higher presence of hyperintensities in bipolar subjects than in control subjects (de Asis et al. 2006; McDonald et al. 1991, 1999). Hyperintensities may be especially important in late-life bipolar disorder because of their effect on treatment response and severity of illness. Their presence in elderly bipolar subjects has been associated with longer hospital stays (Dupont et al. 1990), more frequent rehospitalizations (McDonald et al. 1999), and cognitive changes. Following a review of the literature, Bearden et al. (2001) concluded that hyperintensities play an increasing role in bipolar cognitive impairment with increasing age and chronicity of disorder and may be considered a risk modifier for cognitive dysfunction in bipolar disorder.

Differential Diagnosis

There are five potential presentations of patients with late-life bipolar disorder: 1) those who had an early onset of bipolar disease and have now reached old age; 2) those who previously experienced only episodes of depression but have now switched to a manic episode; 3) those who have never had an affective illness but develop mania because of a specific medical or neurological event (e.g., head trauma, cerebrovascular accident, hyperthyroidism); 4) those who have never been recognized as having bipolar symptoms or who have been misdiagnosed with another disorder; and 5) those who have never had an affective illness but develop mania for unknown reasons. It is unknown how common each presentation may be, although personal experience has shown the most frequently encountered presentation to be of a patient who developed bipolar disorder earlier in life and is now seeking treatment. However, based on findings by Hirschfeld et al. (2003), it is not uncommon for the diagnosis of bipolar illness to have been missed previously.

Since the onset of bipolar disorder in late life is relatively uncommon, every patient who presents with a new onset of mania should have a good medical evaluation, with special emphasis on the neurological examination. Because older adults often are prescribed medications, these should be reviewed for possible temporal association. A laboratory workup consisting of a thyroid panel and basic tests also should be completed. Finally, neuroimaging should be considered, especially if the presentation is associated with psychosis.

Treatment

Lithium

Lithium traditionally has been identified as the gold standard for treatment (Shulman et al. 2003; Umapathy et al. 2000); however, no placebo-controlled efficacy trials have been done in geriatric patients. Young et al. (2004) reviewed four studies (Chen et al. 1999; Himmelhoch et al. 1980; Schaffer and Garvey 1984; van der Velde 1970) that included more than 10 elderly patients in their reports. Overall, 66% of the patients improved with lithium treatment, but concentrations varied widely (0.3–2.0 mEq/L). The recommended lithium level for acute mania in geriatric patients is unclear. Case series have suggested that elderly patients may respond to lower lithium levels (0.5–0.8 mEq/L) than those recommended for younger adults (Chen et al. 1999; Prien et al. 1972; Roose et al. 1979), whereas other reports have not found a difference (DeBattista and Schatzberg 2006; Young et al. 1992).

Special care must be taken in dosing lithium in geriatric patients. With aging, the renal clearance of lithium decreases and the elimination half-life increases (Foster 1992; Shulman et al. 1987; Sproule et al. 2000). Furthermore, commonly prescribed medications such as thiazide diuretics, nonsteroidal anti-inflammatory agents, and angiotensin converting enzyme inhibitors can increase lithium concentrations. Finally, because lithium use can contribute to hypothyroidism and a decline in renal clearance, lithium should be used with caution in patients with kidney problems or thyroid disorders. Because of this, lithium toxicity in elderly patients is not uncommon (Foster 1992). Commonly reported adverse effects of lithium in elderly patients include cognitive impairment, ataxia, urinary frequency, weight gain, edema, tremor, and worsening of psoriasis and arthritis. Because of adverse effects (including neurotoxicity) that can occur even at therapeutic levels, appropriate lithium serum levels in the elderly are largely determined by medical status, frailty, and conservative dosing (Sajatovic et al. 2005b; Young et al. 2004).

Anticonvulsants

Valproate

The past decade has seen a marked increase in the prescription of valproate for bipolar disorder, especially for the elderly. Shulman et al. (2003) noted that prescriptions of valproate for bipolar disorder increased in the late 1990s so that it is now the most prescribed medication treatment for elderly persons with bipolar disorder, despite there being no published data comparing valproate with placebo or lithium in the elderly.

Similar to the published research on lithium, only retrospective and open-label studies of valproate in the geriatric population have been published. Young et al. (2004) reviewed the five published studies that each included more than 10 elderly manic subjects (Chen et al. 1999; Kando et al. 1996; Niedermier and Nasrallah 1998; Noaghiul et al. 1998; Puryear et al. 1995). They found that 59% of the combined sample met the various improvement criteria. Again, however, the dose concentrations varied widely at 25–120 μg/mL. The recommended blood level concentration for valproate in the general population is 50–120 μg/mL (Bowden et al. 2002), and Chen et al. (1999) found that for manic elderly patients, those who had blood level concentrations of 65–

90 μg/mL improved more than patients with lower concentrations.

As patients age, the elimination half-life of valproate may be prolonged and the free fraction of plasma valproate increases. The clinical significance of this is unknown, although it should be noted that usual laboratory tests measure the total valproate level. Thus, the reported level may underrepresent the actual dose in geriatric patients (Sajatovic et al. 2005b; Young et al. 2004). Common medications taken concurrently also may influence the level of valproate: aspirin can increase the valproate free fraction, and phenytoin and carbamazepine may decrease the valproate level. In turn, valproate can inhibit the metabolism of lamotrigine so that the dose of lamotrigine may need to be lowered to minimize side effects, or it may increase the unbound fraction of warfarin necessitating closer monitoring in patients receiving anticoagulation therapy (Panjehshahin et al. 1991).

The most common side effects associated with valproate are nausea, somnolence, and weight gain. Less common side effects that may be particularly important to geriatric patients are the possibility of hair thinning, thrombocytopenia, hepatotoxicity, and pancreatitis (the latter two are less likely to occur with age) (Bowden et al. 2002). Valproate is available in sprinkle and liquid formulations for patients who have difficulty swallowing.

Carbamazepine

Carbamazepine was approved for the treatment of bipolar mania in 1996, and the extended-release formulation was approved in 2005. Some researchers have suggested that carbamazepine may be the preferred mood-stabilizing agent for patients with secondary mania (Evans et al. 1995; Sajatovic 2002); however, very little information is available on the use of carbamazepine for the elderly bipolar patient.

Before initiating carbamazepine, the physician should check liver enzymes, electrolytes, and complete blood cell count. Because carbamazepine also can affect the heart's rhythm, an electrocardiogram should be considered. In elderly patients, carbamazepine may be started at 100 mg either once or twice daily and gradually increased every 3–5 days to 400–800 mg/day (McDonald 2000). Target serum levels are between 6 and 12 µg/L.

Carbamazepine is metabolized in the liver by cytochrome P450 (CYP) enzyme 3A4/5. Because carbamazepine can induce its own metabolism, dose increases may need to be adjusted in the first 1–2 months. Furthermore, carbamazepine clearance is decreased in an age-dependent manner, suggesting (Battino et al. 2003) that elderly patients may require lower doses to achieve therapeutic blood levels. Carbamazepine also may alter the pharmacokinetics of other medications, including oral hormones, calcium channel blockers, cimetidine, terfenadine, and erythromycin (Sajatovic 2002).

Possible adverse effects associated with carbamazepine include sedation, ataxia, nystagmus/blurred vision, leukopenia, hyponatremia (secondary to the syndrome of inappropriate antidiuretic hormone secretion), and agranulocytosis. The U.S. Food and Drug Administration ([FDA] 2007) has recommended that patients of Asian ancestry have a genetic blood test to identify an inherited variant of the gene *HLA=B*1502* (found almost exclusively in people of Asian ancestry) before starting therapy.

Lamotrigine

Lamotrigine was approved by the FDA in 2003 for the maintenance phase of bipolar disorder. Sajatovic et al. (2005a) conducted a retrospective analysis of two placebo-controlled, double-blind clinical trials for maintenance therapy in bipolar disorder focusing on subjects 55 years or older. They found that, similar to the parent study, lamotrigine significantly delayed the time to intervention for any mood episode, whereas lithium and placebo did not. In a subanalysis, the authors found that lamotrigine was significantly more effective than lithium and placebo at increasing time to intervention for depressive recurrences, but lithium performed much better in increasing time to intervention for manic episodes (Sajatovic et al. 2007).

Overall, lamotrigine is well tolerated, although serious skin rashes (Stevens-Johnson syndrome) have been reported. It has been suggested that lamotrigine may have fewer negative effects on cognition compared with other anticonvulsant medications, which may be important for some geriatric patients (Aldenkamp et al. 2003).

Antidepressants

Antidepressants are frequently prescribed for the treatment of bipolar depression in the elderly (Beyer et al. 2008), although the use of antidepressants in bipolar disorder is a point of continued concern among psychiatrists (Ghaemi et al. 2003). Three issues highlight the controversy. First, the literature is ambiguous as to the efficacy of antidepressants in bipolar depression. Second, antidepressants have the potential to precipitate a manic episode. Third, antidepressants also may induce a rapid-cycling course. Thase and Denko (2008) have reviewed the general literature, focusing especially on two large clinical trials from the Stanley Foundation and the National Institute of Mental Health (Systematic Treatment Enhancement for Bipolar Disorders [STEP-BD]) that have attempted to clarify the benefits and risks of antidepressant use in bipolar depression. The results of both trials did not show that antidepressant augmentation of mood stabilizers distinguished itself as more effective than placebo or the use of a second mood stabilizer. However, possible benefit was noted for certain subgroups. On the basis of the data, the authors were neither able to recommend the use of antidepressants nor to conclude that antidepressants should be avoided (Thase 2007).

Given these limitations, the American Psychiatric Association (2002) has maintained its recommendations that primary treatment of bipolar depression should be with a mood stabilizer and that antidepressant augmentation of the mood stabilizer may be considered if the symptoms have limited or no response.

Antipsychotic Agents

The atypical antipsychotic agents are increasingly being used for the treatment of various phases of bipolar disorder. Olanzapine, risperidone, quetiapine, ziprasidone, and aripiprazole are currently approved by the FDA for the treatment of acute mania; olanzapine/fluoxetine and quetiapine are approved for the treatment of acute depression; and olanzapine and aripiprazole are approved for the treatment of the maintenance phase. However, data on their efficacy are limited in the geriatric population.

Beyer et al. (2001) reported on a pooled subanalysis of three double-blind, placebo-controlled acute bipolar mania clinical trials with olanzapine, focusing on subjects older than 50 years. Compared with placebo, olanzapine was found to be efficacious for the treatment of acute mania without any significant change in the side-effect profile. Information on quetiapine, risperidone, clozapine, ziprasidone, and aripiprazole is much more limited. Case reports and open-label studies in

geriatric bipolar treatment are published for quetiapine (Madhusoodanan et al. 2000), risperidone (Madhusoodanan et al. 1995, 1999), and clozapine (Frye et al. 1996; Shulman et al. 1997). No published reports are currently available for ziprasidone or aripiprazole.

In general, a lower-dose strategy in the elderly has been recommended for most atypical antipsychotics (Alexopoulos et al. 2004), although this may be less of a concern in the acute state. A major concern of atypical antipsychotic use is the potential risk of metabolic abnormalities such as obesity, diabetes, and dyslipidemia. This may be less of a concern for elderly patients because they have less propensity for weight gain and other metabolic effects associated with atypical antipsychotics (Meyer 2002). In 2006, a black-box warning was added to each of the atypical antipsychotic agents, warning about an increased risk for death (cardiovascular events) with the use of these agents in the elderly with dementia. No information is available on the incidence in late-life bipolar disorder.

Electroconvulsive Therapy

Electroconvulsive therapy (ECT) has long been known to be effective for the treatment of bipolar disorder. However, data are very limited on the use of ECT in elderly bipolar patients, especially when compared with the literature on ECT for unipolar depression. McDonald and Thompson (2001) reported on a case series of three elderly manic patients who also had some dementia and were resistant to pharmacotherapy but did respond to ECT treatment. Little et al. (2004) reported on a case series of depressed patients that included five elderly bipolar depressed patients treated with bifrontal ECT. They found that this method could be effective, although one-third experienced cognitive side effects.

Key Points

- As with other mental illnesses, the prevalence of bipolar disorder decreases with age. However, bipolar disorder in late life does continue to be a frequent cause for admission to psychiatric inpatient facilities and disruption of patients' lives.

- The mortality rate for older adults with bipolar disorder is significantly higher than that for the general population and for patients with unipolar depression.

- The onset of bipolar disorder at a later age may be associated with fewer genetic associations and more neurological illnesses.

- Treatment guidelines for late-life bipolar disorder are based primarily on case reports and extrapolation from bipolar treatment in younger adults. As in other geriatric treatment recommendations, the maxim "start low and go slow" is applicable to late-life bipolar treatment.

- Elderly patients may require lower doses of lithium because of decreased renal clearance.

References

Aldenkamp AP, De Krom M, Reijs R: Newer antiepileptic drugs and cognitive issues. Epilepsia 44 (suppl 4):21–29, 2003

Alexopoulos GS, Streim J, Carpenter D, et al: Using antipsychotic agents in older patients. J Clin Psychiatry 65 (suppl 2):5–99, 2004

Almeida OP, Fenner S: Bipolar disorder: similarities and differences between patients with illness onset before and after 65 years of age. Int Psychogeriatr 14:311–322, 2002

Altshuler LL, Curran JG, Hauser P, et al: T2 hyperintensities in bipolar disorder: magnetic resonance imaging comparison and literature meta-analysis. Am J Psychiatry 152:1139–1144, 1995

American Psychiatric Association: Diagnostic and Statistical Manual of Mental Disorders, 4th Edition, Text Revision. Washington, DC, American Psychiatric Association, 2000

American Psychiatric Association: Practice guideline for the treatment of patients with bipolar disorder (revision). Am J Psychiatry 159 (4 suppl):1–50, 2002

Aylward EH, Roberts-Twillie JV, Barta PE, et al: Basal ganglia volumes and white matter hyperintensities in patients with bipolar disorder. Am J Psychiatry 151:687–693, 1994

Baron M, Mendlewicz J, Klotz J: Age-of-onset and genetic transmission in affective disorders. Acta Psychiatr Scand 64:373–380, 1981

Battino D, Croci D, Rossini A, et al: Serum carbamazepine concentrations in elderly patients: a case-matched pharmacokinetic evaluation based on therapeutic drug monitoring data. Epilepsia 44:923–929, 2003

Bearden CE, Hoffman KM, Cannon TD: The neuropsychology and neuroanatomy of bipolar affective disorder: a critical review. Bipolar Disord 3:106–150, 2001

Beyer JL, Siegal A, Kennedy JS, et al: Olanzapine, divalproex, and placebo treatment non-head-to-head comparisons of older adult acute mania. Presented at the annual meeting of the International Psychogeriatric Association, Nice, France, September 2001

Beyer JL, Kuchibhatla M, Payne M, et al: Caudate volume measurement in older adults with bipolar disorder. Int J Geriatr Psychiatry 19:109–114, 2004a

Beyer JL, Kuchibhatla M, Payne ME, et al: Hippocampal volume measurement in older adults with bipolar disorder [published erratum appears in Am J Geriatr Psychiatry 13:334, 2005]. Am J Geriatr Psychiatry 12:613–620, 2004b

Beyer JL, Burchitt B, Gersing K, et al: Patterns of pharmacotherapy and treatment response in elderly adults with bipolar disorder. Psychopharmacol Bull 41:102–114, 2008

Botteron KN, Vannier MW, Geller B, et al: Preliminary study of magnetic resonance imaging characteristics in 8- to 16-year-olds with mania. J Am Acad Child Adolesc Psychiatry 34:742–749, 1995

Bowden CL, Lawson DM, Cunningham M, et al: The role of divalproex in the treatment of bipolar disorder. Psychiatr Ann 32:742–750, 2002

Bradley WG, Waluch V, Brant-Zawadzki M, et al: Patchy, periventricular white matter lesions in the elderly: a common observation during NMR imaging. Noninvasive Medical Imaging 1:35–41, 1984

Braffman BH, Zimmerman RA, Trojanowski JQ, et al: Brain MR: pathologic correlation with gross and histopathology, II: hyperintense white-matter foci in the elderly. AJR Am J Roentgenol 151:559–566, 1988

Broadhead J, Jacoby R: Mania in old age: a first prospective study. Int J Geriatr Psychiatry 5:215–222, 1990

Brown FW, Lewine RJ, Hudgins PA, et al: White matter hyperintensity signals in psychiatric and nonpsychiatric subjects. Am J Psychiatry 149:620–625, 1992

Carlson GA, Davenport YB, Jamison K: A comparison of outcome in adolescent- and later-onset bipolar manic depressive illness. Am J Psychiatry 134:919–922, 1977

Cassidy F, Ahearn P, Carroll B: Substance abuse in bipolar disorder. Bipolar Disord 3:181–188, 2001

Chen ST, Altshuler LL, Melnyk KA, et al: Efficacy of lithium vs. valproate in the treatment of mania in the elderly: a retrospective study. J Clin Psychiatry 60:181–185, 1999

Chimowitz MI, Estes ML, Furlan AJ, et al: Further observations on the pathology of subcortical lesions identified on magnetic resonance imaging. Arch Neurol 49:747–752, 1992

de Asis JM, Greenwald BS, Alexopoulos GS, et al: Frontal signal hyperintensities in mania in old age. Am J Geriatr Psychiatry 14:598–604, 2006

DeBattista C, Schatzberg AF: Current psychotropic dosing and monitoring guidelines. Primary Psychiatry 13(6):61–81, 2006

Depp CA, Jeste DV: Bipolar disorder in older adults: a critical review. Bipolar Disord 6:343–367, 2004

Depp CA, Jin H, Mohamed S, et al: Bipolar disorder in middle-aged and elderly adults: is age of onset important? J Nerv Ment Dis 192:796–799, 2004

Depp CA, Lindamer LA, Folsom DP, et al: Differences in clinical features and mental health service use in bipolar disorder across the life span. Am J Geriatr Psychiatry 13:290–298, 2005

Dhingra U, Rabins PV: Mania in the elderly: a 5–7 year follow-up. J Am Geriatr Soc 39:581–583, 1991

Dupont RM, Jernigan TL, Gillin JC, et al: Subcortical signal hyperintensities in bipolar patients detected by MRI. Psychiatry Res 21:357–358, 1987

Dupont RM, Jernigan TL, Butters N, et al: Subcortical abnormalities detected in bipolar affective disorder using magnetic resonance imaging: clinical and neuropsychological significance. Arch Gen Psychiatry 47:55–59, 1990

Dupont RM, Jernigan TL, Heindel W, et al: Magnetic resonance imaging and mood disorders: localization of white matter and other subcortical abnormalities. Arch Gen Psychiatry 52:747–755, 1995

Evans DL, Byerly MJ, Greer RA: Secondary mania: diagnosis and treatment. J Clin Psychiatry 56 (suppl 3):31–37, 1995

Fazekas R, Kleimert R, Offenbacher H, et al: Pathologic correlates of incidental MRI white matter hyperintensities. Neurology 3:1683–1689, 1993

Figiel GS, Krishnan KR, Rao VP, et al: Subcortical hyperintensities on brain magnetic resonance imaging: a comparison of normal and bipolar subjects. J Neuropsychiatry 3:18–22, 1991

Foster JR: Use of lithium in elderly psychiatric patients: a review of the literature. Lithium 3:77–93, 1992

Frye MA, Altshuler LL, Bitran JA: Clozapine in rapid cycling bipolar disorder. J Clin Psychopharmacol 16:87–90, 1996

Fujikawa T, Yanai I, Yamawaki S: Psychosocial stressors in patients with major depression and silent cerebral infarction. Stroke 28:1123–1125, 1997

George AE, de Leon MJ, Kalnin A, et al: Leukoencephalopathy in normal and pathologic aging, 2: MRI of brain lucencies. AJNR Am J Neuroradiol 7:567–570, 1986

Ghaemi SN, Hsu DJ, Soldani F, et al: Antidepressants in bipolar disorder: the case for caution. Bipolar Disord 5:421–433, 2003

Glasser M, Rabins P: Mania in the elderly. Age Ageing 13:210–213, 1984

Goodwin FK, Jamison KR: Manic-Depressive Illness. New York, Oxford University Press, 1990

Hays JC, Krishnan KR, George LK, et al: Age of first onset of bipolar disorder: demographic, family history, and psychosocial correlates. Depress Anxiety 7:76–82, 1998

Himmelhoch J, Neil J, May S, et al: Age, dementia, dyskinesias, and lithium response. Am J Psychiatry 137:941–945, 1980

Hirschfeld RM, Lewis L, Vornik LA: Perceptions and impact of bipolar disorder: how far have we really come? Results of the national depressive and manic-depressive association 2000 survey of individuals with bipolar disorder. J Clin Psychiatry 64:161–174, 2003

Hopkinson G: A genetic study of affective illness in patients over 50. Br J Psychiatry 110:244–254, 1964

James NM: Early and late-onset bipolar affective disorder: a genetic study. Arch Gen Psychiatry 34:715–717, 1977

Kando JC, Tohen M, Castillo J, et al: The use of valproate in an elderly population with affective symptoms. J Clin Psychiatry 57:238–240, 1996

Kessler RC, Rubinow DR, Holmes C, et al: The epidemiology of DSM-III-R bipolar I disorder in a general population survey. Psychol Med 27:1079–1089, 1997

Klap R, Unroe KT, Unutzer J: Caring for mental illness in the United States: a focus on older adults. Am J Geriatr Psychiatry 11:517–524, 2003

Koenig HG, Blazer DG: Epidemiology of geriatric affective disorders. Clin Geriatr Med 8:235–251, 1992

Krabbendam L, Honig A, Wiersma J, et al: Cognitive dysfunctions and white matter lesions in patients with bipolar disorder in remission. Acta Psychiatr Scand 101:274–280, 2000

Laursen TM, Munk-Olsen T, Nordentoft M, et al: Increased mortality among patients admitted with major psychiatric disorders: a register-based study comparing mortality in unipolar depressive disorder, bipolar affective disorder, schizoaffective disorder, and schizophrenia. J Clin Psychiatry 68:899–907, 2007

Little JD, Atkins MR, Munday J, et al: Bifrontal electroconvulsive therapy in the elderly: a 2-year retrospective. J ECT 20:139–141, 2004

Madhusoodanan S, Brenner R, Araujo L, et al: Efficacy of risperidone treatment for psychoses associated with schizophrenia, schizoaffective disorder, bipolar disorder, or senile dementia in 11 geriatric patients: a case series. J Clin Psychiatry 56:514–518, 1995

Madhusoodanan S, Brecher M, Brenner R, et al: Risperidone in the treatment of elderly patients with psychotic disorders. Am J Geriatr Psychiatry 7:132–138, 1999

Madhusoodanan S, Brenner R, Alcantra A: Clinical experience with quetiapine in elderly patients with psychotic disorders. J Geriatr Psychiatry Neurol 13:28–32, 2000

McDonald WM: Epidemiology, etiology, and treatment of geriatric mania. J Clin Psychiatry 61 (suppl 13):3–11, 2000

McDonald WM, Thompson TR: Treatment of mania in dementia with electroconvulsive therapy. Psychopharmacol Bull 35:72–82, 2001

McDonald WM, Krishnan KR, Doraiswamy PM, et al: Occurrence of subcortical hyperintensities in elderly subjects with mania. Psychiatry Res 40:211–220, 1991

McDonald WM, Tupler LA, Marsteller FA, et al: Hyperintense lesions on magnetic resonance images in bipolar disorder. Biol Psychiatry 45:965–971, 1999

Mendlewicz J, Fieve RR, Rainer JD, et al: Manic-depressive illness: a comparative study of patients with and without a family history. Br J Psychiatry 120:523–530, 1972

Meyer JM: A retrospective comparison of weight, lipid, and glucose changes between risperidone- and olanzapine-treated inpatients: metabolic outcomes after 1 year. J Clin Psychiatry 63:425–433, 2002

Niedermier JA, Nasrallah HA: Clinical correlates of response to valproate in geriatric inpatients. Ann Clin Psychiatry 10:165–168, 1998

Noaghiul S, Narayan M, Nelson JC: Divalproex treatment of mania in elderly patients. Am J Geriatr Psychiatry 6:257–262, 1998

Panjehshahin MR, Bowman CJ, Yates MS: Effect of valproic acid, its unsaturated metabolites and some structurally related fatty acids on the binding of warfarin and dansylsacrosine to human albumin. Biochem Pharmacol 41:1227–1233, 1991

Post F: The factor of ageing in affective illness, in Recent Developments in Affective Disorders, Special Publication 2. Edited by Coppen A, Walk A. London, Royal Medico-Psychological Association, 1968, pp 105–116

Prien RF, Caffey EM, Klett CJ: Relationship between serum lithium level and clinical response in acute mania treated with lithium. Br J Psychiatry 120:409–414, 1972

Puryear LJ, Kunik ME, Workman R: Tolerability of divalproex sodium in elderly psychiatric patients with mixed diagnoses. J Geriatr Psychiatry Neurol 8:234–237, 1995

Regenold WT, Thapar RK, Marano C, et al: Increased prevalence of type 2 diabetes mellitus among psychiatric inpatients with bipolar I affective and schizoaffective disorders independent of psychotropic drug use. J Affect Disord 70:19–26, 2002

Roose SP, Bone S, Haidorfer C, et al: Lithium treatment in older patients. Am J Psychiatry 136:843–844, 1979

Sajatovic M: Treatment of bipolar disorder in older adults. Int J Geriatr Psychiatry 17:865–873, 2002

Sajatovic M, Popli A, Semple W: Health resource utilization over a ten-year period by geriatric veterans with schizophrenia and bipolar disorder. J Geriatr Psychiatry Neurol 15:128–133, 1996

Sajatovic M, Gyulai L, Calabrese JR, et al: Maintenance treatment outcomes in older patients with bipolar I disorder. Am J Geriatr Psychiatry 13:305–311, 2005a

Sajatovic M, Madhusoodanan S, Coconcea N: Managing bipolar disorder in the elderly: defining the role of the newer agents. Drugs Aging 22:39–54, 2005b

Sajatovic M, Blow FC, Ignacio RV: Psychiatric comorbidity in older adults with bipolar disorder. Int J Geriatr Psychiatry 21:582–587, 2006

Sajatovic M, Ramsay E, Nanry K, et al: Lamotrigine therapy in elderly patients with epilepsy, bipolar disorder or dementia. Int J Geriatr Psychiatry 22:945–950, 2007

Schaffer CB, Garvey MJ: Use of lithium in acutely manic elderly patients. Clin Gerontol 3:58–60, 1984

Shulman K, Post F: Bipolar affective disorder in old age. Br J Psychiatry 136:26–32, 1980

Shulman KI, Mackenzie S, Hardy B: The clinical use of lithium carbonate in old age: a review. Prog Neuropsychopharmacol Biol Psychiatry 11:159–164, 1987

Shulman KI, Tohen M, Satlin A, et al: Mania compared with unipolar depression in old age. Am J Psychiatry 149:341–345, 1992

Shulman KI, Rochon P, Sykora K, et al: Changing prescription patterns for lithium and valproic acid in old age: shifting practice without evidence. BMJ 326:960–961, 2003

Shulman RW, Singh A, Shulman KI: Treatment of elderly institutionalized bipolar patients with clozapine. Psychopharmacol Bull 33:113–118, 1997

Snowdon J: A retrospective case-note study of bipolar disorder in old age. Br J Psychiatry 158:485–490, 1991

Speer DC: Differences in social resources and treatment history among diagnostic groups of older adults. Hosp Community Psychiatry 43:270–274, 1992

Sproule BA, Hardy BG, Shulman KI: Differential pharmacokinetics of lithium in elderly patients. Drugs Aging 16:165–177, 2000

Stenstedt A: Study in manic-depressive psychosis: clinical, social, and genetic investigations. Acta Psychiatr Neurol Scand Suppl 79:1–111, 1952

Stone K: Mania in the elderly. Br J Psychiatry 155:220–224, 1989

Strakowski SM, Woods BT, Tohen M, et al: MRI subcortical signal hyperintensities in mania at first hospitalization. Biol Psychiatry 33:204–206, 1993

Swayze VW, Andreasen NC, Alliger RJ, et al: Structural brain abnormalities in bipolar affective disorder. Arch Gen Psychiatry 47:1054–1059, 1990

Tariot P, Podgorski C, Blazina L, et al: Mental disorders in the nursing home: another perspective. Am J Psychiatry 150:1063–1069, 1993

Taylor M, Abrams R: Manic states: a genetic study of early and late onset affective disorders. Arch Gen Psychiatry 28:656–658, 1973

Thase ME: STEP-BD and bipolar depression: what have we learned. Curr Psychiatry Rep 9:497–503, 2007

Thase ME, Denko T: Pharmacotherapy of mood disorders. Ann Rev Clin Psychol 4:53–91, 2008

Tohen M, Shulman KI, Satlin A: First-episode mania in late life. Am J Psychiatry 151:130–132, 1994

Tsai S, Kuo C, Chen C, et al: Risk factors for completed suicide in bipolar disorder. J Clin Psychiatry 63:469–476, 2002

Umapathy C, Mulsant BH, Pollock BG: Bipolar disorder in the elderly. Psychiatr Ann 30:473–480, 2000

Unutzer J, Simon G, Pabiniak C, et al: The treated prevalence of bipolar disorder in a large staff-model HMO. Psychiatr Serv 49:1072–1078, 1998

U.S. Food and Drug Administration: Carbamazepine prescribing information to include recommendation of genetic test for patients with Asian ancestry. FDA News, December 12, 2007. Available at: http://www.fda.gov/bbs/topics/NEWS/2007/NEW01755.html. Accessed February 17, 2008.

van der Velde CD: Effectiveness of lithium carbonate in the treatment of manic-depressive illness. Am J Psychiatry 123:345–351, 1970

Videbech P: MRI findings in patients with affective disorder: a meta-analysis. Acta Psychiatr Scand 96:157–168, 1997

Weissman MM, Leaf PJ, Tischler GL, et al: Affective disorders in five United States communities. Psychol Med 18:141–153, 1988

Weissman MM, Bland RC, Canino GJ, et al: Cross-national epidemiology of major depression and bipolar disorder. JAMA 276:293–299, 1996

Wylie M, Mulsant B, Pollock B, et al: Age at onset in geriatric bipolar disorder. Am J Geriatr Psychiatry 7:77–83, 1999

Young RC, Kalayam B, Tsuboyama G, et al: Mania: response to lithium across the age spectrum (abstract). Society for Neuroscience 18:669, 1992

Young RC, Nambudiri DE, Jain H, et al: Brain computed tomography in geriatric manic disorder. Biol Psychiatry 45:1063–1065, 1999

Young RC, Gyulai L, Mulsant BH, et al: Pharmacotherapy of bipolar disorder in old age: review and recommendations. Am J Geriatr Psychiatry 12:342–357, 2004

Suggested Readings

Beyer JL, Burchitt B, Gersing K, et al: Patterns of pharmacotherapy and treatment response in elderly adults with bipolar disorder. Psychopharmacol Bull 41:102–114, 2008

Depp CA, Jeste DV: Bipolar disorder in older adults: a critical review. Bipolar Disord 6:343–367, 2004

Sajatovic M, Madhusoodanan S, Coconcea N: Managing bipolar disorder in the elderly: defining the role of the newer agents. Drugs Aging 22:39–54, 2005

Young RC, Gyulai L, Mulsant BH, et al: Pharmacotherapy of bipolar disorder in old age: review and recommendations. Am J Geriatr Psychiatry 12:342–357, 2004

CHAPTER 10

SCHIZOPHRENIA AND PARANOID DISORDERS

IPSIT V. VAHIA, M.D.
NICOLE M. LANOUETTE, M.D.
DILIP V. JESTE, M.D.

Delusions, hallucinations, and other psychotic symptoms in late life may be more common than previously thought; a recent Swedish investigation (Ostling et al. 2007) found that the prevalence of any psychotic symptom in a nondemented population-based sample of 95-year-old individuals was 7.1%, with 6.7% experiencing hallucinations, 10.4% having delusions, and 0.6% experiencing paranoid ideation. In this chapter, we review the epidemiology, presentation, and treatment of chronic late-life psychotic disorders not secondary to a mood disorder or a general medical condition other than dementia. Thus, we discuss early-onset schizophrenia, late-onset schizophrenia, very-late-onset schizophrenia-like psychosis (with onset after age 60),

delusional disorder, psychosis of Alzheimer's disease (AD), and psychosis associated with other dementias.

Schizophrenia

Early-Onset Schizophrenia

The prevalence of schizophrenia among adults between ages 45 and 64 is approximately 0.6%, and prevalence estimates for schizophrenia among elderly individuals range from 0.1% to 0.5%. Typically, individuals with schizophrenia develop the disease in the second or third decade of life (American Psychiatric Association 1994). Although mortality rates in general, and suicide and homicide rates in particular, are

163

higher among individuals with schizophrenia than in the general population, many of these patients with early-onset schizophrenia are now living into older adulthood. Thus, most older adults with schizophrenia typically have had an early onset of the disease and have a chronic course of illness spanning several decades.

Longitudinal follow-up of schizophrenia patients indicates considerable heterogeneity of outcome. A minority of patients experience remission of both positive and negative symptoms. Auslander and Jeste (2004) reported that approximately 10% of patients may meet criteria for remission, and while the course of illness over time is unchanged in the majority of patients, there is generally an improvement in positive symptoms.

Factors associated with poor prognosis for early-onset schizophrenia include chronicity, insidious onset, premorbid psychosocial or functional deficits, and prominent negative symptoms.

Cognition in Older Schizophrenia Patients

The pattern of cognitive deficits in schizophrenia differs significantly from that in AD; patients with AD have less efficient learning and more rapid forgetting than do patients with schizophrenia. Among community-dwelling older outpatients, cognitive functioning seems to remain relatively stable other than the changes expected from normal aging (Harvey et al. 1999; Heaton et al. 2001). In general, cognitive functioning is better in persons with later ages at onset (Rajji et al. 2009).

Depression in Older Schizophrenia Patients

Studies have shown depressive symptoms to be distinct from negative symptoms. De-

pression is also a major predictor of suicidality in this population. Recent studies of depression in the older schizophrenia patients highlight the role of subsyndromal depression in increasing morbidity (Zisook et al. 2007).

Functional Capacity

The level of functional impairment varies considerably among older adults with schizophrenia (Palmer et al. 2003). In general, worse neuropsychological test performance, lower educational level, and negative symptoms but not positive symptoms are associated with poorer functional capacity in older outpatients with schizophrenia.

Successful Aging and Schizophrenia in Late Life

Some recent literature has assessed whether successful aging may be possible in older adults with schizophrenia (Cohen et al. 2009; Ibrahim et al. 2010). Little consensus exists on definitions of successful aging (Depp and Jeste 2006). However, preliminary evidence based on available definitions and models suggests that older adults with schizophrenia are unlikely to achieve the same levels of successful aging or community integration as comparable subjects without schizophrenia (Abdallah et al. 2009; Ibrahim et al. 2010). Improving physical health (Ibrahim et al. 2010; Vahia et al. 2008) and focusing on spiritual or religious involvement have been suggested as ways to improve the possibility of successful aging in this population (Cohen et al. 2010).

Late-Onset Schizophrenia

A literature review found that approximately 23% of patients with schizophrenia reportedly had onset after age 40, with 3%

being older than 60 (Harris and Jeste 1988). One investigation of first-contact patients reported that 29% of the patients had an onset after age 44, with 12% reporting onset after age 64 (Jeste et al. 1997).

The consensus statement by the International Late-Onset Schizophrenia Group (Howard et al. 2000) suggested that schizophrenia with an onset after age 40 should be called "late-onset schizophrenia" and considered a subtype of schizophrenia rather than a related disorder.

Risk factors and clinical presentation are similar between individuals with early- and late-onset schizophrenia. The self-reported proportion of individuals with a positive family history of schizophrenia (10%–15%), genetic risk, and levels of childhood maladjustment are similar in earlier and late-onset patients (Sachdev et al. 1999). A long-term neuropsychological follow-up of a group of late-onset schizophrenia patients found no evidence of cognitive decline, suggesting a neurodevelopmental rather than a neurodegenerative process (Palmer et al. 2003).

Women predominate among individuals with onset of schizophrenia in middle to late life. It has been speculated that estrogen may serve as an endogenous antipsychotic, masking schizophrenic symptoms in vulnerable women until after menopause, but treatments targeting estrogen have not been found effective (Seeman 1996).

In a study conducted at our research center, we used a comprehensive battery of measurements of psychopathology, cognition, and functioning to compare 110 subjects with late-onset schizophrenia and 744 subjects with early-onset schizophrenia. In our study, we noted that individuals with late-onset schizophrenia were more likely to be women and to have less severe positive symptoms and lower scores on measures of general psychopathology. We also noted that patients with late-onset schizophrenia did better on cognitive tasks measuring abstraction, cognitive flexibility, and verbal memory. Patients with late-onset schizophrenia had better physical and emotional functioning and were receiving lower average doses of antipsychotic medications (Vahia et al. 2010). A recent meta-analysis also noted that cognitive deficits in late-onset schizophrenia are specific rather than just a function of age (Rajji et al. 2009).

Very-Late-Onset Schizophrenia-Like Psychosis

The consensus statement by the International Late-Onset Schizophrenia Group proposed the diagnostic term *very-late-onset schizophrenia-like psychosis* (VLOSLP) for patients whose onset of psychosis is after age 60. Table 10–1 compares risk factors for and clinical features of early-onset schizophrenia, late-onset schizophrenia, and VLOSLP. VLOSLP may be difficult to diagnose clinically because its clinical picture can be confused with other conditions such as delirium or psychosis due to underlying medical illness. Nevertheless, new-onset primary psychotic symptoms have been described in adults as old as 100 (Cervantes et al. 2006).

Factors distinguishing VLOSLP patients from "true" schizophrenia patients include a lower genetic load, less evidence of early childhood maladjustment, a relative lack of thought disorder and negative symptoms (including blunted affect), greater risk of tardive dyskinesia (TD), and evidence of a neurodegenerative rather than a neurodevelopmental process (Moore et al. 2006; Palmer et al. 2003).

In summary, clinical vigilance must be exercised when treating apparent primary-

TABLE 10–1. Comparison of early-onset schizophrenia, late-onset schizophrenia, and very-late-onset schizophrenia-like psychosis (VLOSLP)

	Early-onset schizophrenia	Late-onset schizophrenia	VLOSLP
Age at onset	Before 40	Middle age (~40–60)	Late life (>60)
Female preponderance	–	+	++
Negative symptoms	++	+	–
Minor physical anomalies	+	+	–
Neuropsychological impairment			
Learning	++	+	?++
Retention	–	–	?++
Progressive cognitive deterioration	–	–	++
Brain structure abnormalities (e.g., strokes, tumors)	–	–	++
Family history of schizophrenia	+	+	–
Early childhood maladjustment	+	+	–
Daily antipsychotic dose	++	+	+
Risk of tardive dyskinesia	+	+	++

Note. +=mildly present; ++=strongly present; ?++=probably strongly present, but limited data exist; –=absent.

Source. Adapted from Palmer et al. 2001.

onset psychotic symptoms in older patients, and "organic" causes should be meticulously ruled out.

Delusional Disorder

The essential feature of a delusional disorder is a nonbizarre delusion (e.g., persecutory, somatic, erotomanic, grandiose, or jealous) without prominent auditory or visual hallucinations. Symptoms must be present for at least 1 month. When delusional disorder arises in late life, basic personality features, intellectual performance, and occupational function are preserved, but social functioning is compromised. To diagnose delusional disorder, the clinician must rule out other organic causes (Evans et al. 1996).

The prevalence of delusional disorder according to DSM-IV-TR (American Psychiatric Association 2000) is 0.03% and is slightly higher among women than among men. It typically first appears in middle to late adulthood, with an average age at onset of 40–49 for men and 60–69 for women (Copeland et al. 1998).

Risk factors for delusional disorder include a family history of schizophrenia and avoidant, paranoid, or schizoid personality disorder (Kendler and Davis 1981). Evans and colleagues (1996) compared middle-aged and older patients with schizophrenia and delusional disorder and found no differences in neuropsychological impairment but more severe psychopathology associated with delusional disorder.

Psychosis of Alzheimer's Disease

Ropacki and Jeste (2005) estimated the median prevalence of psychosis in AD to be about 41% (range = 12.2%–74.1%) in their review of 55 studies. Psychosis is associated with more rapid cognitive decline. Some studies have reported a significant association between psychosis and age, age at onset of AD, and illness duration. Paulsen et al. (2000) found a cumulative incidence of psychotic symptoms of 20% at 1 year, 36% at 2 years, 50% at 3 years, and 51% at 4 years in a large sample of patients with probable AD. Active suicidal ideation and history of psychosis are rare. Because psychotic symptoms in dementia patients tend to remit in the late stages of the disease, very-long-term maintenance therapy with antipsychotics is typically unnecessary.

AD patients with and without psychosis differ in several important ways. Neuropsychologically, AD patients with psychosis show greater impairment in executive functioning, more rapid cognitive decline, and a greater prevalence of extrapyramidal symptoms (EPS) than do AD patients without psychosis. Neuropathologically, dementia patients with psychosis showed increased neurodegenerative changes in the cortex, increased norepinephrine in subcortical regions, and reduced serotonin levels in both cortical and subcortical areas.

Jeste and Finkel (2000) have recommended specific diagnostic criteria for psychosis of AD: presence of visual or auditory hallucinations or delusions, a primary diagnosis of AD, and duration (at least 1 month) and time of onset (symptoms of AD preceding those of psychosis) criteria. Alternative causes of psychosis must be excluded, and sufficient functional impairment should be present for this diagnosis to be made.

Psychosis in Other Dementias

Psychosis is also common in other dementias. Visual hallucinations and secondary delusions are common in Lewy body disease, and vascular dementia also may be accompanied by delusions or hallucinations (Schneider et al. 2006). Naimark and colleagues (1996) found psychotic symptoms in approximately one-third of a sample of patients with Parkinson's disease, with hallucinations being more common than delusions. Psychosis in frontotemporal dementias is poorly characterized but may be as common as that in AD.

Treatment

Although conventional agents substantially improved the positive symptoms of schizophrenia (e.g., hallucinations and delusions), several treatment liabilities have been recognized over the years, such as movement disorders, sedation, orthostatic hypotension, elevated prolactin concentrations, and most notably, TD. Atypical antipsychotics have been linked to increased risk of metabolic dysfunction, including diabetes, dyslipidemia, and obesity, leading to a worsened cardiovascular risk profile. In elderly patients with dementia, atypical antipsychotics have been associated with increased risk of cerebrovascular adverse events and mortality compared with placebo, leading pharmaceutical regulatory agencies to issue warnings about their use. However, lack of evidence-based alternatives restricts clinicians to off-label treatments, which must be used with caution and close monitoring. Psychosocial treatments for older adults with psychosis show promise as adjunctive treatments.

Schizophrenia and Delusional Disorder

Pharmacological Treatment

Pharmacotherapy for schizophrenia and delusional disorder in older individuals is restricted by a paucity of randomized placebo-controlled, double-blinded clinical trials in this population. Maintenance pharmacotherapy is usually required for older patients with schizophrenia because of risk of relapse. Older individuals are at higher risk for adverse antipsychotic effects as a result of age-related pharmacokinetic and pharmacodynamic factors, coexisting medical illnesses, and concomitant medications. Therefore, the recommended starting and maintenance doses of antipsychotics in older adults are 50% and 25%–30% lower than the usual younger adult doses, respectively (American Psychiatric Association 1997).

Few efficacy comparisons between conventional and atypical antipsychotics have been done in patients with schizophrenia older than 65 (Jeste et al. 1999). The National Institute of Mental Health Clinical Antipsychotic Trials of Intervention Effectiveness (CATIE) study, which included adults ages 18–65 years, found no significant differences in effectiveness between the conventional antipsychotic perphenazine and the atypical antipsychotics risperidone, olanzapine, quetiapine, or ziprasidone, but it is unknown how these findings would translate to patients older than 65 (Lieberman et al. 2005).

Use of conventional or typical antipsychotics in this population is problematic given the higher incidence of TD in older patients. Aging appears to be the most important risk factor for the development of TD (American Psychiatric Association

2000; Yassa and Nair 1992). Atypical antipsychotics have a less favorable side-effect profile in terms of metabolic function. Common metabolic side effects include excessive weight gain and obesity, glucose intolerance, new-onset type 2 diabetes mellitus, diabetic ketoacidosis, and dyslipidemia (Jin et al. 2004). Although no guidelines are available for management of these side effects specifically in older patients with schizophrenia, the American Diabetes Association et al. (2004) monitoring recommendations are potentially applicable. Because elderly patients tend to be at higher risk for cardiovascular disease than are younger patients, closer monitoring would be necessary for older adults.

The only large-scale randomized, double-blind, controlled trial comparing two atypical antipsychotics in adults older than 60 years was Jeste and colleagues' (2003) multisite international study of risperidone and olanzapine. In that trial, 175 patients with schizophrenia or schizoaffective disorder age 60 years and older were randomly assigned to receive risperidone (1–3 mg/day; median dose = 2 mg/day) or olanzapine (5–20 mg/day; median dose = 10 mg/day). Both groups had significant improvement in symptoms and reduction in EPS rating scale scores. Clinically relevant weight gain was significantly less frequent in patients taking risperidone.

Given the dearth of randomized controlled data, Alexopoulos and colleagues (2004) conducted an expert consensus survey of 48 American experts on antipsychotic treatment in older adults. The consensus first-line recommendation for late-life schizophrenia was risperidone (1.25–3.5 mg/day). The experts' second-line recommendations included quetiapine (100–300 mg/day), olanzapine (7.5–15 mg/day), and aripiprazole

(15–30 mg/day). Support for the use of clozapine, ziprasidone, and high-potency conventional antipsychotics was limited. In one recent trial (Scott et al. 2010), atypical antipsychotics at geriatric doses were effective in treating VLOSLP as well.

Given the data on the increased risk of strokes and mortality in elderly patients with dementia treated with atypical antipsychotics (Gill et al. 2005) and the consequent U.S. Food and Drug Administration black-box warnings (discussed in the "Psychosis of Alzheimer's Disease and Other Dementias" subsection later in this chapter), clinicians should exercise caution when using these drugs in older patients with schizophrenia.

Few data are available specifically on the pharmacological treatment of delusional disorder in late life. Alexopoulos et al.'s (2004) survey of 48 experts in geriatric care concluded that antipsychotics are the only recommended treatment, and their first-line recommendation for older adults with delusional disorder was risperidone (0.75–2.5 mg/day), followed by olanzapine (5–10 mg/day) and quetiapine (50–200 mg/day).

Psychosocial Treatments

Recent years have seen the development and testing of psychosocial interventions for older adults with chronic psychotic disorders. Granholm and colleagues (2005) noted that cognitive-behavioral social skills training (CBSST), which teaches cognitive and behavioral coping techniques, social functioning skills, problem solving, and compensatory aids for neurocognitive impairments, led to significantly increased frequency of performing social functioning activities, greater cognitive insight (more objectivity in reappraising psychotic symptoms), and greater skill mastery. An increase in cognitive insight was significantly correlated with a greater reduction in positive symptoms. At 12-month follow-up (Granholm et al. 2007), the CBSST group had maintained their greater skill acquisition and performance of everyday living skills.

Patterson et al. (2006) conducted a randomized controlled trial of a behavioral group intervention called Functional Adaptation Skills Training (FAST) (a manualized behavioral intervention designed to improve everyday living skills such as medication management, social skills, communication skills, organization and planning, transportation, and financial management). They noted that the FAST group showed significant improvement in daily living skills and social skills but not medication management.

In an examination of employment outcomes among middle-aged and older adults with schizophrenia, Twamley et al. (2005) reported that the highest rates of volunteer or paid work (81%) and competitive or paid work (69%) occurred for the patients who were placed in a job chosen with a vocational counselor and then received individualized on-site support.

Psychosis of Alzheimer's Disease and Other Dementias

Since their introduction over the past decade, the atypical antipsychotics have for the most part replaced conventional antipsychotics in treating psychosis, aggression, and agitation in patients with dementia because of greater tolerability, lower risk for acute EPS, and comparatively lower risk of TD (Kindermann et al. 2002). Most antipsychotic prescriptions in older adults are for behavioral disturbances associated with dementia, despite the fact that atypicals lack this FDA–approved indication (Ballard and Waite 2006).

In the CATIE-AD trial (Schneider et al. 2006), which was the largest ($N=421$) non-industry-sponsored trial of atypical antipsychotics for psychosis or agitation/aggression in people with dementia, olanzapine, quetiapine, and risperidone were no better than placebo for the primary outcome (time to discontinuation for any reason). Time to discontinuation due to lack of efficacy favored olanzapine and risperidone, whereas time to discontinuation due to adverse events favored placebo.

Only a few randomized controlled trials have compared the two classes of antipsychotics for dementia, and results have been inconclusive (De Deyn et al. 1999).

In addition to the liabilities described earlier, use of atypical antipsychotics in elderly dementia patients has been associated with both cerebrovascular adverse events and death, leading to black-box warnings by the FDA in the past few years.

Retrospective database reviews did not find any difference in incidence of cerebrovascular adverse events for typical versus atypical antipsychotic use, although none of these studies were originally designed to examine cerebrovascular adverse event risk.

In May 2004, the FDA also issued a black-box warning that elderly patients with dementia taking atypical antipsychotic drugs are at an increased risk for death compared with those taking placebo. The data on risk of mortality associated with typical versus atypical antipsychotics have been mixed (Jeste et al. 2008).

Unfortunately, data are also insufficient to support systematic use of any of the alternatives to antipsychotics, and few well-designed randomized controlled trials of behavioral and psychosocial interventions have been done in patients with dementia, but there are promising possibilities (e.g., behavioral management techniques, caregiver education; Ayalon et al. 2006; Cohen-Mansfield 2001; Livingston et al. 2005). However, when strict inclusion criteria are used, such as those of the American Psychological Association. very few of these can be considered evidenced-based because the results are often inconclusive.

Patients with Lewy body dementia and parkinsonian dementia are especially sensitive to side effects such as EPS and anticholinergic effects, so very low doses and slow titration schedules should be used to avoid worsening of motor symptoms (Chou et al. 2007; Masand 2000). Low-dose clozapine has shown efficacy in reducing symptoms of psychosis, and clozapine does not worsen and can even improve the parkinsonian tremor.

Key Points

- Schizophrenia may be classified by age at onset into early-onset schizophrenia (onset before age 40), late-onset schizophrenia (onset between ages 40 and 60), and very-late-onset schizophrenia-like psychosis (onset after age 60).

- Patients with late-onset schizophrenia are similar to patients with early-onset schizophrenia in terms of risk factors, clinical presentation, family history of schizophrenia, and response to medications. However, women are overrepresented among late-onset patients. Late-onset schizophrenia is marked by higher rates of delusional symptoms and lower rates of negative symptoms.

- Very-late-onset schizophrenia-like psychosis is a heterogeneous entity with varied etiology.

- Patients with psychosis of Alzheimer's disease tend to have paranoid delusions; visual or auditory hallucinations; and a greater risk of agitation, faster cognitive decline, and institutionalization than patients with Alzheimer's disease without psychosis.

- Older adults are at much higher risk for developing tardive dyskinesia (TD) than are younger patients; atypical antipsychotics are associated with significantly lower risk of TD than conventional agents but have problematic metabolic liabilities.

- Psychosocial treatments have an important place as an adjunctive treatment for older adults with schizophrenia.

- No treatments for psychosis and agitation in dementia are currently approved by the U.S. Food and Drug Administration; however, off-label use of medications, as well as certain psychosocial interventions, may be appropriate.

- In recent years, use of atypical antipsychotics in elderly patients with dementia has been associated with increased risk of cerebrovascular adverse events and mortality, leading to U.S. Food and Drug Administration black-box warnings for this population.

References

Abdallah C, Cohen CI, Sanchez-Almira M, et al: Community integration and associated factors among older adults with schizophrenia. Psychiatr Serv 60:1642–1648, 2009

Alexopoulos GS, Streim JE, Carpenter D: Expert consensus guidelines for using antipsychotic agents in older patients. J Clin Psychiatry 65:5–99, 2004

American Diabetes Association, American Psychiatric Association, American Association of Clinical Endocrinologists, et al: Consensus development conference on antipsychotic drugs and obesity and diabetes. Diabetes Care 27:596–601, 2004

American Psychiatric Association: Diagnostic and Statistical Manual of Mental Disorders, 4th Edition. Washington, DC, American Psychiatric Association, 1994

American Psychiatric Association: Practice guideline for the treatment of patients with schizophrenia. Am J Psychiatry 154 (4 suppl):1–63, 1997

American Psychiatric Association: Diagnostic and Statistical Manual of Mental Disorders, 4th Edition, Text Revision. Washington, DC, American Psychiatric Association, 2000

Auslander LA, Jeste DV: Sustained remission of schizophrenia among community-dwelling older outpatients. Am J Psychiatry 161:1490–1493, 2004

Ayalon L, Gum AM, Feliciano L, et al: Effectiveness of nonpharmacological interventions for the management of neuropsychiatric symptoms in patients with dementia: a systematic review. Arch Intern Med 166:2182–2188, 2006

Ballard C, Waite J: The effectiveness of atypical antipsychotics for the treatment of aggression and psychosis in Alzheimer's disease. Cochrane Database of Systematic Reviews 2006, Issue 1. Art. No.: CD003476.

Cervantes AN, Rabins PV, Slavney PR: Onset of schizophrenia at age 100. Psychosomatics 47:356–359, 2006

Chou KL, Borek LL, Friedman JH: The management of psychosis in movement disorder patients. Expert Opin Pharmacother 8:935–943, 2007

Cohen CI, Pathak R, Ramirez PM, et al: Outcome among community dwelling older adults with schizophrenia: results using five conceptual models. Community Ment Health J 45:151–156, 2009

Cohen CI, Jimenez C, Mittal S: The role of religion in the well-being of older adults with schizophrenia. Psychiatr Serv 61:917–922, 2010

Cohen-Mansfield J: Nonpharmacologic interventions for inappropriate behaviors in dementia: a review and critique. Am J Geriatr Psychiatry 9:361–381, 2001

Copeland JRM, Dewey ME, Scott A, et al: Schizophrenia and delusional disorder in older age: community prevalence, incidence, comorbidity and outcome. Schizophr Bull 19:153–161, 1998

De Deyn P, Rabheru K, Rasmussen A, et al: A randomized trial of risperidone, placebo, and haloperidol for behavioral symptoms of dementia. Neurology 53:946–955, 1999

Depp CA, Jeste DV: Definitions and predictors of successful aging: a comprehensive review of larger quantitative studies. Am J Geriatr Psychiatry 14:6–20, 2006

Evans JD, Paulsen JS, Harris MJ, et al: A clinical and neuropsychological comparison of delusional disorder and schizophrenia. J Neuropsychiatry Clin Neurosci 8:281–286, 1996

Gill SS, Rochon PA, Herrmann N, et al: Atypical antipsychotic drugs and risk of ischaemic stroke: population based retrospective cohort study. BMJ 330:445, 2005

Granholm E, McQuaid JR, McClure FS, et al: A randomized, controlled trial of cognitive behavioral social skills training for middle-aged and older outpatients with chronic schizophrenia. Am J Psychiatry 162:520–529, 2005

Granholm E, McQuaid JR, McClure FS, et al: Randomized controlled trial of cognitive behavioral social skills training for older people with schizophrenia: 12-month follow-up. J Clin Psychiatry 68:730–737, 2007

Harris MJ, Jeste DV: Late-onset schizophrenia: an overview. Schizophr Bull 14:39–55, 1988

Harvey PD, Silverman JM, Mohs RC, et al: Cognitive decline in late-life schizophrenia: a longitudinal study of geriatric chronically hospitalized patients. Biol Psychiatry 45:32–40, 1999

Heaton RK, Gladsjo JA, Palmer BW, et al: Stability and course of neuropsychological deficits in schizophrenia. Arch Gen Psychiatry 58:24–32, 2001

Howard R, Rabins PV, Seeman MV, et al: Late-onset schizophrenia and very-late-onset schizophrenia-like psychosis: an international consensus. Am J Psychiatry 157:172–178, 2000

Ibrahim F, Cohen CI, Ramirez PM: Successful aging in older adults with schizophrenia: prevalence and associated factors. Am J Geriatr Psychiatry 18:879–886, 2010

Jeste DV, Finkel SI: Psychosis of Alzheimer's disease and related dementias: diagnostic criteria for a distinct syndrome. Am J Geriatr Psychiatry 8:29–34, 2000

Jeste DV, Symonds LL, Harris MJ, et al: Nondementia non-praecox dementia praecox? Late-onset schizophrenia. Am J Geriatr Psychiatry 5:302–317, 1997

Jeste DV, Rockwell E, Harris MJ, et al: Conventional versus newer antipsychotics in elderly patients. Am J Geriatr Psychiatry 7:70–76, 1999

Jeste DV, Barak Y, Madhusoodanan S, et al: International multisite double-blind trial of the atypical antipsychotics risperidone and olanzapine in 175 elderly patients with chronic schizophrenia. Am J Geriatr Psychiatry 11:638–647, 2003

Jeste DV, Blazer D, Casey DE, et al: ACNP White Paper: Update on the use of antipsychotic drugs in elderly persons with dementia. Neuropsychopharmacology 33:957–970, 2008

Jin H, Meyer JM, Jeste DV: Atypical antipsychotics and glucose dysregulation: a systematic review. Schizophr Res 71:195–212, 2004

Kendler S, Davis KL: The genetics and biochemistry of paranoid schizophrenia and other paranoid psychoses. Schizophr Bull 7:689–709, 1981

Kindermann SS, Dolder CR, Bailey A, et al: Pharmacologic treatment of psychosis and agitation in elderly patients with dementia: four decades of experience. Drugs Aging 19:257–276, 2002

Lieberman JA, Stroup TS, McEvoy JP, et al: Effectiveness of antipsychotic drugs in patients with chronic schizophrenia. N Engl J Med 353:1209–1223, 2005

Livingston G, Johnston K, Katona C, et al: Systematic review of psychological approaches to the management of neuropsychiatric symptoms of dementia. Am J Psychiatry 162:1996–2021, 2005

Masand PS: Atypical antipsychotics for elderly patients with neurodegenerative disorders and medical conditions. Psychiatr Ann 30:203–208, 2000

Moore R, Blackwood N, Corcoran R, et al: Misunderstanding the intentions of others: an exploratory study of the cognitive etiology of persecutory delusions in very late-onset schizophrenia-like psychosis. Am J Geriatr Psychiatry 14:410–418, 2006

Naimark D, Jackson E, Rockwell E, et al: Psychotic symptoms in Parkinson's disease patients with dementia. J Am Geriatr Soc 44:296–299, 1996

Ostling S, Borjesson-Hanson A, Skoog I: Psychotic symptoms and paranoid ideation in a population-based sample of 95-year-olds. Am J Geriatr Psychiatry 15:999–1004, 2007

Palmer BW, Bondi MW, Twamley EW, et al: Are late-onset schizophrenia-spectrum disorders a neurodegenerative condition? Annual rates of change on two dementia measures. J Neuropsychiatry Clin Neurosci 15:45–52, 2003

Patterson TL, McKibbin C, Mausbach BT, et al: Functional Adaptation Skills Training (FAST): a randomized trial of a psychosocial intervention for middle-aged and older patients with chronic psychotic disorders. Schizophr Res 86:291–299, 2006

Paulsen JS, Salmon DP, Thal LJ, et al: Incidence of and risk factors for hallucinations and delusions in patients with probable AD. Neurology 54:1965–1971, 2000

Rajji TK, Ismail Z, Mulsant BH: Age at onset and cognition in schizophrenia: a meta-analysis. Br J Psychiatry 195:286–293, 2009

Ropacki SA, Jeste DV: Epidemiology of and risk factors for psychosis of Alzheimer's disease: a review of 55 studies published from 1990 to 2003. Am J Psychiatry 162:2022–2030, 2005

Sachdev P, Brodaty H, Rose N, et al: Schizophrenia with onset after age 50 years, 2: neurological, neuropsychological and MRI investigation. Br J Psychiatry 175:416–421, 1999

Schneider LS, Tariot PN, Dagerman KS, et al: Effectiveness of atypical antipsychotic drugs in patients with Alzheimer's disease. N Engl J Med 355:1525–1538, 2006

Scott J, Greenwald BS, Kramer E, et al: Atypical (second generation) antipsychotic treatment response in very late-onset schizophrenia-like psychosis. Int Psychogeriatr 1:1–7, 2010

Seeman MV: The role of estrogen in schizophrenia. J Psychiatr Neurosci 21:123–127, 1996

Twamley EW, Padin DS, Bayne KS, et al: Work rehabilitation for middle-aged and older people with schizophrenia: a comparison of three approaches. J Nerv Ment Dis 193:596–601, 2005

Vahia IV, Diwan S, Bankole AO, et al: Adequacy of medical treatment among older persons with schizophrenia. Psychiatr Serv 59:853–859, 2008

Vahia IV, Palmer BW, Depp C, et al: Is late-onset schizophrenia a subtype of schizophrenia? Acta Psychiatr Scand 122:414–426, 2010

Yassa R, Nair NPV: A 10-year follow-up study of tardive dyskinesia. Acta Psychiatr Scand 86:262–266, 1992

Zisook S, Montross L, Kasckow J, et al: Subsyndromal depressive symptoms in middle-aged and older persons with schizophrenia. Am J Geriatr Psychiatry 15:1005–1014, 2007

CHAPTER 11

Anxiety Disorders

Eric J. Lenze, M.D.
Julie Loebach Wetherell, Ph.D.
Carmen Andreescu, M.D.

Anxiety disorders are common in older adults and cause considerable distress and functional impairment. However, they are typically not assessed or managed properly. In this chapter, we discuss the epidemiology and neurobiology, neuropsychiatry, and neuropsychology of anxiety disorders in late life. We then review treatment outcome studies and discuss guidelines for assessment and management.

Epidemiology

Prevalence

Epidemiological studies have produced wide variation in prevalence estimates of anxiety disorders in elderly persons (Bryant et al. 2008), ranging from 1.2% to 15% in community samples and from 1% to 28% in medical settings. Likewise, the prevalence of clinically relevant anxiety symptoms ranges from 15% to 52% in community samples and 15% to 56% in medical settings. Some have questioned whether diagnostic criteria, and the methods used to observe them, are adequate in detecting mental disorders in older adults (Jeste et al. 2005). This issue may be particularly relevant for anxiety disorders because measures developed for young adults may not capture fear or anxiety as reported by older adults (Kogan and Edelstein 2004). For example, older adults commonly have fear of falling (Gagnon et al. 2005; Nagaratnam et al. 2005), which may not be discerned by standard epidemiological assessments or methodology.

The one anxiety disorder that seems to commonly present in late life is generalized anxiety disorder (GAD): approximately one-half of older adults with GAD have onset later in life (Chou 2009; Le Roux et al. 2005; Lenze et al. 2005a). Otherwise, anxiety disorders are usually considered to have onset in childhood or early adulthood, particularly social phobia and panic disorder. Some have suggested that the onset of anxiety in old age is rare and likely caused by an underlying medical problem such as hyperthyroidism (Flint 2005). Thus, older adults may have reduced propensity for panic or other highly autonomic responses (Flint et al. 2002).

On the contrary, several anxiogenic stressors are associated with aging, such as chronic illness and disability, caregiver status, or bereavement, and clinical samples of elderly anxiety disorder patients reported that many have late onset of illness (Le Roux et al. 2005; Lenze et al. 2005a; Sheikh et al. 2004b). Also, many common conditions in older adults could exacerbate anxiety. Dementia can cause anxiety that often presenting as agitation (Mintzer and Brawman-Mintzer 1996), hoarding syndrome (Saxena et al. 2002), or other atypical symptoms (Starkstein et al. 2007). Many common medical conditions are anxiogenic such as heart disease (Todaro et al. 2007), lung disease (Yohannes et al. 2006), or neurological disease such as Parkinson's disease. Comorbid anxiety is extremely common in late-life depression (Beekman et al. 2000; Lenze et al. 2000).

Course

The few longitudinal studies that have been carried out in older adults with anxiety suggest that it is persistent in this age group (Schuurmans et al. 2005). Of the anxious older adults in epidemiological and treatment-seeking samples, 60%–70% retrospectively reported an onset in or before early adulthood (Blazer et al. 1991; Le Roux et al. 2005; Lenze et al. 2005a; Sheikh et al. 1991).

Anxiety increases disability (Brenes et al. 2005) and potentially elevates mortality risk (Brenes et al. 2007a). Significant quality of life impairment has been noted in GAD in older adults, similar to that seen in late-life depression (Porensky et al. 2009; Wetherell et al. 2004).

Comorbidity With Depression

Depressed elderly patients with comorbid anxiety have greater somatic symptoms, greater likelihood of suicidal ideation (Jeste et al. 2006; Lenze et al. 2000), and a higher risk of suicide (Allgulander and Lavori 1993).

Longitudinally, anxiety symptoms appear to be more stable over time than depressive symptoms and more likely to lead to depressive symptoms than vice versa (Wetherell et al. 2001). Conversely, the combination of anxiety and depression may appear simultaneously (Lenze et al. 2005a); in this case, anxiety symptoms often persist after remission of depression and increase risk for depressive relapse (Dombrovski et al. 2007; Flint and Rifat 1997b). Thus, the greater persistence over time of anxiety symptoms may lead to the poorer outcomes seen in late-life depression comorbid with anxiety.

Many studies have reported a longer time to response in depression, and/or a reduced response rate, in association with anxiety symptoms or disorders (Andreescu et al. 2007; Flint and Rifat 1997a; Steffens and McQuoid 2005), although other research disputes this finding (Nelson et al. 2009). Additionally, comorbid anxiety predicts greater decline in memory during long-term follow-up of late-life depression (DeLuca et al. 2005). In summary, anxious depression is a severe, treatment-relevant subtype of late-life depression.

Neurobiology, Neuropsychiatry, and Neuropsychology

Neurobiology of Anxiety

Understanding the neuropsychiatry of anxiety in older adults requires an understanding of the neuroanatomy of anxiety. Midlife studies have found amygdala hyperactivation in panic disorders and specific phobias; insula hyperactivation in GAD, phobias, and posttraumatic stress disorder (PTSD); and right prefrontal hyperactivation and altered coupling of the amygdala-prefrontal circuit in anxious arousal (Bishop 2007). The amygdala-prefrontal circuit enables both representations of salient emotions and implementation of top-down control mechanisms to influence interpretative processes. Disruption of this circuitry, including deficient recruitment of prefrontal control mechanisms and amygdala hyperresponsivity to threat, leads to a sustained threat-related processing bias in anxious individuals.

Excessive anxiety triggers various anxiety-regulation strategies, ranging from simple attentional control to higher-level cognitive restructuring used to modulate emotion perception and response. Most often, anxiety-regulation strategies involve higher-level cognitive restructuring through the medial prefrontal cortex (mPFC). Top-down conscious reinterpretation reappraises potentially threatening stimuli as less threatening (Arce et al. 2008; Bishop 2007) through the activation of the cingulate cortex and the mPFC.

From the large area of the mPFC involved in the top-down reappraisal of threatening stimuli, recent research has delineated the subgenual anterior cingulate cortex (sACC; the affective division of ACC) as a key region in assessing the salience of emotional information and the regulation of emotional response (Bissiere et al. 2008). Inappropriate recruitment of the sACC during emotional events is one of the functional neuroanatomical bases of clinical anxiety (Simmons et al. 2008a).

One other brain region frequently described in anxiety studies is the insula, which is associated with the discomfort of one's own physiological responses to emotionally salient stimuli. Several reports have described increased insula activation in young, anxiety-prone adults (Arce et al. 2008; Simmons et al. 2008b; Stein et al. 2007). Abnormalities in the prefrontal and limbic-paralimbic cortex likely exist in anxiety disorders, although it is not clear if these findings are disorder specific or reflect common etiological and vulnerability factors that result in common pathophysiological profiles that span through all anxiety disorders.

Neuropsychiatric Conditions in Older Adults That Are Associated With Anxiety

Age-related impairment in functioning brain regions associated with adaptive responses to anxiety may reduce the ability to modulate the anxious response, thus causing the onset or maintenance of an anxiety disorder. In patients with neurodegenerative disease that results in pathological anxiety, the pathophysiology is likely to be network dysregulation, including centrally the dysregulation of the sACC-amygdala axis (Bissiere et al. 2008). Given this disconnectivity hypothesis, neuropsychiatric conditions that affect subcortical white matter, or the functioning of cortical and subcortical components of this network, are likely to be anxiogenic. Of course, the anxiety that frequently arises in stroke and other medical conditions also may reflect their status as anxiogenic life stressors (e.g., leading to sudden or chronic loss of control).

Parkinson's disease may be a particularly anxiogenic neurodegenerative illness because of its association not only with subcortical disease but also with autonomic dysfunction (potentially leading to panic attacks or similar autonomic symptoms) and because of the uncontrollability over basic movements and activities it causes (Lauterbach et al. 2003; Marsh 2000; Richard et al. 1996). Huntington's disease is another subcortical neurodegenerative disease with a high prevalence of anxiety symptoms (Paulsen et al. 2001). Traumatic brain injury can result in diffuse axonal injury, likely leading to the high observed prevalence of post–traumatic brain injury anxiety symptoms (Jorge et al. 1993).

Stroke can cause anxiety symptoms (De Wit et al. 2008), GAD (Astrom 1996; Castillo et al. 1995), or obsessive-compulsive disorder (Swoboda and Jenike 1995). As with depression, some evidence indicates that left hemisphere lesions may be more likely to cause anxiety (Barker-Collo 2007), although the pathophysiology underlying this link is unclear.

Dementing illness (see Lyketsos, Chapter 7, "Dementia and Milder Cognitive Syndromes," in this volume) can cause anxiety symptoms (Ballard et al. 2000; Lyketsos et al. 2002) or GAD (Starkstein et al. 2007). Consistent with the disconnectivity hypothesis is evidence that amyloid binding in the posterior cingulate region is associated with increased anxiety symptoms in nondemented older adults (Lavretsky et al. 2009). Finally, epilepsy is associated with anxiety (Marsh and Rao 2002).

Anxiety may cause or accelerate neurodegeneration in older adults because aging increases vulnerability to adverse effects of stress when homeostatic mechanisms preventing an excessive biological stress response and its deleterious effects are diminished (Lenze and Wetherell 2009; Urry et al. 2006). Anxiety symptoms or disorders in elderly adults are associated with accelerated cognitive decline (DeLuca et al. 2005; Palmer et al. 2007; Sinoff and Werner 2003). Several potential mechanisms exist for anxiety-induced neurodegeneration. Pathological anxiety in late life is associated with activation of the hypothalamic-pituitary-adrenal axis leading to higher cortisol levels, which may adversely affect hippocampal and prefrontal function (Lenze et al. 2011; Mantella et al. 2008). Anxiety may induce cerebrovascular disease via insulin resistance, endothelial reactivity, and impaired autonomic function (Narita et al. 2008). Chronic mood disorders lead, via oxidative stress, to decreased telomerase activity and telomere shrinking, resulting in accelerated cellular aging (Simon et al. 2006). Finally, altering serotonin function in an aging model modifies not only stress responsivity but also age-related neurodegeneration (Sibille et al. 2007).

Neuropsychological Impairments in Late-Life Anxiety

Anxiety and cognitive impairment have a consistent and bidirectional relation in older adults (Beaudreau and O'Hara 2008). Recent investigations have found a variety of memory and executive impairments in geriatric GAD, including poorer short-term memory and executive dysfunction (Butters et al. 2011; Caudle et al. 2007; Mantella et al. 2007; Mohlman and Gorman 2005). Some evidence indicates that cognitive impairment predicts poorer long-term psychotherapy outcome with cognitive-behavioral therapy (CBT) for geriatric GAD (Caudle et al. 2007). In this analysis, errors in temporal orientation predicted poorer maintenance of treatment gains at 6-month follow-up. Overall, these data suggest that mild cognitive impairment may act as a maintenance factor for anxiety in elderly patients, preventing its improvement during treatment or naturalistically.

Treatment Outcome Studies

Both psychotherapy and pharmacotherapy appear to be effective treatment options in this age group (Wetherell et al. 2005b). One meta-analysis and one direct randomized comparison of pharmacotherapy and psychotherapy found medications to be more effective than CBT in the acute phase of treatment (Pinquart and Duberstein 2007; Schuurmans et al. 2006). Nevertheless, the patient's and provider's preference most likely will determine whether to initiate pharmacotherapy or psychotherapy.

Psychotherapy

CBT is currently the dominant formal psychotherapy for anxiety disorders; it might be particularly effective for anxiety disorders in older adults who are able to learn new skills in CBT and use them effectively (Wetherell et al. 2005a). As such, consideration of cognition, motivation, and ability to practice skills should be part of an evaluation for psychotherapy.

CBT for late-life anxiety typically involves psychoeducation, relaxation, cognitive therapy, problem-solving skills training, exposure exercises (i.e., exposure and habituation to anxiogenic situations), and sleep hygiene when necessary for the common problem of insomnia (Brenes et al. 2009), similar to treatment in younger adults (Stanley et al. 2004). In elderly persons, the most effective ingredient of CBT may be

relaxation (Thorp et al. 2009). CBT has been shown to be effective in the primary care setting (Stanley et al. 2009), although the lack of highly skilled CBT therapists with experience in late-life anxiety may be a barrier to widespread implementation.

Modular treatment, a newer personalized approach in psychotherapy research, can use any or all of these components, depending on the patient's presenting problems or symptoms (Wetherell and Stein 2009; Wetherell et al. 2005c).

Booster sessions to prevent loss of efficacy during maintenance treatment are particularly important for older adults because aging is associated with poorer performance on attention and memory tasks for which internally generated and maintained strategies are required (Prull et al. 2006). Booster sessions are also responsive to life events, which appear to play a role in long-term outcomes from late-life GAD (Wetherell and Stein 2009). Booster therapy sessions use the same format as is used for general skills practice during CBT, with an emphasis on skills most applicable to the situation the patient is currently facing. When patients are scheduled for a follow-up booster session, they are assigned at-home practice to complete between the sessions. With respect to long-term management, follow-up studies of older patients with GAD treated with CBT have reported maintenance of gains for up to 1 year following discontinuation of treatment (Barrowclough et al. 2001; Stanley et al. 2003).

Adaptations for older adults include a slower pace with increased repetition, less abstract cognitive restructuring techniques and correspondingly more focus on behavior change, more focus on health-related problems, and a family session reflecting the importance of engaging family in geriatric mental health treatment. In addition to in-session discussion and a written summary of material, we audiotape sessions for participants to consolidate learning. Another possible adaptation is the integration of religion into CBT (Paukert et al. 2009).

Another promising treatment is bibliotherapy (Brenes et al. 2007b). A recent study of late-life anxiety and depression prevention used a stepped-care approach, in which bibliotherapy, the first intervention, was effective at preventing anxiety and depressive episodes (van't Veer-Tazelaar et al. 2009). Many self-help workbooks exist for anxiety disorders, although none to our knowledge are focused on older adults. There is increasing indication that many patients are using the Internet as a guide for treatment, although it is unknown how much this is the case for older adults. Internet-based self-help may play an increasing role in the future.

Pharmacotherapy

The evidence base for pharmacotherapy in older adults is limited and consists mainly of small clinical trials. Benzodiazepines are still commonly used for geriatric anxiety (Benitez et al. 2008), despite the association of these medications with falls (Landi et al. 2005) and cognitive impairment and decline (Paterniti et al. 2002). Generally, their long-term use for late-life anxiety is discouraged.

Two small randomized controlled trials (RCTs; Lenze et al. 2005b; Schuurmans et al. 2006) and a full-scale RCT (Lenze et al. 2009) showed the efficacy of selective serotonin reuptake inhibitors (SSRIs) in the acute treatment of anxiety disorders, predominantly GAD, in older adults. In the latter study, which involved 177 older adults with GAD, escitalopram was superior to

placebo in cumulative response (69% vs. 51%). The effect size for most outcome measures in that study was in the low to medium range.

With respect to serotonin-norepinephrine reuptake inhibitors (SNRIs), retrospective examinations of venlafaxine extended release and duloxetine studies found them to be efficacious in adults 60 years or older (Davidson et al. 2008; Katz et al. 2002). Additionally, a large-scale study with pregabalin found it to be efficacious in geriatric GAD (Montgomery et al. 2008). Note that pregabalin is not approved by the U.S. Food and Drug Administration to treat anxiety disorders.

In addition to the studies of mainly GAD, some other medication studies should be noted: one supported the use of citalopram in PTSD (English et al. 2006), another supported superiority of mirtazapine over an SSRI (Chung et al. 2004), and a third found evidence that the α-adrenergic antagonist prazosin was efficacious for sleep-related concerns in PTSD (Raskind et al. 2007). Additionally, in late-life panic disorder, one study found evidence for the superiority of escitalopram over citalopram in time to response (Rampello et al. 2006), and a small open-label study found evidence of benefit from sertraline (Sheikh et al. 2004a). Finally, nortriptyline was efficacious in a merged dataset of several RCTs of post-stroke depression, in which patients with comorbid GAD were analyzed (Kimura et al. 2003).

The only published augmentation study in late-life anxiety disorders was a small study with risperidone (Morinigo et al. 2005). The use of atypical antipsychotics in elderly patients is problematic given concerns about higher mortality with antipsychotics compared with placebo in older patients with dementia. It remains unclear whether these risks apply to nondemented elderly persons.

The long-term or maintenance treatment of late-life anxiety with medication has not been studied, and no augmentation strategies can be recommended with confidence, although a pilot study has suggested benefits of sequencing SSRI with CBT (Wetherell et al. 2011), and two RCTs are under way to test this combination in late-life GAD.

No data exist on the efficacy and safety of complementary and alternative medications for anxiety in older adults. This is an important issue because it appears that many patients are using such treatments, which may have a potential role in treating anxiety. For example, stress reduction techniques such as Mindfulness-Based Stress Reduction, Tai Chi, yoga, and Qigong reduce cortisol and self-reported stress and anxiety symptoms in other samples. Complementary medicines are used by many patients for the treatment of anxiety, particularly kava kava, valerian, passion flower, and chamomile (Werneke et al. 2006). The safety and effectiveness of these and related treatments have not been rigorously studied in the elderly, however. Indeed, kava is banned in several European countries because of concerns about liver toxicity.

Treatment Guidelines for Assessing and Managing Anxiety in Elderly Persons

- *Assessment should measure severity and provide objective criteria for assessing response, as well as assess comorbidity, prior treatment, cognitive status, and need for a medical workup.* Anxiety assessment is challeng-

ing in older adults, who may not find terms such as *anxiety* or *worry* to be relevant (preferring words like *concern*). A helpful introduction to the topic is to ask about stress; for example, "Older adults often deal with stress; how do you feel in times of stress?" Patients who describe symptoms suggestive of anxiety or worry can then be further queried. Asking directly if anxiety or worry is "excessive" or "uncontrollable" is unhelpful. Nondirective questioning should be used to determine the severity of anxiety symptoms. *Geriatric anxiety disorders* are defined, in presence and severity, by 1) level of distress (how much the anxiety symptoms bother the patient, and what strategies are being used to control or avoid anxiety); 2) amount of time consumed by anxiety symptoms, including associated somatic and psychic symptoms; and 3) avoidance. Avoidance is one of the most disabling components of anxiety disorders that often is not recognized by patients. For example, older adults may downplay changes in behavior patterns as being a result of poor health. Paradoxically, avoidance also may take the form of excessive engagement in activities as a form of distraction or intrusive overinvolvement with family members as an attempt to decrease perceived loss of control.

Inquiring about somatic symptoms is helpful. For example, elderly patients may not endorse "panic attacks" but may admit to brief periods with multiple physical symptoms (particularly autonomic symptoms such as palpitations). Likewise, older patients with GAD may downplay the effects of worrying on their lives but more readily complain about distress from sleep disturbance or difficulty concentrating (regarding the latter, patients typically interpret these as memory problems, and elderly anxious patients often have concerns about Alzheimer's disease).

Although much emphasis has been placed on differentiating anxiety from depression, patients often fail to appreciate such a distinction. In reality, the clinician often must deal with anxiety as well as depression in a patient, sequentially or concurrently.

Most older adults who present with an anxiety disorder describe long-term, often lifelong, anxiety symptoms or anxiety proneness. Thus, a report that "I was never an anxious person, until just recently" should elicit consideration of 1) depression; 2) cognitive impairment (dementia, delirium); 3) anxiety-inducing medications (or recent discontinuation of sedatives); and 4) common and rare medical conditions that could masquerade as an anxiety disorder. Regarding the latter, the clinician should consider thyroid disease, B_{12} deficiency, hypoxia, ischemia, metabolic changes (e.g., hypercalcemia or hypoglycemia), and arrhythmia.

- *No knee-jerk benzodiazepine prescription should be given.* Benzodiazepines, like any sedatives, have a poor risk-benefit ratio in elderly persons. They are associated with an increased risk of falling in elderly persons. Using medications with shorter half-life and less complicated elimination (e.g., lorazepam) has not been shown to reduce the risk of falls or fall-related injuries. Furthermore, benzodiazepines appear to cause cognitive impairment in this age group, particularly in recall (Pomara et al. 1989, 1998a, 1998b). This cognitive problem is more likely with higher doses of benzodiazepines and in elderly persons who are already predisposed to cognitive impairment. Therefore, long-term use of benzodiazepines appears unfavorable in this age group, and patients should be warned about the risks associated with these medications.

  A common recommendation is to use these medications at low doses as a short-term adjunct, in which case they may provide some early relief and improve adherence to the treatment regimen. This short-term adjunctive use of benzodiazepines is typically unnecessary and can reinforce an inappropriate message to patients that anxiety must be immediately relieved (i.e., avoided). Because many patients will require psychotherapy, sending this contradictory message via benzodiazepine use should be minimized.

- *Psychoeducation about anxiety and treatment, including potential health benefits, should be provided.* Psychoeducation may be the most important management step because most older adults, even those with a lifelong history of anxiety, have never received the diagnosis before. Providers should inform patients that they have a treatable condition and should address stigma, misinformation, and other common and entirely remediable barriers to treatment. Of paramount importance (because it will improve treatment adherence) are the implications of treating anxiety for improving quality of life, health, and cognition.

- *Choice of first-line treatment should be based on patient preference, provider preference and competence, and treatment availability.* The patient's preference and the provider's competence should dictate the choice of first-line treatment. First-line options include one or more of the following: an SSRI, an SNRI, relaxation training, and CBT. Bibliotherapy can be recommended alongside any of these options, as well as more generic lifestyle changes regarding sleep, exercise, physical activity, and social engagement.

- *Frequent follow-up, particularly within the first month of treatment or dose change, is necessary to encourage adherence and monitor treatment response.* Antidepressants can initially have a stimulating or mildly anxiogenic effect. Older adults with anxiety disorders often report that they are sensitive or intolerant to antidepressant medications, which appears to stem from their anticipatory concern about side effects, their vigilance toward interoceptive stimuli, and their tendency to catastrophize about any sensations they detect. Thus, the anxiety itself interferes with adherence to pharmacotherapy.

Overcoming patient fears related to the medication's potentially negative effects is not an easy task. The management of this fear is part of the process of engaging the patient in treatment. The clinician should describe how such antidepressant medications have established efficacy and good tolerability in his or her experience. He or she should state that side effects are possible, but no particular side effect is inevitable, and most patients will have either no side effects or brief, self-limited side effects that subside in a few weeks. The clinician needs to emphasize that the medication is unlikely to be incapacitating. If a patient appears to be focusing on the laundry list of side effects associated with a drug, the clinician must explain that this is a list of all of the symptoms that pa-

tients in studies of this medication have described, however infrequently, and that the medication does not necessarily cause these side effects. When a patient mentions that "I already have that symptom," the clinician should assure the patient that he or she is not more likely to have that as a side effect as a result.

Family involvement can help with adherence. Patients' and families' concerns about medication should be addressed during the initial visit. Nevertheless, patients may have additional concerns between when the medication is prescribed and when they take the first dose. The clinician should explicitly state that it is natural for patients to have questions and should encourage them to call at any time to discuss them; 24-hour contact information should be given so that patients may telephone with concerns (typically they do not, but they are calmed by the knowledge that they can). We recommend weekly visits, or biweekly visits with interim telephone contacts, for the first month of treatment and the month subsequent to a dose increase because this is when patients are most likely to develop concerns about side effects.

At subsequent visits, the clinician should interview patients for concerns about perceived side effects. If such an issue is noted (even if the patient does not bring it up spontaneously or expresses that he or she does not think it is "important"), an immediate contact by the treating psychiatrist should ensue, usually as a same-day telephone call. This reassures the patient that he or she is being monitored closely by experts and that the medication is not causing some sort of severe or worsening problem. We have found that this oversight is helpful in reducing premature discontinuation of pharmacotherapy.

Patients usually get better, but given the fluctuating nature of anxiety disorders and the issues with insight, they often do not realize they are improving. Repeated assessment of symptoms can be helpful in showing improvement to the patient, particularly in the early phase of treatment.

- *Dosing of medications should start low, go slow, but go—as aggressively as required to treat symptoms to remission.* Elderly persons differ from young adults in terms of increased comorbid medical conditions, pharmacokinetic changes, frailty, drug interactions, and side effects. In particular, older and frailer or medically ill individuals need close monitoring (e.g., of gait, vital signs, or any incident medical issues that arise) along with lower starting doses. However, the main acute goal is a treatment course of sufficient intensity and duration to alleviate symptoms. Thus, inadequate treatment is at least as significant a problem as medication intolerance.
- *Clinicians should consider augmentation treatment and refer to experts if necessary.* Monotherapy is usually inadequate, and persistence is required. If a good trial does not help enough, another should be added. After the clinician has exhausted all options, he or she should refer the patient to someone with expertise in geriatrics or in other empirically supported forms of treatment for anxiety (e.g., a psychotherapist skilled at treating anxiety disorders).
- *The clinician should provide maintenance treatment or evaluate the need for such if treatment is discontinued.* Because anxiety is chronic and waxing or waning, treatment probably will need to be long-term (i.e., maintenance medication, booster therapy sessions). Maintenance pharmacotherapy tends to be simpler, with less frequent oversight required, although continued monitoring of side effects, changes in coprescribed medications, and patient concerns is important.
- *A patient who chooses to taper off a medication may need to resume it at some future point.* A medication taper should be very gradual to avoid symptoms of rebound anxiety. In our experience, relapse following discontinuation of medication typically occurs within the first 3 months, whereas relapse following discontinuation of psychotherapy is often conditional on stressful life events coupled with failure to continue practicing anxiety management skills.

Conclusion

Significant advances have been made in the understanding of anxiety disorders in older adults. The high prevalence of anxiety disorders, and their close and reciprocal relations with cognitive impairment and with disability, highlights their importance for public health. There appears to be a strong bidirectional link between anxiety and neurodegenerative changes in aging. Effective treatments include antidepressants and psychotherapy. Following simple management strategies as outlined earlier in this chapter, clinicians can effectively manage anxiety disorders in older patients.

Key Points

- Epidemiological studies show wide variation of prevalence and suggest that generalized anxiety disorder (GAD) is the most common anxiety disorder in late life.

- Late-onset anxiety disorders are more common than previously thought but may appear qualitatively different from typical DSM-IV-TR disorders.

- Pharmacological and psychotherapeutic treatments are similar to those in young adults.

- Increased vigilance is required of the clinician to detect and manage anxiety in this age group.

- More research is needed to examine the nature, course, and treatment of these common syndromes.

References

Allgulander C, Lavori PW: Causes of death among 936 elderly patients with "pure" anxiety neurosis in Stockholm County, Sweden, and in patients with depressive neurosis or both diagnoses. Compr Psychiatry 34:299–302, 1993

Andreescu C, Lenze EJ, Dew MA, et al: Effect of comorbid anxiety on treatment response and relapse risk in late-life depression: controlled study. Br J Psychiatry 190:344–349, 2007

Arce E, Simmons AN, Lovero KL, et al: Escitalopram effects on insula and amygdala BOLD activation during emotional processing. Psychopharmacology (Berl) 196:661–672, 2008

Astrom M: Generalized anxiety disorder in stroke patients: a 3-year longitudinal study. Stroke 27:270–275, 1996

Ballard C, Neill D, O'Brien J, et al: Anxiety, depression and psychosis in vascular dementia: prevalence and associations. J Affect Disord 59:97–106, 2000

Barker-Collo SL: Depression and anxiety three months poststroke: prevalence and correlates. Arch Clin Neuropsychol 22:519–531, 2007

Barrowclough C, King P, Colville J, et al: A randomized trial of the effectiveness of cognitive-behavioral therapy and supportive counseling for anxiety symptoms in older adults. J Consult Clin Psychol 69:756–762, 2001

Beaudreau SA, O'Hara R: Late-life anxiety and cognitive impairment: a review. Am J Geriatr Psychiatry 16:790–803, 2008

Beekman AT, de Beurs E, van Balkom AJ, et al: Anxiety and depression in later life: co-occurrence and communality of risk factors. Am J Psychiatry 157:89–95, 2000

Benitez CI, Smith K, Vasile RG, et al: Use of benzodiazepines and selective serotonin reuptake inhibitors in middle-aged and older adults with anxiety disorders: a longitudinal and prospective study. Am J Geriatr Psychiatry 16:5–13, 2008

Bishop SJ: Neurocognitive mechanisms of anxiety: an integrative account. Trends Cogn Sci 11:307–316, 2007

Bissiere S, Plachta N, Hoyer D, et al: The rostral anterior cingulate cortex modulates the efficiency of amygdala-dependent fear learning. Biol Psychiatry 63:821–831, 2008

Blazer D, George KL, Hughes D: The epidemiology of anxiety disorders: an age comparison, in Anxiety in the Elderly: Treatment and Research. Edited by Salzman C, Lebowitz BD. New York, Springer, 1991, pp 17–30

Brenes GA, Guralnik JM, Williamson JD, et al: The influence of anxiety on the progression of disability. J Am Geriatr Soc 53:34–39, 2005

Brenes GA, Kritchevsky SB, Mehta KM, et al: Scared to death: results from the Health, Aging, and Body Composition study. Am J Geriatr Psychiatry 15:262–265, 2007a

Brenes GA, McCall WV, Williamson JD, et al: Feasibility and acceptability of bibliotherapy and telephone sessions for the treatment of late-life anxiety disorders. Clin Gerontol 33:62–68, 2007b

Brenes GA, Miller ME, Stanley MA, et al: Insomnia in older adults with generalized anxiety disorder. Am J Geriatr Psychiatry 17:465–472, 2009

Bryant C, Jackson H, Ames D: The prevalence of anxiety in older adults: methodological issues and a review of the literature. J Affect Disord 109:233–250, 2008

Butters MA, Bhalla RK, Andreescu C, et al: Changes in neuropsychological functioning following treatment for late-life generalised anxiety disorder. Br J Psychiatry 199:211–218, 2011

Castillo CS, Schultz SK, Robinson RG: Clinical correlates of early onset and late-onset poststroke generalized anxiety. Am J Psychiatry 152:1174–1179, 1995

Caudle DD, Senior AC, Wetherell JL, et al: Cognitive errors, symptom severity, and response to cognitive behavior therapy in older adults with generalized anxiety disorder. Am J Geriatr Psychiatry 15:680–689, 2007

Chou KL: Age at onset of generalized anxiety disorder in older adults. Am J Geriatr Psychiatry 17:455–464, 2009

Chung MY, Min KH, Jun YJ, et al: Efficacy and tolerability of mirtazapine and sertraline in Korean veterans with posttraumatic stress disorder: a randomized open label trial. Hum Psychopharmacol 19:489–494, 2004

Davidson J, Allgulander C, Pollack MH, et al: Efficacy and tolerability of duloxetine in elderly patients with generalized anxiety disorder: a pooled analysis of four randomized, double-blind, placebo-controlled studies. Hum Psychopharmacol 23:519–526, 2008

De Wit L, Putman K, Baert I, et al: Anxiety and depression in the first six months after stroke: a longitudinal multicentre study. Disabil Rehabil 30:1858–1866, 2008

DeLuca AK, Lenze EJ, Mulsant BH, et al: Comorbid anxiety disorder in late life depression: association with memory decline over four years. Int J Geriatr Psychiatry 20:848–854, 2005

Dombrovski AY, Mulsant BH, Houck PR, et al: Residual symptoms and recurrence during maintenance treatment of late-life depression. J Affect Disord 103:77–82, 2007

English BA, Jewell M, Jewell G, et al: Treatment of chronic posttraumatic stress disorder in combat veterans with citalopram: an open trial. J Clin Psychopharmacol 26:84–88, 2006

Flint AJ: Anxiety and its disorders in late life: moving the field forward. Am J Geriatr Psychiatry 13:3–6, 2005

Flint AJ, Rifat SL: Anxious depression in elderly patients: response to antidepressant treatment. Am J Geriatr Psychiatry 5:107–115, 1997a

Flint AJ, Rifat SL: Two-year outcome of elderly patients with anxious depression. Psychiatry Res 66:23–31, 1997b

Flint A, Bradwejn J, Vaccarino F, et al: Aging and panicogenic response to cholecystokinin tetrapeptide: an examination of the cholecystokinin system. Neuropsychopharmacology 27:663–671, 2002

Gagnon N, Flint AJ, Naglie G, et al: Affective correlates of fear of falling in elderly persons. Am J Geriatr Psychiatry 13:7–14, 2005

Jeste DV, Blazer DG, First M: Aging-related diagnostic variations: need for diagnostic criteria appropriate for elderly psychiatric patients. Biol Psychiatry 58:265–271, 2005

Jeste ND, Hays JC, Steffens DC: Clinical correlates of anxious depression among elderly patients with depression. J Affect Disord 90:37–41, 2006

Jorge RE, Robinson RG, Starkstein SE, et al: Depression and anxiety following traumatic brain injury. J Neuropsychiatry Clin Neurosci 5:369–374, 1993

Katz IR, Reynolds CF 3rd, Alexopoulos GS, et al: Venlafaxine ER as a treatment for generalized anxiety disorder in older adults: pooled analysis of five randomized placebo-controlled clinical trials. J Am Geriatr Soc 50:18–25, 2002

Kimura M, Tateno A, Robinson RG: Treatment of poststroke generalized anxiety disorder comorbid with poststroke depression: merged analysis of nortriptyline trials. Am J Geriatr Psychiatry 11:320–327, 2003

Kogan JN, Edelstein BA: Modification and psychometric examination of a self-report measure of fear in older adults. J Anxiety Disord 18:397–409, 2004

Landi F, Onder G, Cesari M, et al: Psychotropic medications and risk for falls among community-dwelling frail older people: an observational study. J Gerontol A Biol Sci Med Sci 60:622–626, 2005

Lauterbach EC, Freeman A, Vogel RL: Correlates of generalized anxiety and panic attacks in dystonia and Parkinson disease. Cogn Behav Neurol 16:225–233, 2003

Lavretsky H, Siddarth P, Kepe V, et al: Depression and anxiety symptoms are associated with cerebral FDDNP-PET binding in middle-aged and older nondemented adults. Am J Geriatr Psychiatry 17:493–502, 2009

Le Roux H, Gatz M, Wetherell JL: Age at onset of generalized anxiety disorder in older adults. Am J Geriatr Psychiatry 13:23–30, 2005

Lenze EJ, Wetherell JL: Bringing the bedside to the bench, and then to the community: a prospectus for intervention research in late-life anxiety disorders. Int J Geriatr Psychiatry 24:1–14, 2009

Lenze EJ, Mulsant BH, Shear MK, et al: Comorbid anxiety disorders in depressed elderly patients. Am J Psychiatry 157:722–728, 2000

Lenze EJ, Mulsant BH, Mohlman J, et al: Generalized anxiety disorder in late life: lifetime course and comorbidity with major depressive disorder. Am J Geriatr Psychiatry 13:77–80, 2005a

Lenze EJ, Mulsant BH, Shear MK, et al: Efficacy and tolerability of citalopram in the treatment of late-life anxiety disorders: results from an 8-week randomized, placebo-controlled trial. Am J Psychiatry 162:146–150, 2005b

Lenze EJ, Rollman BL, Shear MK, et al: Escitalopram for older adults with generalized anxiety disorder: a placebo-controlled trial. JAMA 301:296–303, 2009

Lenze EJ, Mantella RC, Shi P, et al: Elevated cortisol in older adults with generalized anxiety disorder is reduced by treatment: a placebo-controlled evaluation of escitalopram. Am J Geriatr Psychiatry 19:482–490, 2011

Lyketsos CG, Lopez O, Jones B, et al: Prevalence of neuropsychiatric symptoms in dementia and mild cognitive impairment: results from the cardiovascular health study. JAMA 288:1475–1483, 2002

Mantella RC, Butters MA, Dew MA, et al: Cognitive impairment in late-life generalized anxiety disorder. Am J Geriatr Psychiatry 15:673–679, 2007

Mantella RC, Butters MA, Amico JA, et al: Salivary cortisol is associated with diagnosis and severity of late-life generalized anxiety disorder. Psychoneuroendocrinology 33:773–781, 2008

Marsh L: Neuropsychiatric aspects of Parkinson's disease. Psychosomatics 41:15–23, 2000

Marsh L, Rao V: Psychiatric complications in patients with epilepsy: a review. Epilepsy Res 49:11–33, 2002

Mintzer JE, Brawman-Mintzer O: Agitation as a possible expression of generalized anxiety disorder in demented elderly patients: toward a treatment approach. J Clin Psychiatry 57 (suppl 7):55–63; discussion 73–75, 1996

Mohlman J, Gorman JM: The role of executive functioning in CBT: a pilot study with anxious older adults. Behav Res Ther 43:447–465, 2005

Montgomery S, Chatamra K, Pauer L, et al: Efficacy and safety of pregabalin in elderly people with generalised anxiety disorder. Br J Psychiatry 193:389–394, 2008

Morinigo A, Blanco M, Labrador J, et al: Risperidone for resistant anxiety in elderly persons. Am J Geriatr Psychiatry 13:81–82, 2005

Nagaratnam N, Ip J, Bou-Haidar P: The vestibular dysfunction and anxiety disorder interface: a descriptive study with special reference to the elderly. Arch Gerontol Geriatr 40:253–264, 2005

Narita K, Murata T, Hamada T, et al: Associations between trait anxiety, insulin resistance, and atherosclerosis in the elderly: a pilot cross-sectional study. Psychoneuroendocrinology 33:305–312, 2008

Nelson JC, Delucchi K, Schneider LS: Anxiety does not predict response to antidepressant treatment in late life depression: results of a meta-analysis. Int J Geriatr Psychiatry 24:539–544, 2009

Palmer K, Berger AK, Monastero R, et al: Predictors of progression from mild cognitive impairment to Alzheimer disease. Neurology 68:1596–1602, 2007

Paterniti S, Dufouil C, Alperovitch A: Long-term benzodiazepine use and cognitive decline in the elderly: the Epidemiology of Vascular Aging Study. J Clin Psychopharmacol 22:285–293, 2002

Paukert AL, Phillips L, Cully JA, et al: Integration of religion into cognitive-behavioral therapy for geriatric anxiety and depression. J Psychiatr Pract 15:103–112, 2009

Paulsen JS, Ready RE, Hamilton JM, et al: Neuropsychiatric aspects of Huntington's disease. J Neurol Neurosurg Psychiatry 71:310–314, 2001

Pinquart M, Duberstein PR: Treatment of anxiety disorders in older adults: a meta-analytic comparison of behavioral and pharmacological interventions. Am J Geriatr Psychiatry 15:639–651, 2007

Pomara N, Deptula D, Medel M, et al: Effects of diazepam on recall memory: relationship to aging, dose, and duration of treatment. Psychopharmacol Bull 25:144–148, 1989

Pomara N, Tun H, DaSilva D, et al: Benzodiazepine use and crash risk in older patients. JAMA 279:113–114; author reply 115, 1998a

Pomara N, Tun H, DaSilva D, et al: The acute and chronic performance effects of alprazolam and lorazepam in the elderly: relationship to duration of treatment and self-rated sedation. Psychopharmacol Bull 34:139–153, 1998b

Porensky EK, Dew MA, Karp JF, et al: The burden of late-life generalized anxiety disorder: effects on disability, health-related quality of life, and healthcare utilization. Am J Geriatr Psychiatry 17:473–482, 2009

Prull MW, Dawes LL, Martin AM 3rd, et al: Recollection and familiarity in recognition memory: adult age differences and neuropsychological test correlates. Psychol Aging 21:107–118, 2006

Rampello L, Alvano A, Raffaele R, et al: New possibilities of treatment for panic attacks in elderly patients: escitalopram versus citalopram. J Clin Psychopharmacol 26:67–70, 2006

Raskind MA, Peskind ER, Hoff DJ, et al: A parallel group placebo controlled study of prazosin for trauma nightmares and sleep disturbance in combat veterans with post-traumatic stress disorder. Biol Psychiatry 61:928–934, 2007

Richard IH, Schiffer RB, Kurlan R: Anxiety and Parkinson's disease. J Neuropsychiatry Clin Neurosci 8:383–392, 1996

Saxena S, Maidment KM, Vapnik T, et al: Obsessive-compulsive hoarding: symptom severity and response to multimodal treatment. J Clin Psychiatry 63:21–27, 2002

Schuurmans J, Comijs HC, Beekman AT, et al: The outcome of anxiety disorders in older people at 6-year follow-up: results from the Longitudinal Aging Study Amsterdam. Acta Psychiatr Scand 111:420–428, 2005

Schuurmans J, Comijs H, Emmelkamp PM, et al: A randomized, controlled trial of the effectiveness of cognitive-behavioral therapy and sertraline versus a waitlist control group for anxiety disorders in older adults. Am J Geriatr Psychiatry 14:255–263, 2006

Sheikh JI, King RJ, Taylor CB: Comparative phenomenology of early onset versus late-onset panic attacks: a pilot survey. Am J Psychiatry 148:1231–1233, 1991

Sheikh JI, Lauderdale SA, Cassidy EL: Efficacy of sertraline for panic disorder in older adults: a preliminary open-label trial. Am J Geriatr Psychiatry 12:230, 2004a

Sheikh JI, Swales PJ, Carlson EB, et al: Aging and panic disorder: phenomenology, comorbidity, and risk factors. Am J Geriatr Psychiatry 12:102–109, 2004b

Sibille E, Su J, Leman S, et al: Lack of serotonin1B receptor expression leads to age-related motor dysfunction, early onset of brain molecular aging and reduced longevity. Mol Psychiatry 12:1042–1056, 1975, 2007

Simmons A, Matthews SC, Feinstein JS, et al: Anxiety vulnerability is associated with altered anterior cingulate response to an affective appraisal task. Neuroreport 19:1033–1037, 2008a

Simmons A, Matthews SC, Paulus MP, et al: Intolerance of uncertainty correlates with insula activation during affective ambiguity. Neurosci Lett 430:92–97, 2008b

Simon NM, Smoller JW, McNamara KL, et al: Telomere shortening and mood disorders: preliminary support for a chronic stress model of accelerated aging. Biol Psychiatry 60:432–435, 2006

Sinoff G, Werner P: Anxiety disorder and accompanying subjective memory loss in the elderly as a predictor of future cognitive decline. Int J Geriatr Psychiatry 18:951–959, 2003

Stanley MA, Beck JG, Novy DM, et al: Cognitive-behavioral treatment of late-life generalized anxiety disorder. J Consult Clin Psychol 71:309–319, 2003

Stanley MA, Diefenbach GJ, Hopko DR: Cognitive behavioral treatment for older adults with generalized anxiety disorder: a therapist manual for primary care settings. Behav Modif 28:73–117, 2004

Stanley MA, Wilson NL, Novy DM, et al: Cognitive behavior therapy for generalized anxiety disorder among older adults in primary care: a randomized clinical trial. JAMA 301:1460–1467, 2009

Starkstein SE, Jorge R, Petracca G, et al: The construct of generalized anxiety disorder in Alzheimer disease. Am J Geriatr Psychiatry 15:42–49, 2007

Steffens DC, McQuoid DR: Impact of symptoms of generalized anxiety disorder on the course of late-life depression. Am J Geriatr Psychiatry 13:40–47, 2005

Stein MB, Simmons AN, Feinstein JS, et al: Increased amygdala and insula activation during emotion processing in anxiety-prone subjects. Am J Psychiatry 164:318–327, 2007

Swoboda KJ, Jenike MA: Frontal abnormalities in a patient with obsessive-compulsive disorder: the role of structural lesions in obsessive-compulsive behavior. Neurology 45:2130–2134, 1995

Thorp SR, Ayers CR, Nuevo R, et al: Meta-analysis comparing different behavioral treatments for late-life anxiety. Am J Geriatr Psychiatry 17:105–115, 2009

Todaro JF, Shen BJ, Raffa SD, et al: Prevalence of anxiety disorders in men and women with established coronary heart disease. J Cardiopulm Rehabil Prev 27:86–91, 2007

Urry HL, van Reekum CM, Johnstone T, et al: Amygdala and ventromedial prefrontal cortex are inversely coupled during regulation of negative affect and predict the diurnal pattern of cortisol secretion among older adults. J Neurosci 26:4415–4425, 2006

van't Veer-Tazelaar PJ, van Marwijk HW, van Oppen P, et al: Stepped-care prevention of anxiety and depression in late life: a randomized controlled trial. Arch Gen Psychiatry 66:297–304, 2009

Werneke U, Turner T, Priebe S: Complementary medicines in psychiatry: review of effectiveness and safety. Br J Psychiatry 188:109–121, 2006

Wetherell JL, Stein MB: Geriatric psychiatry: anxiety disorders, in Comprehensive Textbook of Psychiatry, 9th Edition. Edited by Kaplan BJ, Sadock VA, Ruiz P. Baltimore, MD, Wolters Kluwer, 2009, pp 4040-4046

Wetherell JL, Gatz M, Pedersen NL: A longitudinal analysis of anxiety and depressive symptoms. Psychol Aging 16:187–195, 2001

Wetherell JL, Thorp SR, Patterson TL, et al: Quality of life in geriatric generalized anxiety disorder: a preliminary investigation. J Psychiatr Res 38:305–312, 2004

Wetherell JL, Hopko DR, Diefenbach GJ, et al: Cognitive-behavioral therapy for late-life generalized anxiety disorder: who gets better? Behav Ther 36:147–156, 2005a

Wetherell JL, Lenze EJ, Stanley MA: Evidence-based treatment of geriatric anxiety disorders. Psychiatr Clin North Am 28:871–896, ix, 2005b

Wetherell JL, Sorrell JT, Thorp SR, et al: Psychological interventions for late-life anxiety: a review and early lessons from the CALM study. J Geriatr Psychiatry Neurol 18:72–82, 2005c

Wetherell JL, Stoddard JA, White KS, et al: Augmenting antidepressant medication with modular CBT for geriatric generalized anxiety disorder: a pilot study. Int J Geriatr Psychiatry 26:869–875, 2011

Yohannes AM, Baldwin RC, Connolly MJ: Depression and anxiety in elderly patients with chronic obstructive pulmonary disease. Age Ageing 35:457–459, 2006

Suggested Readings

Beaudreau SA, O'Hara R: Late-life anxiety and cognitive impairment: a review. Am J Geriatr Psychiatry 16:790–803, 2008

Bryant C, Jackson H, Ames D: The prevalence of anxiety in older adults: methodological issues and a review of the literature. J Affect Disord 109:233–250, 2008

Lenze EJ, Wetherell JL: Bringing the bedside to the bench, and then to the community: a prospectus for intervention research in late-life anxiety disorders. Int J Geriatr Psychiatry 24:1–14, 2009

Lenze EJ, Rollman BL, Shear MK, et al: Escitalopram for older adults with generalized anxiety disorder: a placebo-controlled trial. JAMA 301:296–303, 2009

Stanley MA, Wilson NL, Novy DM, et al: Cognitive behavior therapy for generalized anxiety disorder among older adults in primary care: a randomized clinical trial. JAMA 301:1460–1467, 2009

van't Veer-Tazelaar PJ, van Marwijk HW, van Oppen P, et al: Stepped-care prevention of anxiety and depression in late life: a randomized controlled trial. Arch Gen Psychiatry 66:297–304, 2009

Wetherell JL, Lenze EJ, Stanley MA: Evidence-based treatment of geriatric anxiety disorders. Psychiatr Clin North Am 28:871–896, ix, 2005

CHAPTER 12

BEREAVEMENT

MORIA J. SMOSKI, PH.D.
LARRY W. THOMPSON, PH.D.

Late-life bereavement is an important topic that is affecting a growing number of individuals as the population ages. We begin this chapter with a review of the demographics of bereavement, followed by theoretical and empirical perspectives on adjustment to the loss of a loved one. Finally, we review considerations in the diagnosis and treatment of complicated grief.

Late-Life Bereavement

Who Are the Elderly Bereaved?

The terms *bereavement* and *grief reaction* have been used to refer to any number of losses.

These losses include (but are not limited to) the death of a spouse, an adult child, another family member, or a close personal friend; divorce (Cain 1988); prolonged caregiving for a severely impaired relative (Bass et al. 1991); and a significant decline in one's own health, attractiveness, capabilities, opportunities, and so forth (Kalish 1987). When used in its narrowest sense, *bereavement* refers to the reaction or process that results after the death of someone close. Indeed, death of a spouse is generally accepted as the most common and traumatic life event that older people experience (Jacobs and Ostfeld 1977).

In the United States, the mean age at which widowhood or widowerhood occurs is 69 years for men and 66 years for women.

This work was supported in part by grant R01-AG01959 from the National Institute on Aging and grants R01-MH36834 and R01-MH37196 from the National Institute of Mental Health. In addition, author M.J.S. was supported by grant K23-MH087754.

Forty-five percent of women and 15% of men older than 65 have lost a spouse (Federal Interagency Forum on Aging Related Statistics 2000). The mean duration of widowhood or widowerhood is approximately 14 years for women versus only 7 years for men (U.S. Census Bureau 2001). These data, plus the fact that widowers are more likely to remarry after losing their wives, have often led to the interpretation that widowhood is a women's issue. However, research has shown that after the loss of a spouse, older men are at higher risk for mortality than are women. For example, in the University of Southern California longitudinal study of spousal bereavement, the first year after bereavement saw a mortality rate of 12% in men but only about 1% in women (Gallagher-Thompson et al. 1993; Thompson et al. 1991).

The rates of widowhood among persons age 65 years or older are similar for whites and Hispanics and are slightly higher for African Americans (U.S. Census Bureau 2001). Given the prediction that the elderly population in each of these ethnic groups will increase considerably over the next 20 years (Federal Interagency Forum on Aging Related Statistics 2000), there is a clear need to understand how the processes of bereavement are mediated by cultural factors.

Theories About Adjustment to Permanent Losses

Numerous theoretical perspectives on the function and process of bereavement have been developed over the years. For a more comprehensive review, the interested reader is referred to articles by Osterweis et al. (1984) and, more recently, Stroebe and Schut (1999) and Stroebe et al. (2001a).

Early work emphasized that mourning was a process whereby the bereaved gradu-

ally "surrendered" their attachment to the lost loved one by engaging in certain specific psychological and behavioral tasks that occurred at appropriate time points during the bereavement (Freud 1917 [1915]/1957; Lindemann 1944). This process was thought to be necessary for the individual to develop new constructive attachments to other people entering his or her life. Failure to complete these tasks would result in the development of a psychiatric disorder. Bowlby (1961) offered a somewhat different interpretation of grief behaviors. He posited that any involuntary separation, including bereavement, gives rise to many forms of attachment behavior (such as separation anxiety and pining) that reflect the person's desire to reunite with the lost person. Thus, the function of bereavement is not a surrendering of attachment but rather an attempt to regain a sense of connection with the lost object of attachment. With time, these behaviors were thought to dissipate through a series of stages, including shock, protest, despair, and finally breakage of the bond and adjustment to a new self.

Parkes (1972) and Horowitz (1976) proposed models that involve phases or stages of reaction to the death of a loved one. These models are similar to Kübler-Ross's (1969) seminal stage model of the reactions of individuals facing a terminal illness. Shock and disbelief, combined with emotional numbness and cognitive confusion, characterize the initial period, with intense free-floating anxiety and sharp mood fluctuations. The second phase generally begins as the numbness and anxiety start to decrease. During this period, family and friends gradually become less available and often convey the message that the bereaved person should be getting on with life and should be getting over his or her grief, although the individual is far from ready to do so. Specific symptoms such as frequent crying, chronic sleep disturbance, blue mood, poor appetite, low energy, feelings of fatigue, loss of interest in daily living, and problems with attention and concentration are common. Nevertheless, most individuals do not develop major depression, even though certain symptoms of grief and depression overlap. This second phase is described as a time of "yearning and protest," during which the bereaved may actively or implicitly search for the deceased (Parkes 1972). Although these seeking experiences may be startling to an outside observer (e.g., hallucinations of the lost loved one), they are common (approximately half of bereaved individuals in one study reported seeing, hearing, or sensing their deceased spouse within 13 months of their death) and sometimes are reported as positive or comforting (Carlsson and Nilsson 2007). The final phase is often referred to as "identity reconstruction" (Lopata 1996). During this period, the bereaved person gradually reinvests the psychic energy that has been completely focused on the lost loved one into new relationships and activities. Lopata (1996) estimated that identity reconstruction most often takes a year or more, depending on what she refers to as the "centrality of roles" involved and the complexity of new learning that must occur in developing a new sense of self.

Although stage theories of adaptation have been widely accepted by health care professionals, little empirical evidence exists to support these theories. For example, although stage theories would predict an eventual end stage in which grieving ceases, grief symptoms often do not abate in elderly widows and widowers (Bierhals et al. 1995). To expect that grief will resolve or end is now considered erroneous by some

theorists (Stroebe et al. 2001b). Bereavement, as Rosenblatt (1996) contended, is a dynamic process that may continue for several years and even for the remainder of one's life. Also, bereaved individuals do not proceed from one clearly identifiable phase to another in an orderly fashion, a fact particularly true of older adults. Maciejewski and colleagues (2007) provided one of the few empirical attempts to test a stage theory when they tested Jacobs's (1993) stage theory, in which the bereaved pass through stages of disbelief, yearning, anger, depression, and acceptance. Results were mixed. Across indicators, acceptance was the most frequent response given and yearning the second most frequent response at all time points across 2 years postloss. However, when examining the peak frequency within each indicator, peaks occurred in the predicted order. Disbelief was at its highest immediately postloss and declined over time; yearning peaked at approximately 4 months postloss and then declined; and all other indicators peaked in the predicted order (Maciejewski et al. 2007). Thus, although participants did not complete a stage before moving to a new one, the stage model did provide potentially useful information about the ebb and flow of a given characteristic of grief. Although the specific process of moving through stages has not been supported, the stage models provide a useful descriptive overview of many commonly recognized facets of the bereavement process.

Another trend in bereavement theory has been to consider environmental changes and role adaptation along with individual emotional and psychological adjustments. Whereas earlier positions focused solely on intrapsychic processes (e.g., Bowlby 1961), more recently theorists have incorporated interpersonal and social processes into their models (e.g., Neimeyer 1998). Grieving is not just a process involving preoccupation with the deceased, accepting the loss and trying to make sense of what has happened, and so on; it also involves attempts to construct meaning of the loss and reduce the chaos associated with such traumatic events. As Stroebe and Schut (1999, 2010) address with their dual-process model, the bereaved oscillate between dealing with *loss-oriented stressors* and dealing with *restoration-oriented stressors.* The former focus on the specific components of the loss leading to emotional, behavioral, and cognitive symptoms and how to deal with these; the latter pertain to how one must interact constructively with social/environmental systems to maintain adaptive function in social, vocational, and avocational activities. Grief "tasks" usually have included confronting the loss, restructuring thoughts and memories about the deceased person, and emotionally withdrawing from (but not forgetting) the deceased person. Restoration tasks include accepting the changed world, spending time away from grieving, and developing new relationships and identities. Stroebe and Schut (1999) argued that alternation or "oscillation" in dealing with these two types of stressors is critical in the adjustment process. Psychological mechanisms that help the individual avoid or minimize the massive effect of the loss are helpful in the adjustment process, provided that they are not persistently implemented and are not the only coping efforts used. Periodically engaging in restoration coping tasks serves to interrupt the process of coping with the loss, and this may in turn facilitate a gradual habituation to the loss. Balance in dealing with the two types of stressors as a result of oscillation thus precludes the preoccupation with one or the other that may lead to prolonged and complicated bereavement. Limited empirical support for this model is emerging, with individuals reporting actively dealing with both loss–oriented stressors and restoration-oriented stressors showing the best psychological outcomes (Bennett et al. 2010).

Course of Bereavement Symptoms and Clinical Definitions

Results from several longitudinal studies are consistent in their descriptions of the course of depressed mood, anxiety, well-being, and level of grief following a loss. Grief is separable from depression and can include components of nonacceptance of loss, emotional responses to the loss, and thoughts about the loss (Futterman et al. 2010). Generally, significant differences between bereaved and nonbereaved individuals are readily apparent during the first 6 months after the loss. However, at approximately 12 months post-loss, levels of reported distress in the bereaved are substantially reduced, and often the difference between bereaved individuals and nonbereaved control subjects may be difficult to detect (Harlow et al. 1991; Thompson et al. 1991). Although considerable recovery has occurred, many symptoms are still present (Harlow et al. 1991; Thompson et al. 1984).

Although a period of distress followed by gradual abatement may be the most common course following a loss, it is not the only pattern. Several recent prospective and retrospective studies have identified other common patterns, including *resilience* and *chronic grief*. Individuals identified as resilient show consistent low levels of depression or negative affect across the postloss period.

This pattern is perhaps surprisingly common, with estimates of the percentage of bereaved individuals following the resilient pattern ranging from 34% (Ott et al. 2007) to 45% (Bonanno et al. 2004). Resilient individuals were found not to differ from common or chronic grief groups in either relationship quality or interviewer ratings of interpersonal skill or warmth (Bonanno et al. 2004; Ott et al. 2007) and were more likely to use religious coping (Ott et al. 2007). Follow-up analyses found that the resilient group reported the most comfort from positive memories of their spouse and the least from search for meaning in the death (Bonanno et al. 2004). Identifying the characteristics of individuals following a resilient course is an active area of current research (Coifman et al. 2007a, 2007b).

Chronic grief (also referred to as *complicated bereavement* or *traumatic grief*) occurs in 10%–15% of individuals (Bonnano et al. 2002; Ott et al. 2007) and is characterized by unremitting distress that lasts for an extended period following a loss. Differential diagnostic criteria for normal and chronic grief, depression, and other stress disorders remain controversial at present. For abnormal grief, Horowitz et al. (1997) emphasized the importance of both *intrusive symptoms* and signs of *avoidance and failure to adapt*. Intrusive symptoms include unbidden memories, strong spells of severe emotion related to the lost relationship, and distressingly strong yearnings for the deceased. Signs of avoidance and poor adjustment are characterized by feelings of emptiness or of being very much alone; avoidance of people, places, or activities that remind one of the deceased person; unusual levels of sleep disturbance; and loss of interest and decreased engagement in social, occupational, or recreational activities. Evidence of these signs and symptoms must be present for 14 months af-

ter the loss. Similarly, Prigerson et al. (1999) have defined a category of "traumatic grief." Primary symptoms include yearning and searching for the deceased person, loneliness, and intrusive thoughts about the deceased person. These are accompanied by traumatic distress that includes purposelessness; numbness or detachment; disbelief; feelings of meaninglessness; loss of a sense of trust, security, or control; and excessive irritability, bitterness, or anger related to the death. Prigerson et al. (1999) indicated that traumatic grief does not include symptoms of avoidance, and the symptoms must be present for only 2 months.

Although no consensus is yet apparent, the groundwork is being laid for specific criteria to distinguish normal and abnormal (i.e., complicated or traumatic) grief reactions. Continued research is indicated to help refine and solidify what cognitive, affective, and behavioral features characterize these two forms. As data are accumulated, theories and therapies will continue to be modified. For example, as noted earlier, it is becoming increasingly apparent that continued attachment often can be comforting (Stroebe et al. 2010; Wortman and Silver 1987). Variations in grief practices across cultures also have emphasized the effect that cultural traditions and beliefs can have on bereavement practices and have widened the scope of what can be termed as *normal* grief reactions. Thus, one might wonder if it is necessary to minimize one's attachment to a deceased individual in order to resolve one's grief, or if grief resolution itself should be the goal. Other issues include what constitutes a reasonable time period for a "normal" grief reaction and what constitute the indisputable signs of abnormal bereavement patterns predictive of poor adjustment. Until these issues are resolved, the best the clinician can do is to use currently available guidelines, as noted in this chapter, to help evaluate the individual patient.

DSM Definitions

In DSM-IV-TR (American Psychiatric Association 2000a), bereavement is in the V Code section, meaning that it is a condition that may be the focus of attention or treatment but is not directly attributable to a psychiatric disorder. Bereavement within the first 2 months following a loss is also a specific rule-out for a major depressive episode in DSM-IV-TR, unless the episode is characterized by "marked functional impairment, morbid preoccupation with worthlessness, suicidal ideation, psychotic symptoms, or psychomotor retardation" (American Psychiatric Association 2000a, p. 356). Based in part on recent studies showing that the symptom severity and clinical course of individuals experiencing depressive symptoms that would otherwise meet major depressive episode criteria postloss do not differ significantly from individuals with symptoms meeting major depressive episode criteria not in the context of bereavement (e.g., Corruble et al. 2009; Karam et al. 2009), the bereavement rule-out for major depressive episode is proposed for removal from DSM-5. At present, it does not appear that a separate diagnosis of complicated, chronic, or traumatic grief will be included in DSM-5, although work continues on the development of consensus criteria and empirical support for such a diagnosis.

Risk Factors for Intensification of Grief

Grief has been characterized by many as not only a highly charged emotional state but also a significant risk factor for a wide range of negative outcomes, including mortality and major physical and mental health disturbances. On the contrary, some clinicians and researchers have been struck by the ability of many older adults to survive and cope quite well overall with the profound losses of old age. In their 10-year follow-up study of a national sample of bereaved men and women, McCrae and Costa (1993) found that the great majority of individuals showed considerable ability to adapt to this major life stress (although length of recovery seemed to vary considerably). Nevertheless, an attempt to identify elderly people at risk for negative outcomes after spousal loss is an important mental health objective (for a thorough review, see Sanders 1993 and Stroebe et al. 2001a). Variables often associated with prolonged or complicated bereavement include 1) age and gender of the survivor, 2) the mode of death, 3) presence of significant depression shortly after the death, 4) prior relationship satisfaction, and 5) social support. Strength of religious commitment and involvement, participation in culturally appropriate mourning rituals, and redistribution of roles within the family after the death also may affect the grief process, although these findings are not as consistent.

Gender differences in bereavement are complex. Stroebe and colleagues (2001b) concluded that "widowers are indeed at relatively higher risk [of death] than widows, and, given that death is the most extreme consequence of bereavement, much weight may be attached to this finding" (p. 69). Bowling (1988–1989) followed up 500 elderly widows and widowers for 6 years after their loss and found that men age 75 years or older had excessive mortality compared with men at the same age in the general population. Gallagher-Thompson and colleagues (1993) found that widowers who died within the first year of spousal bereavement had reported more often than survivors that their wives were their main confidants and that they had minimal involvement in activities with other persons after their wives' deaths. The differential psychological effect of bereavement on men and women also appears unbalanced. Several studies have found a greater effect of bereavement on depression scores in men than in women (van Grootheest et al. 1999; Williams 2003) or that men may begin to experience greater depression before the loss of their wives, which is maintained in bereavement (Lee and DeMaris 2007). Women have been found to have less life satisfaction than men following the loss of a spouse (Lichtenstein et al. 1996; Williams 2003) but also may experience more personal growth after the loss (Carr 2004). Referring to their dual-process model, Stroebe and colleagues (2001b) hypothesized that women are more focused on psychological aspects of coping with the loss, whereas men are more focused on restoring their life pattern without the loved one. However, societal and structural demands prompt flexible coping in women (e.g., in addition to loss-focused coping, women must adjust to new financial and domestic circumstances), whereas less pressure exists for men to engage with their nonpreferred coping focus. Further research is needed to determine whether less flexibility in coping focus mediates the relation between gender and psychological outcomes.

Violent, stigmatized (as in the case of AIDS), or unexpected deaths generally are associated with poorer adaptation (Farberow et al. 1987; Osterweis et al. 1984; Parkes and Weiss 1983; van der Houwen et al. 2010; Worden 2002), although comparisons between the effect of long-term ill-ness and the effect of unexpected loss have been inconsistent (Burton et al. 2006; Kitson 2000).

Clinically significant symptoms of depression within the first 2 months postloss are a significant risk factor for poor outcome over time. Lund and colleagues (1993) found that intense negative emotions at 2 months postloss—such as a desire to die and frequent crying—were associated with poor coping 2 years later. Wortman and Silver (1989) reviewed several studies indicating that depression confounds successful resolution of grief. Both early loss and preloss depression may play a significant role in adjustment. In a prospective longitudinal study of the course of bereavement outcomes, it appears that a higher proportion of individuals with preloss depression remained depressed at 18 months postloss (43%) than those without depression preloss (21%, based on Bonanno et al. 2002). In our own work investigating the relation between depression and later bereavement outcome (Gilewski et al. 1991), we found that individuals with self-reported depression in the moderate to severe range were at greatest risk for all other psychopathological symptoms, such as increased anxiety, hostility, interpersonal sensitivity, and other indices of global psychiatric distress. This result occurred whether their spouses had committed suicide or died of natural causes. However, subjects whose spouses had committed suicide and who were moderately to severely depressed at the outset had the highest mean score of any subgroup on the depression measure that was used, maintained higher mean levels of depression over time, and were more likely to score high on other distress measures. These data suggest that, again, the interaction of one or more risk factors may contribute to the greatest distress.

The effects of preloss relationship characteristics as a risk factor remain unclear (Parkes and Weiss 1983; Worden 2002). More positive ratings of satisfaction were associated with more severe depression initially, but this relationship was lower at 30 months postloss. Bonanno et al. (2002) found that poor relationship quality rated preloss was most strongly associated with either a pattern of preloss depression followed by an improvement in symptoms postloss or chronic depression beginning preloss and continuing throughout bereavement. Follow-up analyses did find increased idealization of the relationship in bereaved individuals, but the degree of idealization did not differ based on level of adjustment (Bonanno et al. 2004). Relationship dependency was associated with risk of chronic grief (Ott et al. 2007). Thus, relationship variables may interact with several other variables, including general psychological health and a change in perspective on the relationship over the course of the bereavement process.

The role of social support is less ambiguous overall. Since the publication of Cobb's (1976) seminal paper on the stress-buffering effects of social support, it has been widely recognized as a moderator of many kinds of life stress. Across bereavement types (e.g., spousal, parental) and ages, social support is predictive of grief, depressive symptoms, and positive mood (van der Houwen et al. 2010). In a comprehensive review of the role of social support in mitigating the effects of late-life spousal bereavement, Dimond et al. (1987) found in their longitudinal study that the total size of the reported support network at baseline was positively correlated with perceived coping skills and life satisfaction at later times of measurement. They also found that the quality of the network was inversely related to later depression and was positively correlated with later measures of life satisfaction. Finally, through a series of multiple regression analyses, they found that several baseline social network factors made independent contributions to the variance accounted for in predicting depression at later times of measurement. This finding suggests that social support mitigates severe negative reactions to the loss of a spouse in older individuals.

On the basis of these data, it is apparent that several risk factors are associated with a more difficult subsequent grief process in elderly individuals. It is noteworthy, however, that the available research was conducted with volunteer subjects typically with higher educational levels and often from higher socioeconomic levels. Furthermore, the response rate from this segment of our population tends to be extremely low (approximately 30%–40%), which clearly limits the generality of these findings. Greater efforts should be made to engage elderly persons who are economically disadvantaged, in poor health, with low social support systems and low community involvement. In addition, more studies are needed on the interactive effect of several of these risk factors (particularly because they may change over time in relative intensity or salience to the individual) as well as on whether the same risk factors apply to bereavement from other causes, such as divorce and death of a parent or an adult child. Clearly, more research is needed on risk factors among ethnically and culturally diverse elders as well.

Interventions for Late-Life Bereavement

Many clinical comments throughout the bereavement literature indicate that treatment can be immensely helpful to some individuals. The extent to which a treatment might be effective depends in large measure on the intensity and pattern of symptoms present. In some situations, it appears that intervention above the usual family and community support is not called for and indeed may even be counterproductive. In others, medication, psychotherapy, or a combination of the two would be advised. Decisions about treatment strategy are facilitated by knowing whether the symptom pattern is consistent with what would be termed a *normal grief reaction* for the particular cultural group with which the person is identified or if it appears that the severity, type of symptoms present, and risk factor profile suggest a complicated course. In particular, it is important to determine whether the symptom picture is consistent with the diagnostic criteria for some other psychiatric disorder, such as depression or posttraumatic stress disorder. This distinction is critical for making appropriate intervention choices (Raphael et al. 2001). Although the literature is not conclusive on diagnostic issues, the distinction between complicated and normal bereavement is often made, and given this, it seems reasonable to review treatments that have been used for individuals in one or the other of these categories.

Treatment of Complicated Bereavement

A thorough assessment of any comorbid psychological conditions should be conducted before beginning treatment for bereavement. This is especially important for conditions with similar symptoms to bereavement, such as depression. Clinical levels of depression should be treated with

medication and/or psychotherapy before the focus of treatment can effectively shift to bereavement (National Institutes of Health Consensus Conference 1992; Parkes and Weiss 1983; Raphael et al. 2001; Reynolds 1992). Reynolds (1992) stated, "Our clinical practice has been to intervene as early as 2 months, and certainly by 4 months, in the presence of clear syndromal major depression" (p. 50). Remission will enable the focus of treatment to return to the bereavement. Careful attention to the grief process can often then determine whether additional interventions are required. In particular, risk factors may become an important focus for remediation. For example, considerable evidence now indicates that older widowers may not thrive if they do not have a constructive support system. Isolation is a documented risk factor, and men undergoing stress may not have the requisite skills to build or implement a nourishing social network. It may become necessary to provide specific assistance with this problem. Once accomplished, other interventions may not be necessary.

Other common complications that are particularly significant in older bereaved persons (Rosenzweig et al. 1997) and that require treatment include posttraumatic stress disorder, anxiety disorders (that may or may not be related to the bereavement), and subsyndromal depression (Reynolds et al. 1999). A combination of medication and psychotherapy appears to be more effective than either alone when attempting to reduce psychiatric symptoms that occur with bereavement. For example, the late-life depression research group at the Western Psychiatric Institute tested the efficacy of nortriptyline therapy, interpersonal psychotherapy, and combined treatment in elderly patients with bereavement-related major depression and reported that combined treatment was superior to either intervention alone, particularly among patients age 70 or older (Miller et al. 1997; Reynolds et al. 1999).

In some instances, older persons either cannot or refuse to use psychotropic medications. Although recent data have suggested that "counseling" of various kinds may not be all that helpful with individuals undergoing a normal grief reaction, evidence indicates that various psychological treatments can have a positive effect in treating complicated bereavement (Currier et al. 2008; Neimeyer 2000). Both individual and group psychotherapies reflecting different theoretical perspectives have been used in treating complicated bereavement with mixed results (Raphael et al. 1993; Schut et al. 2001).

One of the more common psychodynamic therapies used with complicated bereavement is Horowitz's (1976) time-limited psychodynamic therapy. This 12-session phase-oriented strategy is designed to help individuals work through emotional reactions to traumatic life events. Careful attention is also paid to tailor treatment to the patient's particular personality type. Abreaction, clarification, and interpretation of defenses and affects are used to facilitate realistic appraisals of the implications of a death and to explore the effect of the loss of a relationship on the bereaved person's self-concept. Empirical data confirming its effectiveness are available (Horowitz et al. 1981, 1984).

Cognitive and cognitive-behavioral therapies of various forms are effective in treating patients with complex bereavement reactions (Currier et al. 2010). One such strategy focuses on core constructs known to be disrupted during intense grief (Viney 1990). As these disrupted constructs are identified through self-monitoring and Socratic questioning during treatment sessions, the patient learns methods of reconstructing shattered beliefs about the self, the present surroundings, and future events. A blend of cognitive and behavioral techniques (such as challenging dysfunctional thoughts and teaching specific behavioral skills for use in resolving interpersonal problems) has been applied successfully with individual patients (see Florsheim and Gallagher-Thompson 1990 for an example).

Another treatment for complicated grief involves principles similar to those featured in the treatment of posttraumatic stress disorder (Frank et al. 1997; Shear et al. 2005). The treatment for complicated grief included a series of cognitive-behavioral techniques such as imaginal exposure to the death scene; in vivo, graded exposure to avoided death-related circumstances; mindful breathing; reminiscence of positive and negative memories of the loved one; and writing good-bye letters to the deceased person. Also integral to the treatment were homework assignments involving listening to tapes of imaginal exposure. Following the dual-process model, the treatment also involved motivational enhancement and goal setting to facilitate restorative goals. The results of this treatment were encouraging: complicated grief, anxiety, and depressive symptoms were significantly reduced. In a randomized controlled trial, individuals undergoing complicated grief treatment showed a greater response than did those undergoing interpersonal psychotherapy (Shear et al. 2005).

Prigerson and Jacobs (2001) suggested that for bereavement-related major depression, interventions should follow the practice guideline for depression (American

Psychiatric Association 2000b), whereas for bereavement complications, use of selective serotonin reuptake inhibitors combined with cognitive-behavioral interventions is probably most effective. However, few empirical studies have focused on the efficacy of specific treatment programs. Open-label trials of bupropion (Zisook et al. 2001), nortriptyline (Pasternak et al. 1991), antidepressant treatment with either nortriptyline or sertraline (Oakley et al. 2002), and paroxetine (Zygmont et al. 1998) for bereavement-related major depression in older adults have shown promise. As Hensley (2006) noted in her review of medication treatments for bereavement-related depression, antidepressant medications appear to have a larger effect on depressive symptoms than on grief-specific symptoms.

Finally, several recent interventions have targeted caregivers both to reduce distress during caregiving and to attempt to prevent complications during bereavement. A caregiver support intervention targeting caregivers of patients with Alzheimer's disease reduced depressive symptoms both pre- and postloss compared with no-treatment control subjects (Haley et al. 2008). Another intervention for caregivers of patients with Alzheimer's disease was found to reduce grief symptoms, although its effect on depression symptoms was less clear (Holland et al. 2009). Given that preloss psychopathology, including depression, is a predictor of chronic grief, interventions for at-risk populations such as caregivers have promise in altering the course of symptoms postloss.

Treatment of Normal Grief Reactions

There is a long history of formal and informal interventions for normal grief reactions, including self-help groups and individual and group counseling. Most bereaved persons (particularly elders) do not seek professional assistance for their grief. Self-help support groups for bereaved persons are often used by those who find the experience too painful and the loneliness overwhelming. Despite conceptual and anecdotal support for the effectiveness of these programs, relatively little empirical support has been found. Several reviews have examined the literature on counseling for normal grief reactions and have concluded that these interventions by and large do not reduce grief or depressive symptoms above and beyond the effects of time, nor do they facilitate better adjustment postintervention (Currier et al. 2008; Jordan and Neimeyer 2003; Schut et al. 2001). In fact, individuals experiencing uncomplicated bereavement may experience an iatrogenic effect of treatment, appearing worse off at the end of the treatment than if they had not participated (Neimeyer 2000).

Furthermore, the use of medication for the treatment of uncomplicated grief (other than for specific symptoms such as insomnia) has been questioned. Many clinicians believe that medication, if used at all, should be minimal and brief. For example, Raphael et al. (2001) argued that if depression is not evident, then antidepressants should not be prescribed to reduce symptoms of grief. There are concerns that medication may impede recovery by masking the full experience of bereavement (Parkes 1972; Worden 2002) and that prescribing medication pathologizes a natural human process. Others believe that the provider should intervene sooner rather than later, given the tendency of depressive symptoms to persist throughout the first year of spousal bereavement (Reynolds 1992). It has been noted that empirical evidence is limited that one must go through a difficult grieving process in order to resume one's life effectively (Bonanno et al. 2002); therefore, it is argued that pharmacological (and other) treatments for pain and suffering should be available to those who request them (Wortman and Silver 1987). Further research is necessary to determine the optimum level of pharmacological intervention to both ease suffering and allow the natural process of bereavement to take its course.

Key Points

- *Bereavement* can refer to a person's reactions to any set of significant losses but typically refers to the loss of a loved one such as a spouse.

- Among persons age 65 and older, 45% of women and 15% of men have experienced the loss of a spouse.

- The *dual-process model* of bereavement outlined by Strobe and Schut focuses on the interplay of loss-oriented stressors and restoration-oriented stressors. These are stressors related to the loss of the presence of the loved one in a person's life (e.g., loneliness, loss of support) as well as stressors related to building a new life without the presence of the loved one (e.g., taking on roles previously performed by the spouse, changing one's identity from one of wife to widow). Bereaved persons oscillate in their focus on these two stressors, and this is thought to promote more healthy adjustment.

- Culture can play a key role in the expected course of grief and should be taken into account when assessing or designing interventions for complicated grief.

- Research by Bonnano and colleagues highlights different potential patterns of adaptation after the loss of a spouse. It is notable that many individuals show resilience to or recovery from depressive symptoms within 18 months after the loss of a spouse. However, symptoms of grief such as missing the deceased person and engaging in fond remembrances of the lost loved one may continue indefinitely, even in individuals who show minimal depressive symptoms.

- Postloss adjustment among bereaved individuals can vary widely. Several risk factors are predictive of poor adjustment. These include male gender; loss through a violent, stigmatized, or unexpected death; the presence of significant depressive symptoms early in the loss; poor coping skills and low self-esteem; and poor breadth and quality of social support.

- Bereavement reactions can be categorized as "normal" or "complicated" grief. Most people experience "normal" grief, which can include the experience of sadness, loneliness, or longing for the deceased; experiencing the "presence" of the deceased; and disruptions in sleep and appetite. Although no single standard set of criteria exists for a diagnosis of complicated grief, typical definitions include an element of prolonged duration of symptoms, marked distress, and avoidance of or failure to adapt to new life roles.

- Several empirically validated treatments are available for complicated bereavement, including cognitive-behavioral therapy and a complicated-grief treatment based on the principles of treating posttraumatic stress disorder.

- Normal bereavement typically resolves without the need for treatment beyond targeted interventions for specific symptoms (e.g., disturbed sleep). In fact, some common interventions for normal bereavement have been found to lead to a worsening of symptoms and are not recommended.

References

American Psychiatric Association: Diagnostic and Statistical Manual of Mental Disorders, 4th Edition, Text Revision. Washington, DC, American Psychiatric Association, 2000a

American Psychiatric Association: Practice Guideline for the Treatment of Patients With Major Depressive Disorder, 2nd Edition. Washington, DC, American Psychiatric Association, 2000b

Bass DM, Bowman K, Noelker LS: The influence of caregiving and bereavement support on adjusting to an older relative's death. Gerontologist 31:32–42, 1991

Bennett KM, Gibbons K, Mackenzie-Smith S: Loss and restoration in later life: an examination of dual process model of coping with bereavement. Omega (Westport) 61:315–332, 2010

Bierhals AJ, Prigerson HG, Fasiczka A, et al: Gender differences in complicated grief among the elderly. Omega (Westport) 32:303–317, 1995

Bonanno GA, Wortman CB, Lehman DR, et al: Resilience to loss and chronic grief: a prospective study from pre-loss to 18 months post-loss. J Pers Soc Psychol 83:1150–1164, 2002

Bonanno GA, Wortman CB, Nesse RM: Prospective patterns of resilience and maladjustment during widowhood. Psychol Aging 19:260–271, 2004

Bowlby J: Processes of mourning. Int J Psychoanal 42:317–340, 1961

Bowling A: Who dies after widow(er)hood? a discriminant analysis. Omega (Westport) 19:135–153, 1988–1989

Burton AM, Haley WE, Small BJ: Bereavement after caregiving or unexpected death: effects on elderly spouses. Aging Ment Health 10:319–326, 2006

Cain BS: Divorce among elderly women: a growing social phenomenon. Soc Casework 69:563–568, 1988

Carlsson ME, Nilsson IM: Bereaved spouses' adjustment after the patients' death in palliative care. Palliat Support Care 5:397–404, 2007

Carr D: Gender, preloss marital dependence, and older adults' adjustment to widowhood. J Marriage Fam 66:220–235, 2004

Cobb S: Presidential Address—1996: social support as a moderator of life stress. Psychosom Med 3:300–314, 1976

Coifman KG, Bonanno G, Rafaeli E: Affect dynamics, bereavement and resilience to loss. Journal of Happiness Studies 8:371–392, 2007a

Coifman KG, Bonanno GA, Ray RD, et al: Does repressive coping promote resilience? Affective-autonomic response discrepancy during bereavement. J Pers Soc Psychol 92:745–758, 2007b

Corruble E, Chouinard VA, Letierce A, et al: Is DSM-IV bereavement exclusion for major depressive episode relevant to severity and pattern of symptoms? A case-control, cross-sectional study. J Clin Psychiatry 70:1091–1097, 2009

Currier JM, Neimeyer RA, Berman JS: The effectiveness of psychotherapeutic interventions for bereaved persons: a comprehensive quantitative review. Psychol Bull 134:648–661, 2008

Currier JM, Holland JM, Neimeyer RA: Do CBT-based interventions alleviate distress following bereavement? A review of the current evidence. International Journal of Cognitive Therapy 3:77–93, 2010

Dimond M, Lund DA, Caserta MS: The role of social support in the first two years of bereavement in an elderly sample. Gerontologist 27:599–604, 1987

Farberow NL, Gallagher DE, Gilewski MJ, et al: An examination of the early impact of bereavement on psychological distress in survivors of suicide. Gerontologist 27:592–598, 1987

Federal Interagency Forum on Aging Related Statistics: Older Americans 2000: Key Indicators of Well-Being. Washington, DC, Federal Interagency Forum on Aging Related Statistics, 2000

Florsheim M, Gallagher-Thompson D: Cognitive/behavioral treatment of atypical bereavement: a case study. Clin Gerontol 10:73–76, 1990

Frank E, Prigerson HG, Shear MK, et al: Phenomenology and treatment of bereavement related distress in the elderly. Int Clin Psychopharmacol 12(suppl):S25–S29, 1997

Freud S: Mourning and melancholia (1917 [1915]), in The Standard Edition of the Complete Psychological Works of Sigmund Freud, Vol 14. Translated and edited by Strachey J. London, Hogarth, 1957, pp 237–260

Futterman A, Holland JM, Brown PJ, et al: Factorial validity of the Texas Revised Inventory of Grief-Present scale among bereaved older adults. Psychol Assess 22:675–687, 2010

Gallagher-Thompson D, Futterman A, Farberow N, et al: The impact of spousal bereavement on older widows and widowers, in Handbook of Bereavement. Edited by Stroebe MS, Stroebe W, Hansson R. Cambridge, UK, Cambridge University Press, 1993, pp 227–239

Gilewski MJ, Farberow NL, Gallagher DE, et al: Interaction of depression and bereavement on mental health in the elderly. Psychol Aging 6:67–75, 1991

Haley WE, Bergman EJ, Roth DL, et al: Long-term effects of bereavement and caregiver intervention on dementia caregiver depressive symptoms. Gerontologist 48:732–740, 2008

Harlow SD, Goldberg EL, Comstock GW: A longitudinal study of the prevalence of depressive symptomatology in elderly widowed and married women. Arch Gen Psychiatry 48:1065–1068, 1991

Hensley PL: Treatment of bereavement-related depression and traumatic grief. J Affect Disord 92:117–124, 2006

Holland JM, Currier JM, Gallagher-Thompson D: Outcomes from the Resources for Enhancing Alzheimer's Caregiver Health (REACH) program for bereaved caregivers. Psychol Aging 24:190–202, 2009

Horowitz MJ: Stress Response Syndromes. New York, Jason Aronson, 1976

Horowitz MJ, Krupnick J, Kaltreider N, et al: Initial response to parental death. Arch Gen Psychiatry 38:316–323, 1981

Horowitz MJ, Weiss DS, Kaltreider N, et al: Reactions to the death of a parent: results from patients and field subjects. J Nerv Ment Dis 172:383–392, 1984

Horowitz MJ, Siegel B, Holen A, et al: Diagnostic criteria for complicated grief disorder. Am J Psychiatry 154:904–910, 1997

Jacobs S: Pathologic Grief: Maladaptation to Loss. Washington, DC, American Psychiatric Press, 1993

Jacobs SC, Ostfeld AM: An epidemiological review of the mortality of bereavement. Psychosom Med 39:344–357, 1977

Jordan JR, Niemeyer RA: Does grief counseling work? Death Stud 27:765–786, 2003

Kalish RA: Older people and grief. Generations 11:33–38, 1987

Karam EG, Tabet CC, Alam D, et al: Bereavement related and nonbereavement related depressions: a comparative field study. J Affect Disord 112:102–110, 2009

Kitson GC: Adjustment to violent and natural deaths in later and earlier life for black and white widows. J Gerontol B Psychol Sci Soc Sci 55:S341–S351, 2000

Kübler-Ross E: On Death and Dying. New York, Simon & Schuster, 1969

Lee GR, DeMaris A: Widowhood, gender, and depression: a longitudinal analysis. Res Aging 29:56–72, 2007

Lichtenstein P, Gatz M, Pedersen NL, et al: A co-twin-control study of response to widowhood. J Gerontol B Psychol Sci Soc Sci 51B:P279–P289, 1996

Lindemann E: Symptomatology and management of acute grief. Am J Psychiatry 101:141–148, 1944

Lopata HZ: Current Widowhood: Myths and Realities. Thousand Oaks, CA, Sage, 1996

Lund DA, Caserta M, Dimond M: The course of spousal bereavement in later life, in Handbook of Bereavement. Edited by Stroebe MS, Stroebe W, Hansson R. Cambridge, UK, Cambridge University Press, 1993, pp 240–254

Maciejewski PK, Zhang B, Block SD, et al: An empirical examination of the stage theory of grief. JAMA 297:716–723, 2007

McCrae RR, Costa PT: Psychological resilience among widowed men and women: a 10-year follow-up of a national sample, in Handbook of Bereavement. Edited by Stroebe MS, Stroebe W, Hansson R. Cambridge, UK, Cambridge University Press, 1993, pp 196–207

Miller MD, Wolfson L, Frank E, et al: Using interpersonal psychotherapy (IPT) in a combined psychotherapy/medication research protocol with depressed elders: a descriptive report with case vignettes. J Psychother Pract Res 7:47–55, 1997

National Institutes of Health Consensus Conference: Diagnosis and treatment of depression in late life. JAMA 268:1018–1024, 1992

Neimeyer RA: The Lessons of Loss: A Guide to Coping. Raleigh, NC, McGraw-Hill, 1998

Neimeyer RA: Searching for the meaning of meaning: grief therapy and the process of reconstruction. Death Stud 24:531–558, 2000

Oakley F, Khin NA, Parks L, et al: Improvement in activities of daily living in elderly following treatment for post-bereavement depression. Acta Psychiatr Scand 105:231–234, 2002

Osterweis M, Solomon F, Green M (eds): Bereavement: Reactions, Consequences, and Care. Washington, DC, National Academy Press, 1984

Ott CH, Lueger RJ, Kelber ST, et al: Spousal bereavement in older adults: common, resilient, and chronic grief with defining characteristics. J Nerv Ment Dis 195:332–341, 2007

Parkes CM: Bereavement: Studies of Grief in Adult Life. New York, International Universities Press, 1972

Parkes CM, Weiss RS: Recovery From Bereavement. New York, Basic Books, 1983

Pasternak RE, Reynolds CF 3rd, Schlernitzauer M, et al: Acute open-label trial of nortriptyline therapy of bereavement-related depression in late life. J Clin Psychiatry 52:307–310, 1991

Prigerson HG, Jacobs SC: Perspectives on care at the close of life: caring for bereaved patients: "all the doctors just suddenly go." JAMA 286:1369–1376, 2001

Prigerson HG, Shear MK, Jacobs SC, et al: Consensus criteria for traumatic grief: a preliminary empirical test. Br J Psychiatry 174:67–73, 1999

Raphael B, Middleton W, Martinek N, et al: Counseling and therapy of the bereaved, in Handbook of Bereavement. Edited by Stroebe MS, Stroebe W, Hansson R. Cambridge, UK, Cambridge University Press, 1993, pp 427–453

Raphael B, Minkov C, Dobson M: Psychotherapeutic and pharmacological intervention for bereaved persons, in Handbook of Bereavement Research: Consequences, Coping, and Care. Edited by Stroebe MS, Hansson RO, Stroebe W, et al. Washington, DC, American Psychological Association, 2001, pp 587–612

Reynolds CF 3rd: Treatment of depression in special populations. J Clin Psychiatry 53 (suppl):45–53, 1992

Reynolds CF 3rd, Miller MD, Pasternak RE, et al: Treatment of bereavement-related major depressive episodes in later life: a controlled study of acute and continuation treatment with nortriptyline and interpersonal psychotherapy. Am J Psychiatry 156:202–208, 1999

Rosenblatt PC: Grief that does not end, in Continuing Bonds: New Understandings of Grief (Series in Death Education, Aging, and Health Care, 0275–3510). Edited by Klass D, Silverman PR, Nickman SL. Washington, DC, Taylor & Francis, 1996, pp 45–58

Rosenzweig A, Prigerson H, Miller MD, et al: Bereavement and late-life depression: grief and its complications in the elderly. Annu Rev Med 48:421–428, 1997

Sanders CM: Risk factors in bereavement outcome, in Handbook of Bereavement. Edited by Stroebe MS, Stroebe W, Hansson R. Cambridge, UK, Cambridge University Press, 1993, pp 255–267

Schut H, Stroebe MS, van den Bout J, et al: The efficacy of bereavement interventions: determining who benefits, in Handbook of Bereavement Research: Consequences, Coping, and Care. Edited by Stroebe MS, Hansson RO, Stroebe W, et al. Washington, DC, American Psychological Association, 2001, pp 705–737

Shear [M]K, Frank E, Houck PR, et al: Treatment of complicated grief: a randomized controlled trial. JAMA 293:2601–2608, 2005

Stroebe M, Schut H: The Dual Process Model of Coping With Bereavement: rationale and description. Death Stud 23:197–224, 1999

Stroebe M, Schut H: The Dual Process Model of Coping With Bereavement: a decade on. Omega (Westport) 61:273–289, 2010

Stroebe MS, Hansson RO, Stroebe W, et al: Introduction: concepts and issues in contemporary research on bereavement, in Handbook of Bereavement Research: Consequences, Coping, and Care. Edited by Stroebe MS, Hansson RO, Stroebe W, et al. Washington, DC, American Psychological Association, 2001a, pp 3–22

Stroebe MS, Stroebe W, Schut H: Gender differences in adjustment to bereavement: an empirical and theoretical review. Rev Gen Psychol 5:62–83, 2001b

Stroebe M, Schut H, Boerner K: Continuing bonds in adaptation to bereavement: toward theoretical integration. Clin Psychol Rev 30:259–268, 2010

Thompson LW, Breckenridge JN, Gallagher D, et al: Effects of bereavement on self-perceptions of physical health in elderly widows and widowers. J Gerontol 39:309–314, 1984

Thompson LW, Gallagher-Thompson D, Futterman A, et al: The effects of late-life spousal bereavement over a 30-month interval. Psychol Aging 6:434–441, 1991

U.S. Census Bureau: Marital status of people 15 years and over, by age, sex, personal earnings, race, and Hispanic origin, March 2000. Released June 29, 2001. Available at: http://www.census.gov/population/www/socdemo/hh-fam/cps2001.html. Accessed August 12, 2008.

van der Houwen K, Stroebe M, Stroebe W, et al: Risk factors for bereavement outcome: a multivariate approach. Death Stud 34:195–220, 2010

van Grootheest DS, Beekman ATF, Broese van Groenou MI, et al: Sex differences in depression after widowhood: do men suffer more? Soc Psychiatry Psychiatr Epidemiol 34:391–398, 1999

Viney L: The construing widow: dislocation and adaptation in bereavement. Psychotherapy Patient 6:207–222, 1990

Williams K: Has the future of marriage arrived? A contemporary examination of gender, marriage, and psychological well-being. J Health Soc Behav 44:470–487, 2003

Worden JW: Grief Counseling and Grief Therapy, 3rd Edition. New York, Springer, 2002

Wortman C, Silver RC: Coping with irrevocable loss, in Cataclysms, Crises, and Catastrophes: Psychology in Action (The Master Lectures). Edited by VandenBos G, Bryant BK. Washington, DC, American Psychological Association, 1987, pp 185–235

Wortman C, Silver RC: The myths of coping with loss. J Consult Clin Psychol 57:349–357, 1989

Zisook S, Shuchter SR, Pedrelli P, et al: Bupropion sustained release for bereavement: results of an open trial. J Clin Psychiatry 62:227–230, 2001

Zygmont M, Prigerson HG, Houck PR, et al: A post hoc comparison of paroxetine and nortriptyline for symptoms of traumatic grief. J Clin Psychiatry 59:241–245, 1998

Suggested Readings

Bonanno GA, Wortman CB, Lehman DR, et al: Resilience to loss and chronic grief: a prospective study from pre-loss to 18 months post-loss. J Pers Soc Psychol 83:1150–1164, 2002

Breckenridge J, Gallagher D, Thompson LW, et al: Characteristic depressive symptoms of bereaved elders. J Gerontol 41:163–168, 1986

Currier JM, Neimeyer RA, Berman JS: The effectiveness of psychotherapeutic interventions for bereaved persons: a comprehensive quantitative review. Psychol Bull 134:648–661, 2008

Horowitz MJ, Siegel B, Holen A, et al: Diagnostic criteria for complicated grief disorder. Am J Psychiatry 154:904–910, 1997

Maciejewski PK, Zhang B, Block SD, et al: An empirical examination of the stage theory of grief. JAMA 297:716–723, 2007

Neimeyer R: Searching for the meaning of meaning: grief therapy and the process of reconstruction. Death Stud 24:531–558, 2000

Ott CH, Lueger RJ, Kelber ST, et al: Spousal bereavement in older adults: common, resilient, and chronic grief with defining characteristics. J Nerv Ment Dis 195:332–341, 2007

Prigerson HG, Shear MK, Jacobs SC, et al: Consensus criteria for traumatic grief: a preliminary empirical test. Br J Psychiatry 174:67–73, 1999

Stroebe M, Schut H: The dual process model of coping with bereavement: rationale and description. Death Stud 23:197–224, 1999

Worden JW: Grief Counseling and Grief Therapy, 3rd Edition. New York, Springer, 2002

Wortman C, Silver RC: Coping with irrevocable loss, in Cataclysms, Crises, and Catastrophes: Psychology in Action (The Master Lectures). Edited by VandenBos G, Bryant BK. Washington, DC, American Psychological Association, 1987, pp 185–235

CHAPTER 13

Sleep and Circadian Rhythm Disorders

Andrew D. Krystal, M.D., M.S.
Jack D. Edinger, Ph.D.
William K. Wohlgemuth, Ph.D.

Sleep disorders are an important aspect of geriatric psychiatry. In the United States, more than half of noninstitutionalized individuals older than 65 years report chronic sleep difficulties (Foley et al. 1995; National Institutes of Health Consensus Development Conference Statement 1991; Prinz et al. 1990), which affect quality of life, increase the risk of accidents and falls, and may lead to long-term care placement (Pollak and Perlick 1991; Pollak et al. 1990; Sanford 1975). Working effectively with elderly individuals requires expertise in the diagnosis and treatment of sleep disorders.

Sleep disorders are typically divided into 1) insomnias, 2) disorders of excessive daytime sleepiness, and 3) disorders of circadian rhythm. Insomnias are characterized by complaints of sustained difficulty in initiating or maintaining sleep and/or complaints of nonrestorative sleep, along with significant distress or impairment in daytime function (American Psychiatric Association 2000; American Sleep Disorders Association 1997). The insomnias include primary insomnia and comorbid insomnia (in which a psychiatric or medical disorder occurs along with the sleep disturbance) (American Psychiatric Association 2000).

Disorders of excessive daytime sleepiness are characterized by persistent daytime sleepiness that causes significant distress or impairment in function (American Psychiatric Association 2000; American Sleep Disorders Association 1997). The most important disorders of excessive sleepiness are sleep apnea, periodic limb movement disorder (PLMD), and narcolepsy.

Circadian rhythm disorders manifest as a misalignment between an individual's sleep-wake cycle and the pattern that is desired or required (American Psychiatric Association 2000; American Sleep Disorders Association 1997). The circadian rhythm is important for function because it is a cycle not only of sleep and wakefulness but also of many physiological processes and phenomena, including body temperature, alertness, cognitive performance, and hormone release (Czeisler et al. 1990; Folkard and Totterdell 1994; Minors et al. 1994).

The incidence of nearly all these sleep disorders increases with age. In addition, evidence shows that changes in sleep and the circadian rhythm occur even in healthy elderly individuals without such disorders (Bliwise 1993; Foley et al. 1995; Gislason and Almqvist 1987; Prinz 1995; Prinz et al. 1990). However, sleep and circadian rhythm disturbances are not an inevitable consequence of aging. A complication in this regard is that sleep disturbance that is linked to symptoms in younger individuals may not be associated with symptoms in elderly persons. Furthermore, clinical care of the elderly population requires a heightened awareness of and expertise in identifying underlying medical and psychiatric disorders.

Although these challenges can be formidable, they are not insurmountable. In this chapter, we review the changes in sleep and circadian rhythm that occur in individuals without medical and psychiatric disorders. We then review the disorders that can cause disturbances of sleep and chronobiology and whose likelihood increases with age. Finally, we discuss the treatment of a sleep complaint or suspected sleep-related dysfunction in elderly individuals.

Influence of Aging on Sleep and Circadian Functions

Extensive research has shown that marked changes in the duration, continuity, and depth of nocturnal sleep accompany normal aging (Hirshkowitz et al. 1992). Nocturnal sleep time steadily decreases across the life span, and nocturnal wake time increases because of an increase in arousals (Figure 13–1). Accompanying these changes are marked reductions in stages 3 and 4 sleep ("deeper" stages of non–rapid eye movement [NREM] sleep). Although the clinical significance of these changes is unknown, they may relate to the reported reduction in subjective sleep quality and lowering of the arousal threshold with age (Riedel and Lichstein 1998; Zepelin et al. 1984).

The amplitudes of both the sleep-wake cycle and the 24-hour body temperature rhythm appear to decrease with aging as well (Bliwise 2000; Czeisler et al. 1999). Older adults also tend to awaken at an earlier phase and show a greater propensity to awaken during the later portions of their sleep episodes (Dijk et al. 1997; Duffy et al. 1998). Furthermore, psychosocial changes that accompany aging may alter important *zeitgebers* ("time markers") for the circadian system and promote the onset of sleep difficulties.

Disorders Associated With Sleep and Circadian Rhythm Disturbances

Several medical and psychiatric conditions are associated with sleep difficulties, and these conditions occur more frequently with increasing age. The long-standing

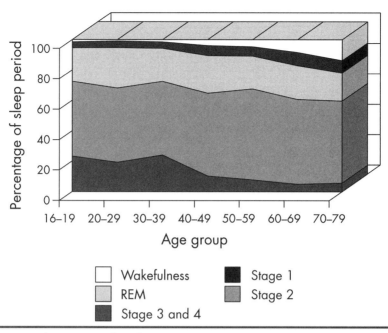

FIGURE 13–1. **Sleep-stage distributions across age groups.**

Note. REM=rapid eye movement.

view was that such conditions caused disorders of sleep and circadian rhythm (National Institutes of Health Consensus Conference 1984). More recent data suggest that the relation is often more complex than previously believed, and in some cases the causality appears to be bidirectional (Krystal 2006; National Institutes of Health 2005). The emerging view is that sleep disorders occurring with medical and psychiatric disorders have been undertreated and that the sleep problems are best thought of as *comorbid* and not *secondary* conditions (National Institutes of Health 2005).

Primary Sleep Disorders

Sleep Apnea

In sleep apnea, breathing ceases for periods of 10 seconds or more (Aldrich 2000), either because no effort is made to breathe (central sleep apnea) or because the oro-

pharynx collapses (obstructive sleep apnea). The frequency of obstructive sleep apnea increases with age (Ancoli-Israel 1989; Ancoli-Israel et al. 1991; Dickel and Mosko 1990; Roehrs et al. 1983). Apnea generally causes sleepiness, although mild to moderate apnea can be associated with insomnia. Referral to a sleep disorders specialist is required for diagnosis and treatment. The treatment of choice for obstructive sleep apnea is continuous positive airway pressure (CPAP). This treatment involves blowing air through the nose at night to increase pressure within the upper airway, thereby preventing the collapse that leads to apnea. Individuals with anatomical anomalies predisposing them to apnea are treated with upper airway surgery. Central sleep apnea is relatively rare (4%–10% of apnea cases) (White 2000) and has many causes, including alveolar hypoventilation, congestive heart failure, neurological disorders, and nasal and upper airway obstruction. Therapy should be targeted to the underlying process. When no such problem can be identified, CPAP is usually attempted (White 2000).

PLMD and Restless Legs Syndrome

In PLMD, repetitive muscular contractions occur during sleep; these contractions most commonly involve the legs and often cause sleep disturbances. The frequency of these events is characterized in terms of the number of movements associated with arousal per hour of sleep (the movement-arousal index). Thresholds for abnormality ranging from 5 to 15 movements per hour have been suggested (Ancoli-Israel et al. 1991; Dickel and Mosko 1990). Some authors have suggested that a higher threshold for abnormality should be applied to elderly patients (Ancoli-Israel 1989). PLMD is more prevalent in the elderly (Roehrs et al. 1983). Several studies indicate that clinically significant PLMD is seen in 30%–45% of adults age 60 years or older, compared with 5%–6% of all adults (Ancoli-Israel et al. 1991).

Individuals with PLMD may complain of leg kicks, cold feet, excessive daytime sleepiness, and insomnia (Ancoli-Israel 1989; Ancoli-Israel et al. 1991; Roehrs et al. 1983). The insomnia may be characterized by difficulty in falling asleep or staying asleep (Ancoli-Israel 1989). Unfortunately, PLMD is difficult to predict reliably on the basis of the history (Ancoli-Israel 1989; Dickel and Mosko 1990). Furthermore, a high level of confidence in the diagnosis is needed before institution of treatment because treatment typically involves long-term use of medications that can have significant side effects. Therefore, when a history is suggestive of PLMD, standard practice is to make a referral for a polysomnogram for definitive diagnosis (Ancoli-Israel 1989). Polysomnography (PSG) is also indicated when an individual has significant insomnia or hypersomnia that does not respond to usual treatment. Such a patient may have significant undetected PLMD.

Restless legs syndrome (RLS) is often associated with PLMD and is described as an uncomfortable feeling in the lower extremities that creates an irresistible urge to move. RLS occurs in 6% of the adult population and is present in up to 28% of patients older than 65 years (Clark 2001). PSG is not needed for a diagnosis of RLS.

RLS and PLMD have been associated with anemia (O'Keeffe et al. 1994). Ferritin levels less than 45 μg/L are associated with an increased risk of RLS, and such patients often benefit from administration of supplemental iron (O'Keeffe et al. 1994). Also associated with PLMD and RLS are diabetes mellitus, pregnancy, iron deficiency anemia, and use of certain medications, including antidepressants (Bliwise et al. 1985). The same medications are effective for both RLS and PLMD. The primary treatment for these conditions is dopaminergic agonists (Bliwise et al. 2005; Montplaisir et al. 1999). Second-line treatment options include anticonvulsants (gabapentin) and benzodiazepines (clonazepam). Opiates are typically reserved for patients whose symptoms do not respond to these other drugs.

Neuropsychiatric Disorders

Bereavement

Psychological factors that most commonly affect sleep in elderly persons are reactions to loss. Although bereavement is normal, it is often associated with substantial sleep disturbance (American Psychiatric Association

2000). Antidepressant medication may be helpful. A short course of sedative-hypnotic therapy may provide substantial symptomatic relief. If all symptoms of bereavement have resolved except insomnia, cognitive-behavioral therapy for insomnia should be considered. Grief counseling also should be considered.

Major Depression

Depression is frequently associated with sleep disruption in individuals older than 60 years. Approximately 10%–15% of individuals older than 65 years experience clinically significant depressive symptoms (Hoch et al. 1989). The most frequent sleep complaints in affected individuals are 1) experiencing a decrease in total sleep time and 2) waking earlier than desired.

Major depression is the condition for which the evidence is strongest for a complex bidirectional relation with sleep disturbance (Krystal 2006). Although insomnia has long been viewed as a secondary symptom of underlying depression, the results of a series of studies are inconsistent with this point of view (National Institutes of Health Consensus Conference 1984). The findings include evidence that those with insomnia have an increased future risk of major depression, that insomnia is an independent risk factor for suicide in depressed individuals, that antidepressant treatment frequently does not result in resolution of insomnia, and that this residual insomnia is associated with an increased risk of depression relapse (Breslau et al. 1996; Fawcett et al. 1990; Livingston et al. 1994; Reynolds et al. 1997).

The strongest evidence of the importance of depression is a study indicating that adding an insomnia medication (eszopiclone) to fluoxetine not only improved sleep but also led to greater and more rapid improvement in non-sleep-related depression symptoms (Fava et al. 2006; Krystal et al. 2007). However, the available research literature provides little guidance on the optimal management of insomnia occurring in this setting.

Alzheimer's Disease

People with Alzheimer's disease have been found to experience an increased number of arousals and awakenings, to take more daytime naps, and to have a diminished amount of rapid eye movement (REM) sleep and slow-wave sleep (Prinz et al. 1982). Individuals with dementia often experience evening or nocturnal agitation and confusion. This phenomenon, called *sundowning,* is among the leading reasons that individuals with dementia become institutionalized (Pollak and Perlick 1991; Pollak et al. 1990; Sanford 1975). Several features appear to increase the risk of sundowning, including greater dementia severity, pain, fecal impaction, malnutrition, polypharmacy, infections, REM sleep behavior disorder, PLMD, and environmental sleep disruptions (Bliwise 2000).

Treatment of sundowning should begin with an assessment for such conditions. If no causative condition can be found, or if attempts to eliminate the cause are unsuccessful, treatment such as light therapy, melatonin, structured activity programs, and eliminating naps should be considered. In terms of medications, benzodiazepines are ineffective (Bliwise 2000). Antipsychotic medications have the most evidence supporting efficacy (Bliwise 2000). Most studies involved older agents. The newer antipsychotics may have fewer side effects (Bliwise 2000), but they have been linked to an increased risk of mortality in this population (Kales et al. 2007).

Parkinson's Disease

Sleep complaints are noted in 60%–90% of individuals with Parkinson's disease (Trenk-walder 1998). Most Parkinson's disease patients experience difficulty in initiating and maintaining sleep, daytime fatigue, RLS, and an inability to turn over in bed. Another sleep problem seen in patients with Parkinson's disease is REM sleep behavior disorder, in which the patient acts out dreams because the paralysis that usually occurs during REM sleep is absent (Claren-bach 2000). No study findings indicate how to manage sleep difficulties in patients with Parkinson's disease.

Medical Conditions

Pain

Pain is a central feature of many conditions that occur with increased frequency in elderly individuals, including arthritis, neuropathies, angina, reflux esophagitis, and peptic ulcer disease (Aldrich 2000), and pain frequently disrupts sleep (Pilowsky et al. 1985). Attempts to ameliorate the condition causing the pain should be the first step. When these attempts fail, treatment for the pain should be instituted. Often, combined behavioral and pharmacological treatment is needed. Some evidence indicates that, as with depression, pain may have a bidirectional relation with sleep disturbance in that the treatment of insomnia improves pain (Edinger et al. 2005; Walsh et al. 1996).

Chronic Obstructive Pulmonary Disease

Individuals with chronic obstructive pulmonary disease (COPD) have been found to have both subjective and objective evidence of disturbed sleep (Douglas 2000). PSG is not routinely indicated for individuals with COPD who have sleep difficulties (Connaughton et al. 1988). Nocturnal oxygen may be needed in some patients (Connaughton et al. 1988). Oral theophyllines, which are frequently used in COPD treatment, are adenosine-receptor antagonists and may have a disruptive effect on sleep (Douglas 2000). Also, patients with COPD should be instructed to avoid alcohol, which can exacerbate hypoxemia and promote other complications. In severe COPD, the benzodiazepines triazolam and flunitrazepam, but not the nonbenzodiazepine zolpidem, adversely affected oxygenation (Murciano et al. 1993). However, in patients with mild to moderate COPD, both zolpidem and triazolam improved awakenings compared with placebo, and neither had an adverse effect on respiration compared with placebo (Steens et al. 1993). The melatonin receptor agonist ramelteon also has been found to improve sleep without adversely affecting respiration in patients with mild to moderate COPD (Kryger et al. 2008).

Cerebrovascular Disease

The sleep pathology associated with cerebrovascular disease depends on which areas of the brain are affected by the condition. Hypersomnia has been associated with lesions of the midbrain and paramedian region of the thalamus (Bassetti and Chervin 2000). Insomnia directly related to damage of specific areas of the brain is uncommon (Bassetti and Chervin 2000).

Nocturia

Nocturia (excessive urination at night) is the most common explanation given by elderly individuals for difficulty in maintaining sleep (Middelkoop et al. 1996). The most common causes of nocturia are conditions that increase in frequency with age: benign prostatic hypertrophy in men and decreased urethral resistance due to decreased estrogen levels in women (Bliwise 2000). Sleep apnea can also lead to nocturia (Bliwise 2000). Thus, when evaluating elderly individuals with complaints of sleep maintenance, the clinician should assess for nocturia and the associated conditions that increase the risk for nocturia.

Menopause

Evidence shows that many menopausal women experience sleep disruption in association with vasomotor symptoms (night sweats and hot flashes) that are caused by decreased levels of circulating estrogen and progesterone (Bliwise 2000; Krystal et al. 1998).

Elderly women with insomnia should be evaluated for underlying causes of sleep disturbance (e.g., medical and psychiatric conditions, primary sleep disorders), and clinicians should determine whether an association exists between changes in menstrual periods, vasomotor symptoms, and insomnia symptoms. If an association between insomnia and menopausal changes appears to exist, a trial of hormone replacement therapy could be considered. If hormone replacement therapy ameliorates vasomotor symptoms but insomnia complaints persist, behavioral therapy should be considered. If hormone replacement therapy is contraindicated or if use of this treatment is not preferred, other treatments such as pharmacological management of insomnia or cognitive-behavioral sleep therapy should be considered. Two studies (Dorsey et al. 2004; Soares et al. 2006) documented the efficacy of zolpidem 10 mg and eszopiclone 3 mg for improving sleep difficulties that occur in association with hot flashes.

Loss of Hearing, Vision, and Mobility

Many elderly individuals experience decrements in hearing, vision, and mobility (e.g., walking, driving). Changes in these vital functions can have a profound effect on sleep, which stems from a loss of activities in which the affected individual can engage. The person then takes unplanned naps or tries to sleep more than he or she is physiologically able to in order to pass the time. The result is fragmentation of sleep and loss of circadian rhythmicity. Although this problem should be easily solved by increasing activity and developing new activity options, in practice, making these changes is difficult to achieve.

Treatment of Insomnia

Cognitive-Behavioral Treatment

Myriad lifestyle changes that accompany aging increase risks of insomnia among older adults (Morgan 2000). Currently, a range of behavioral interventions are available for treating insomnia in these patients, including relaxation therapies, cognitive therapies, and treatments that target disruptive sleep habits. Among the more effective of these interventions is stimulus control therapy, developed by Bootzin (1972). This treatment is particularly useful for older adults who have fallen out of a normal sleep–wake routine and for those who compromise their nighttime sleep by excessive daytime napping. Stimulus control therapy addresses such problems by curtailing daytime napping and by enforcing a consistent sleep–wake schedule. In addition, this treatment enhances sleep-inducing qualities of the bedroom by eliminating sleep-incompatible behaviors in bed. The patient with insomnia is instructed to go to bed only when sleepy; establish a standard wake-up time; get out of bed whenever he or she is awake for more than 15–20 minutes; avoid reading, watching television, eating, worrying, and engaging in other sleep-incompatible behaviors in the bed and bedroom; and refrain from daytime napping.

Because older adults appear to have a reduced homeostatic sleep drive (Dijk et al. 1997) as well as a propensity to spend excessive time in bed (Carskadon et al. 1982), measures are often needed to reduce the amount of time older patients with insomnia allot for nocturnal sleep. Such a reduction is the aim of sleep restriction therapy (Spielman et al. 1987; Wohlgemuth and Edinger 2000). Typically, this treatment begins with the patient maintaining a sleep log. After 2–3 weeks, the average total sleep time (TST) is calculated. Subsequently, an initial time-in-bed (TIB) prescription may be set either at the average TST or at a value equal to the average TST plus an amount of time that is deemed to represent normal nocturnal wakefulness (e.g., 30 minutes). The TIB prescription is increased by 15- to 20-minute increments after weeks in which the person with insomnia sleeps more than 85%–90% of the TIB, on average, and continues to report daytime sleepiness. Conversely, TIB is usually reduced by similar increments after weeks in which the individual sleeps less than 80% of the time spent in bed, on average. Research suggests that stimulus-control and sleep-restriction therapies are more effective than most other nonpharmacological interventions (Morin et al. 1999, 2006; Murtagh and Greenwood 1995). Results of clinical trials also have generally suggested that therapies combining stimulus control, sleep restriction, and

cognitive strategies to alter dysfunctional sleep-related beliefs hold particular promise for treatment of the sleep maintenance difficulties so common in older age groups (Edinger et al. 2001, 2007; Morin et al. 1999).

Pharmacological Treatment

Studies of treatment for up to 2 weeks have established the risk-benefit profile for seven agents available in the United States for the treatment of insomnia. These are the benzodiazepines flurazepam, triazolam, and temazepam; the nonbenzodiazepines eszopiclone, zaleplon, and zolpidem; and the melatonin agonist ramelteon (Krystal 2009). Some of the benzodiazepines have half-lives that are too long for them to be suitable insomnia treatment agents, because of inevitable daytime impairment. Only triazolam and temazepam have half-lives in a range that makes them reasonable to use in the treatment of insomnia. Of the medications most frequently used to treat insomnia, the nonbenzodiazepine hypnotic zaleplon and the melatonin receptor agonist ramelteon have the shortest half-lives (approximately 1 hour), making them well suited for treating problems falling asleep. Because of its short half-life, zaleplon also may be useful in the middle of the night for individuals who sometimes wake up at that time (Stone et al. 2002). Zolpidem, with a half-life of approximately 2.5 hours, is another agent approved for the treatment of difficulties falling asleep. Although the agent with the shortest half-life that effectively treats the sleep difficulty should always be used to minimize risks, individuals with difficulty staying asleep generally need longer-acting agents. Of the agents available in the United States, eszopiclone is the only one shown to improve the ability to fall and stay asleep in older adults with insomnia (McCall et al. 2006). The tricyclic antidepressant doxepin (3 mg) recently was found to have significant benefit for sleep maintenance and early-morning awakening in older adults and a very favorable side-effect profile (Krystal et al. 2010). Although other antidepressants are widely used to treat insomnia in the United States (most notably, trazodone, mirtazapine, and amitriptyline), there has yet to be a study of any of these agents in older adults with insomnia (Walsh 2004).

The primary adverse effects of the benzodiazepines and nonbenzodiazepines are motor and cognitive impairment. Many older adults may be particularly vulnerable to adverse outcomes because of these effects. In terms of motor impairment, these agents might be expected to increase the risks for falls in older adults. Although evidence indicates an association of falls with benzodiazepines, nonbenzodiazepines, and medications with anticholinergic and antiadrenergic effects (includes antihistamines and antidepressants), studies also suggest that untreated insomnia increases the risks for falls (Allain et al. 2005; Avidan et al. 2005; Brassington et al. 2000; Koski et al. 1998; Nebes et al. 2007; Neutel et al. 2002; Suzuki et al. 1992). Further research will be needed to provide guidance, when managing insomnia in clinical practice, as to how to take into account the risks of falls caused by being awake at night versus the risks of falls caused by medications.

In summary, although cognitive-behavioral therapy always should be considered for the treatment of insomnia, medications may be needed in some cases. In general, it is best to use agents with relatively short half-lives to minimize risks of daytime im-

pairment. However, some older adults require an agent that addresses difficulty staying asleep. Several medications have been reported to have a favorable risk-benefit profile for the treatment of insomnia in older individuals and can be used in such cases. However, it is important to be cognizant of the risks of treatment in this highly vulnerable population. More studies of insomnia therapies in older adults and, in particular, of longer-term trials of treatment are needed.

Conclusion

Management of sleep disorders in elderly patients is challenging. Although sleep disorders are not an inevitable consequence of aging, elderly persons are more prone to primary sleep disorders and medical and psychiatric conditions that cause sleep difficulties. Therefore, evaluation of a sleep complaint in an elderly individual should include a thorough workup to determine whether primary sleep pathology and associated psychiatric and medical disorders are present. Effective behavioral and medication treatments exist for treating sleep and circadian rhythm disorders in elderly patients, but these treatments have significant limitations. More research is needed to develop and assess nonmedication therapies that are effective in treating insomnia and normalizing the circadian rhythm. Particularly promising areas in this regard include cognitive-behavioral sleep therapy and exercise programs.

In addition, research to improve medication treatment is needed. More medications are needed that can help elderly individuals stay asleep without causing next-day sedation. Furthermore, medications are needed that do not cause motor or cognitive impairment or anticholinergic side effects and that have been evaluated in trials of long-term treatment in older adults. Studies of the efficacy and safety of antidepressants in the treatment of insomnia in older adults are also needed. Finally, a better understanding of sundowning is needed, as are more effective treatments for this common condition.

Key Points

- More than one-half of noninstitutionalized individuals older than 65 years report chronic sleep difficulties.

- Although disturbed sleep is not an inevitable consequence of aging, the elderly are at increased risk for experiencing several sleep disorders and are uniquely vulnerable to the consequences of these disorders, which include insomnia, restless legs syndrome, sleep apnea, and disorders of circadian rhythm.

- Effective behavioral and medication treatments exist for treating sleep and circadian rhythm disorders in elderly patients, but more research is needed to develop improved treatments and to establish the risk-benefit profiles of some of the most commonly administered therapies.

References

Aldrich MS: Cardinal manifestations of sleep disorders, in Principles and Practice of Sleep Medicine, 3rd Edition. Edited by Kryger MH, Roth T, Dement WC. Philadelphia, PA, WB Saunders, 2000, pp 526–534

Allain H, Bentué-Ferrer D, Polard E, et al: Postural instability and consequent falls and hip fractures associated with use of hypnotics in the elderly: a comparative review. Drugs Aging 22:749–765, 2005

American Psychiatric Association: Diagnostic and Statistical Manual of Mental Disorders, 4th Edition, Text Revision. Washington, DC, American Psychiatric Association, 2000

American Sleep Disorders Association: The International Classification of Sleep Disorders: Diagnostic and Coding Manual, Revised Edition. Rochester, MN, American Sleep Disorders Association, 1997

Ancoli-Israel S: Epidemiology of sleep disorders. Clin Geriatr Med 5:347–362, 1989

Ancoli-Israel S, Kripke DF, Klauber MR, et al: Periodic limb movements in sleep in community-dwelling elderly. Sleep 14:496–500, 1991

Avidan AY, Fries BE, James ML, et al: Insomnia and hypnotic use, recorded in the minimum data set, as predictors of falls and hip fractures in Michigan nursing homes. J Am Geriatr Soc 53:955–962, 2005

Bassetti C, Chervin R: Cerebrovascular diseases, in Principles and Practice of Sleep Medicine, 3rd Edition. Edited by Kryger MH, Roth T, Dement WC. Philadelphia, PA, WB Saunders, 2000, pp 1072–1086

Bliwise DL: Sleep in normal aging and dementia. Sleep 16:40–81, 1993

Bliwise DL: Normal aging, in Principles and Practice of Sleep Medicine, 3rd Edition. Edited by Kryger MH, Roth T, Dement WC. Philadelphia, PA, WB Saunders, 2000, pp 26–42

Bliwise DL, Petta D, Seidel W, et al: Periodic leg movements during sleep in the elderly. Arch Gerontol Geriatr 4:273–281, 1985

Bliwise DL, Freeman A, Ingram CD, et al: Randomized, double-blind, placebo-controlled, short-term trial of ropinirole in restless legs syndrome. Sleep Med 6:141–147, 2005

Bootzin RR: A stimulus control treatment for insomnia. Proc Am Psychol Assoc 7:395–396, 1972

Brassington GS, King AC, Bliwise DL: Sleep problems as a risk factor for falls in a sample of community-dwelling adults aged 64–99 years. J Am Geriatr Soc 48:1234–1240, 2000

Breslau N, Roth T, Rosenthal L, et al: Sleep disturbance and psychiatric disorders: a longitudinal epidemiological study of young adults. Biol Psychiatry 39:411–418, 1996

Carskadon MA, Brown ED, Dement WC: Sleep fragmentation in the elderly: relationship to daytime sleep tendency. Neurobiol Aging 3:321–327, 1982

Clarenbach P: Parkinson's disease and sleep. J Neurol 247 (suppl 4):IV20–IV23, 2000

Clark MM: Restless legs syndrome. J Am Board Fam Pract 14:368–374, 2001

Connaughton JJ, Catterall JR, Elton RA, et al: Do sleep studies contribute to the management of patients with severe chronic obstructive pulmonary disease? Am Rev Respir Dis 138:341–344, 1988

Czeisler CA, Johnson MP, Duffy JF, et al: Exposure to bright light and darkness to treat physiologic maladaptation to night work. N Engl J Med 322:1253–1259, 1990

Czeisler CA, Duffy JF, Shanahan TL, et al: Stability, precision, and near-24-hour period of the human circadian pacemaker. Science 284:2177–2181, 1999

Dickel MJ, Mosko SS: Morbidity cut-offs for sleep apnea and periodic leg movements in predicting subjective complaints in seniors. Sleep 13:155–166, 1990

Dijk DJ, Duffy JF, Riel E, et al: Altered interaction of circadian and homeostatic aspects of sleep propensity results in awakening at an earlier circadian phase in older people. Sleep Res 26:710, 1997

Dorsey CM, Lee KA, Scharf MB: Effect of zolpidem on sleep in women with perimenopausal and postmenopausal insomnia: a 4-week, randomized, multicenter, double-blind, placebo-controlled study. Clin Ther 26:1578–1586, 2004

Douglas NJ: Chronic obstructive pulmonary disease, in Principles and Practice of Sleep Medicine, 3rd Edition. Edited by Kryger MH, Roth T, Dement WC. Philadelphia, PA, WB Saunders, 2000, pp 965–975

Duffy JF, Dijk DJ, Klerman EB, et al: Later endogenous circadian temperature nadir relative to an earlier wake time in older people. Am J Physiol 275:R1478–R1487, 1998

Edinger JD, Wohlgemuth WK, Radtke RA, et al: Cognitive behavioral therapy for treatment of chronic primary insomnia: a randomized controlled trial. JAMA 285:1856–1864, 2001

Edinger JD, Wohlgemuth WK, Krystal AD, et al: Behavioral insomnia therapy for fibromyalgia patients: a randomized clinical trial. Arch Intern Med 165:2527–2535, 2005

Edinger JD, Wohlgemuth WK, Radtke RA, et al: Dose response effects of cognitive-behavioral insomnia therapy: a randomized clinical trial. Sleep 30:203–212, 2007

Fava M, McCall WV, Krystal A, et al: Eszopiclone co-administered with fluoxetine in patients with insomnia co-existing with major depressive disorder. Biol Psychiatry 59:1052–1060, 2006

Fawcett J, Scheftner WA, Fogg L, et al: Time-related predictors of suicide in major affective disorder. Am J Psychiatry 147:1189–1194, 1990

Foley DJ, Monjan AA, Brown SL, et al: Sleep complaints among elderly persons: an epidemiologic study of three communities. Sleep 18:425–432, 1995

Folkard S, Totterdell P: "Time since sleep" and "body clock" components of alertness and cognition. Acta Psychiatr Belg 94:73–74, 1994

Gislason T, Almqvist M: Somatic diseases and sleep complaints: an epidemiological study of 3,201 Swedish men. Acta Med Scand 221:475–481, 1987

Hirshkowitz M, Moore CA, Hamilton CR, et al: Polysomnography of adults and elderly: sleep architecture, respiration, and leg movement. J Clin Neurophysiol 9:56–62, 1992

Hoch CC, Buysse DJ, Reynolds CF: Sleep and depression in late life. Clin Geriatr Med 5:259–272, 1989

Kales HC, Valenstein M, Kim HM, et al: Mortality risk in patients with dementia treated with antipsychotics versus other psychiatric medications. Am J Psychiatry 164:1568–1576, 2007

Koski K, Luukinen H, Laippala P, et al: Risk factors for major injurious falls among the home-dwelling elderly by functional abilities: a prospective population-based study. Gerontology 44:232–238, 1998

Kryger M, Wang-Weigand S, Zhang J, et al: Effect of ramelteon, a selective MT(1)/MT(2)-receptor agonist, on respiration during sleep in mild to moderate COPD. Sleep Breath 12:243–250, 2008

Krystal AD: Sleep and psychiatry: future directions. Psychiatr Clin North Am 29:1115–1130, 2006

Krystal AD: A compendium of placebo-controlled trials of the risks/benefits of pharmacologic treatments for insomnia: the empirical basis for clinical practice. Sleep Med Rev 13:265–274, 2009

Krystal AD, Edinger J, Wohlgemuth W, et al: Sleep in peri-menopausal and post-menopausal women. Sleep Med Rev 2:243–253, 1998

Krystal AD, Fava M, Rubens R, et al: Evaluation of eszopiclone discontinuation after co-therapy with fluoxetine for insomnia with co-existing depression. J Clin Sleep Med 3:48–55, 2007

Krystal AD, Durrence HH, Scharf M, et al: Efficacy and safety of doxepin 1 mg and 3 mg in a 12-week sleep laboratory and outpatient trial of elderly subjects with chronic primary insomnia. Sleep 33:1553–1561, 2010

Livingston G, Blizard B, Mann A: Does sleep disturbance predict depression in elderly people? A study in inner London. Br J Gen Pract 44:445–448, 1994

McCall WV, Erman M, Krystal AD, et al: A polysomnography study of eszopiclone in elderly patients with insomnia. Curr Med Res Opin 22:1633–1642, 2006

Middelkoop HA, Smilde-van den Doel DA, Neven AK, et al: Subjective sleep characteristics of 1,485 males and females aged 50–93: effects of sex and age and factors related to self-evaluated quality of sleep. J Gerontol A Biol Sci Med Sci 51:M108–M115, 1996

Minors DS, Waterhouse JM, Akerstedt T: The effect of the timing, quality, and quantity of sleep upon the depression (masking) of body temperature on an irregular sleep/wake schedule. J Sleep Res 3:45–51, 1994

Montplaisir J, Nicolas A, Denesle R, et al: Restless legs syndrome improved by pramipexole: a double-blind randomized trial. Neurology 52:938–943, 1999

Morgan K: Sleep and aging, in Treatment of Late-Life Insomnia. Edited by Lichstein KL, Morin CM. Thousand Oaks, CA, Sage, 2000, pp 3–36

Morin CM, Colecchi C, Stone J, et al: Behavioral and pharmacological therapies for late-life insomnia: a randomized controlled trial. JAMA 281:991–1035, 1999

Morin CM, Bootzin R, Buysse DJ, et al: Psychological and behavioral treatment for insomnia. Sleep 29:1398–1414, 2006

Murciano D, Armengaud MH, Cramer PH, et al: Acute effects of zolpidem, triazolam and flunitrazepam on arterial blood gases and control of breathing in severe COPD. Eur Respir J 6:625–629, 1993

Murtagh DR, Greenwood KM: Identifying effective psychological treatments for insomnia: a meta-analysis. J Consult Clin Psychol 63:79–89, 1995

National Institutes of Health: National Institutes of Health State of the Science Conference statement on manifestations and management of chronic insomnia in adults, June 13–15, 2005. Sleep 28:1049–1057, 2005

National Institutes of Health Consensus Conference: Drugs and insomnia: the use of medications to promote sleep. JAMA 251:2410–2414, 1984

National Institutes of Health Consensus Development Conference Statement: The treatment of sleep disorders in older people, March 26–28, 1990. Sleep 14:169–177, 1991

Nebes RD, Pollock BG, Halligan EM, et al: Serum anticholinergic activity and motor performance in elderly persons. J Gerontol A Biol Sci Med Sci 62:83–85, 2007

Neutel CI, Perry S, Maxwell C: Medication use and risk of falls. Pharmacoepidemiol Drug Saf 11:97–104, 2002

O'Keeffe ST, Gavin K, Lavan JN: Iron status and restless legs syndrome in the elderly. Age Ageing 23:200–203, 1994

Pilowsky I, Crettenden I, Townley M: Sleep disturbance in pain clinic patients. Pain 23:27–33, 1985

Pollak CP, Perlick D: Sleep problems and institutionalization of the elderly. J Geriatr Psychiatry Neurol 4:204–210, 1991

Pollak CP, Perlick D, Linsner JP, et al: Sleep problems in the community elderly as predictors of death and nursing home placement. J Community Health 15:123–135, 1990

Prinz PN: Sleep and sleep disorders in older adults. J Clin Neurophysiol 12:139–146, 1995

Prinz PN, Peskind ER, Vitaliano PP, et al: Changes in the sleep and waking EEGs of nondemented and demented elderly subjects. J Am Geriatr Soc 30:86–93, 1982

Prinz PN, Vitiello MV, Raskind MA, et al: Geriatrics: sleep disorders and aging. N Engl J Med 323:520–526, 1990

Reynolds CF 3rd, Frank E, Houck PR, et al: Which elderly patients with remitted depression remain well with continued interpersonal psychotherapy after discontinuation of antidepressant medication? Am J Psychiatry 154:958–962, 1997

Riedel BW, Lichstein KL: Objective sleep measures and subjective sleep satisfaction: how do older adults with insomnia define a good night's sleep? Psychol Aging 13:159–163, 1998

Roehrs T, Zorick F, Sicklesteel J, et al: Age-related sleep-wake disorders at a sleep disorder center. J Am Geriatr Soc 31:364–370, 1983

Sanford JRA: Tolerance of debility in elderly dependants by supporters at home: its significance for hospital practice. BMJ 3:471–473, 1975

Soares CN, Joffe H, Rubens R, et al: Eszopiclone in patients with insomnia during perimenopause and early postmenopause: a randomized controlled trial. Obstet Gynecol 108:1402–1410, 2006

Spielman AJ, Saskin P, Thorpy MJ: Treatment of chronic insomnia by restriction of time in bed. Sleep 10:45–55, 1987

Steens RD, Pouliot Z, Millar TW, et al: Effects of zolpidem and triazolam on sleep and respiration in mild to moderate chronic obstructive pulmonary disease. Sleep 16:318–326, 1993

Stone BM, Turner C, Mills SL, et al: Noise-induced sleep maintenance insomnia: hypnotic and residual effects of zaleplon. Br J Clin Pharmacol 53:196–202, 2002

Suzuki M, Okamura T, Shimazu Y, et al: A study of falls experienced by institutionalized elderly. Nippon Koshu Eisei Zasshi 39:927–940, 1992

Trenkwalder C: Sleep dysfunction in Parkinson's disease. Clin Neurosci 5:107–114, 1998

Walsh JK: Drugs used to treat insomnia in 2002: regulatory-based rather than evidence-based medicine. Sleep 27:14441–14442, 2004

Walsh JK, Muehlbach MJ, Lauter SA, et al: Effects of triazolam on sleep, daytime sleepiness, and morning stiffness in patients with rheumatoid arthritis. J Rheumatol 23:245–252, 1996

White DP: Central sleep apnea, in Principles and Practice of Sleep Medicine, 3rd Edition. Edited by Kryger MH, Roth T, Dement WC. Philadelphia, PA, WB Saunders, 2000, pp 827–839

Wohlgemuth WK, Edinger JD: Sleep restriction therapy, in Treatment of Late-Life Insomnia. Edited by Lichstein KL, Morin CM. Thousand Oaks, CA, Sage, 2000, pp 147–184

Zepelin H, McDonald CS, Zammit GK: Effects of age on auditory awakening thresholds. J Gerontol 39:294–300, 1984

Suggested Readings

Ancoli-Israel S, Richardson GS, Mangano RM, et al: Long-term use of sedative hypnotics in older patients with insomnia. Sleep Med 6:107–113, 2005

Bliwise DL: Sleep in normal aging and dementia. Sleep 16:40–81, 1993

National Institutes of Health Consensus Development Conference Statement: The treatment of sleep disorders in older people, March 26–28, 1990. Sleep 14:169–177, 1991

Pollak CP, Perlick D: Sleep problems and institutionalization of the elderly. J Geriatr Psychiatry Neurol 4:204–210, 1991

Pollak CP, Perlick D, Linsner JP, et al: Sleep problems in the community elderly as predictors of death and nursing home placement. J Community Health 15:123–135, 1990

CHAPTER 14

ALCOHOL AND DRUG PROBLEMS

DAVID W. OSLIN, M.D.
SHAHRZAD MAVANDADI, PH.D.

Alcohol and drug misuse are associated with a wide array of negative physical and mental health outcomes that are exacerbated with advancing age, such as functional and cognitive decline, compromised immune function, and depression. Yet relatively little work has examined the correlates and consequences of substance use among older adults. Accordingly, substance misuse in later life has been called an "invisible epidemic" (Widlitz and Marin 2002). Epidemiological work determined that beginning in the mid- to late 20s, overall rates of alcohol and illicit drug use begin to decline, with most older adults reporting no substance use. Nevertheless, changes in demographic and cohort trends suggest that substance misuse in later life is a pressing public health matter and that older adults represent a group in growing need of specialized substance treatment programs and

services (Gfroerer et al. 2003). Most notable among demographic changes is the aging of the "baby boom" generation. The baby boom cohort poses unique challenges; in addition to reporting higher rates of illicit drug and alcohol use and addiction than earlier aging cohorts, the baby boom cohort is significantly larger than previous cohorts (Koenig et al. 1994).

The potential public health effect of these demographic trends is highlighted by examining changes in rates of substance use and misuse in the last several decades. For example, it has been estimated that from the early 1990s until 2002, the prevalence of alcohol abuse or dependence tripled to 3.1% among adults age 65 and older (Grant et al. 2004). Heavy and binge drinking among adults older than 65 also has increased, with recent reports citing rates near 7.6% (Office of Applied Studies 2007). Reports of substance use among the baby boomers are notably higher; 22% of adults ages 50–54 were heavy or binge drinkers in 2006, and rates of illicit drug use among those in this age group increased from 3.4% to 6.0% from 2002 to 2006 (Office of Applied Studies 2007).

Guidelines and Classification: A Spectrum of Use

Proper screening, diagnosis, and treatment of individuals with drug and/or alcohol problems require an understanding of both drinking guidelines and the full range of substance use behavior seen among older adults. Because physiological factors render older adults more sensitive not only to alcohol and illicit drugs but also to over-the-counter and prescription medications, guidelines and recommendations for use of these substances by older adults differ from those applied to younger adults. For example, lean body mass and total water volume decrease relative to total fat volume in later life. As a result, total body volume decreases, thereby increasing the serum concentration, absorption, and distribution of alcohol and drugs in the body (Moore et al. 2007).

Because of these age-related factors, guidelines for alcohol use are lower for older relative to younger adults. Recommendations set forth by the Center for Substance Abuse Treatment's Treatment Improvement Protocol on older adults state that adults age 65 years and older should consume no more than one standard drink per day (Table 14–1) (Blow 1998; National Institute on Alcohol Abuse and Alcoholism 1995). Moreover, older adults should not consume more than two standard drinks on any one occasion (binge drinking). These drinking-limit

recommendations are in accord with data concerning the relation between heavy consumption and alcohol-related problems (Chermack et al. 1996) as well as evidence for the beneficial health effects of low-risk drinking among older adults (Klatsky and Armstrong 1993; Poikolainen 1991).

Recommendations for the appropriate use of prescription and over-the-counter medications must be considered on a case-by-case basis, with special consideration given to the potential benefits relative to the potential risks of medication use for each patient. There are no accepted safe limits for tobacco, marijuana, or other illicit drug use.

In addition to considering the quantity of consumption, diagnostic categories that include clinical effect are considered. The following categories and their definitions, which primarily focus on patterns of alcohol use, reflect both the clinical experience and the research findings of addiction specialists (Blow 1998).

Abstainers is the term used to describe individuals who report drinking fewer than 1–2 drinks in the previous year. This is the most common drinking pattern in later life, with approximately 50%–70% of older adults reporting abstinence (Blow 1998; Kirchner et al. 2007). Nevertheless, determining the reasons for abstinence has important implications for subsequent treatment and counseling of older adults who do not drink. For example, although some individuals may have had lifelong patterns of abstinence, others may not drink because of the onset or presence of acute or chronic illness. Furthermore, some individuals may abstain from alcohol use because of a history of alcohol problems or abuse. Past use may make older adults more vulnerable to other mental health problems such as psychiatric disorders or cognitive declines.

TABLE 14–1. Alcohol conversion chart

"One standard drink"

Beverage type	Quantity
Beer	12 oz.
Wine	5 oz.
Fortified wine	3 oz.
Hard liquor (80-proof distilled spirits)	1½ oz. (i.e., "a shot")
Malt liquor	8 oz.
Liqueur or aperitif	4 oz.

Additional conversions

Beverage type/quantity	No. of standard drinks
Beer	
1 6-pack of 16-oz. cans/bottles	8
1 quart	3
Wine (e.g., red, white, Chianti)	
1 bottle (750 mL)	5
1 magnum	12
½ gallon	16
Fortified wine (e.g., sherry, port; low-end wines [e.g., Thunderbird, "bum wine"])	
1 bottle (750 mL)	8
Hard liquor (e.g., bourbon, rum, gin, tequila, vodka)	
"Fifth" (750 mL)	17
"Pint" (250 mL)	5

Low-risk, social, or moderate drinkers include individuals who drink within the recommended guidelines (i.e., drink no more than one drink per day) and do not have any alcohol-related problems. Older adults in this group also observe caution and do not drink when driving a motor vehicle or boat or when using contraindicated medications.

Low-risk medication/drug use involves adhering to physicians' prescriptions. Nevertheless, it is important to evaluate the number and types of medications being used by low-risk users because harmful medication interactions still may occur among this group.

At-risk or excessive substance users among older adults are those who consume sub-stances above recommended levels yet experience minimal or no substance-related health, social, or emotional problems. Often the danger of drinking at this level relates to exacerbation of an existing medical problem such as diabetes or heart disease. Targeting and identifying older adults in this category are important; although they currently may not be experiencing any substance use–related problems, these individuals may have a high risk of developing alcohol- or medication-related health problems should their substance use remain consistent or increase over time. Nevertheless, because older individuals in this group are at a greater risk for negative consequences such as falls, liver disease, pancreatitis, and harmful interactions between alcohol and medications (Moore et al. 2000), they represent a group that would greatly benefit from screening, identification, and intervention.

Problem use or abuse describes a pattern in older adults in which alcohol or drug consumption is at a level whereby adverse medical, psychological, or social consequences have occurred or are significantly likely to occur. Thus, this category of use is not dependent on the quantity or frequency of use but rather the extent to which substance use impairs physical and psychosocial functioning.

Alcohol or drug dependence or addiction is defined, according to DSM-IV-TR criteria, as a medical disorder marked by clinically significant distress or impairment coupled with preoccupation with alcohol or drugs, loss of control, continued substance use despite adverse consequences, and/or physiological symptoms such as tolerance and withdrawal (American Psychiatric Association 2000). As is the case for substance use, DSM-IV-TR criteria are based mostly on research with young to middle-aged adults and have not been sufficiently validated among older populations; therefore, the symptoms and consequences set forth in DSM may not be sensitive enough to capture dependence in later life. Moreover, determining whether individuals meet diagnostic criteria relies heavily on self-reported behavioral symptoms. This is potentially problematic because self-report is susceptible to bias because of memory impairments, lack of insight or knowledge about the adverse effects of substance use, or unwillingness to admit symptoms. For example, benzodiazepine abuse and dependence may go unnoticed or unreported because of older adults not linking the consequences of medication use to health or social problems.

Epidemiology of Late-Life Substance Use

Alcohol

Even though alcohol misuse is often underreported and thus underestimated in later life, epidemiological work suggests that alcohol problems are common among older individuals. For instance, the most recent National Survey on Drug Use and Health reported that 51.6% of adults ages 60–64 years had consumed alcohol in the past month, with 37.8% reporting current nonbingeing or nonheavy alcohol use, 10.5% reporting bingeing behavior, and 3.3% reporting heavy use (Substance Abuse and Mental Health Services Administration 2011). With respect to alcohol abuse or dependence, epidemiological census-based work estimates that 2.4% of older men and 0.4% of older women meet diagnostic criteria for alcohol abuse, whereas an additional 0.4% and 0.1% of older men and older women, respectively, meet criteria for alcohol dependence (Grant et al. 2004).

Because substance misuse is more likely to be presented in health care settings, rates of alcohol problems and dependence are higher among clinical than among community-based samples. For example, Kirchner et al. (2007) reported that of the 24,863 individuals screened in primary care settings, 21.5% drank within the recommended levels (1–7 drinks per week), 4.1% were at-risk drinkers (8–14 drinks per week), and 4.5% were heavy (>14 drinks per week) or binge drinkers. Rates of abuse and dependence appear to be particularly high among patients in mental health clinics and nursing homes. In their study of 140 patients enrolled in a geriatric mental health outpatient clinic, Holroyd and Duryee (1997) found that 8.6% of patients met DSM-IV (American Psychiatric Association 1994) criteria for alcohol dependence. Oslin et al. (1997b) found that 29% of male nursing home residents had a lifetime diagnosis of alcohol abuse or dependence, with 10% of residents meeting criteria for abuse or dependence within 1 year of admission to the home.

Prescription and Over-the-Counter Medications

The use of pharmaceutical drugs is prevalent in older adulthood, and the risk of misusing prescription and over-the-counter medications, which include substances such as sedatives-hypnotics, narcotic and nonnarcotic analgesics, diet aids, and decongestants, also increases with age. According to a review of the scant literature on this topic, up to 11% of older women misuse prescription drugs, and it is projected that by the year 2020, 2.7 million adults will be using prescription drugs for nonmedical purposes (Simoni-Wastila and Yang 2006). A large proportion of medications prescribed to older adults include psychoactive, mood-altering drugs.

Examination of pharmaceutical data supports the notion that older adults are more likely than younger people to take multiple medications (Golden et al. 1999; Lassila et al. 1996). For instance, in one study of rural, community-dwelling older adults, 71% of the 1,360 participants sampled reported regularly taking at least 1 prescription medication, and 10% reported taking 5 or more medications (Lassila et al. 1996). In fact, it has been estimated that the average older patient takes 5.3 prescription medications each day (Golden et al. 1999). Over-the-counter drug use also is quite common; in one study, 87% of the older adults reported regular use of over-the-counter medications, and 5.7% were taking 5 or more over-the-counter medications concurrently (Stoehr et al. 1997).

Illicit Drugs

Unlike alcohol and prescription/over-the-counter medication use, illicit drug use among older adults is rare. According to the most recent National Household Survey on Drug Use and Health, the percentage of adults ages 55–59 using illicit drugs in the past month increased from 1.9% in 2002 to 4.1% in 2010 (Substance Abuse and Mental Health Services Administration 2011). Although this increase in drug use may not seem significant, it is important to keep in mind that the baby boomers represent the only age group that showed notable increases in illicit substance use during the designated time period.

Correlates and Consequences of Substance Use Problems

Correlates of and Risk Factors for Substance Abuse

Several studies have sought to identify factors that are related to increased vulnerability to substance misuse and the maintenance of problematic substance use patterns in later life. Factors such as gender, medical comorbidity, history of past use, and social and family environment are all correlated with problematic substance use. Longitudinal work, for instance, suggests that older men tend to drink greater quantities of alcohol than do women and are more likely to have alcohol-related problems (Moore et al. 2005). Furthermore, increases in free time coupled with a reduction in role obligations may have a large effect on problem drinking in older women (Wilsnack and Wilsnack 1995). Indeed, age-related losses in social, physical, and occupational/role domains, such as widowhood, the death of family and friends, reduced physical function, and retirement, help contribute to the adoption or maintenance of abusive drinking patterns in later life among men and women (Blow 1998). Finally, longitudinal work has found that additional social context and life history factors, such as friends' approval of drinking and a history of heavy drinking or alcohol problems, also are related to a higher likelihood of late-life drinking problems (Moos et al. 2004).

With respect to prescription and over-the-counter drugs, factors such as declining physical health and physiological changes that accompany the aging process increase exposure and reactivity to medications and, thus, the potential for misuse of these substances in later life. Women are less likely than men to use and abuse alcohol but are more likely than men to use and misuse psychoactive medications (Simoni-Wastila and Yang 2006), particularly if they are divorced or widowed, have lower socioeconomic status (e.g., education and income), or have received a mood disorder diagnosis such as depression or anxiety (Closser and Blow 1993). Comorbid psychiatric diagnoses, in general, increase the risk for prescription drug abuse and dependence, regardless of gender (Simoni-Wastila and Yang 2006). When considering the full range of factors associated with drug misuse, it also is important to recognize factors such as inappropriate prescribing practices and insufficient monitoring of drug reactions and patient adherence by health care providers (Montamat and Cusack 1992).

Consequences of Substance Use

Although the literature presented thus far has alluded to the adverse effects of problematic substance use and dependence, some evidence suggests that low-risk or moderate alcohol consumption may have a positive effect on physical health and mental well-being. For example, low-risk or moderate alcohol consumption is associated with a reduced risk of cardiovascular disease in both men and women and a reduced risk of cardiovascular disease–related disability (Rimm et al. 1991; Stampfer et al. 1988). With respect to functional decline, findings from cross-sectional studies suggest that among older men, low to moderate alcohol consumption is associated with lower odds of reporting physical limitations when compared with abstinence or heavy use (Cawthon et al. 2007). Finally, light to moderate alcohol use has beneficial effects on subjective well-being for both men and women (Lang et al. 2007) and improves self-esteem, reduces stress, and provides relaxation, particularly in social situations (Dufour et al. 1992).

Although the literature cited previously does suggest that low to moderate use of alcohol can lead to various health benefits among older adults, it is important to recognize that no evidence supports the notion that recommending that nondrinkers initiate drinking will translate into reduced health risks. Moreover, no evidence suggests that an individual with a medical condition, such as cardiovascular disease, will benefit from continued drinking or the initiation of drinking. In fact, abstinence should still be recommended for individuals who are taking certain medications, those who have been diagnosed with certain acute or chronic conditions (e.g., diabetes and cardiovascular disease), and those who present with a history of alcohol or drug abuse because substance use is detrimental in these cases. Indeed, low to moderate consumption of alcohol also has been shown to impair one's ability to drive and may increase the risk of accidents and fatal injuries caused by falls, motor vehicle crashes, and suicides (Sorock et al. 2006). Depression, memory problems, liver disease, cardiovascular disease, cognitive changes, and sleep problems also have been linked to moderate alcohol use (Gambert and Katsoyannis 1995; Liberto et al. 1992), whereas alcohol dependence is associated with an increased probability of morbidity and mortality from disease-specific disorders such as acute pancreatitis, alcohol-induced cirrhosis, or alcohol-related cardiomyopathy. When assessing and treating older adults, it is pertinent not only that clinicians take the previously mentioned factors into account but also that they consider the potential interaction between alcohol and both prescribed and over-the-counter medications, especially psychoactive medications such as benzodiazepines, barbiturates, and antidepressants. Finally, mental health providers should be well versed in the effect of moderate alcohol consumption on other mental health disorders. In a study of more than 2,000 elderly patients, Oslin et al. (2000) reported that reducing moderate alcohol use (defined as 1–7 drinks per week) while treating a depressive disorder enhanced treatment outcomes. Results further indicated that the greater the alcohol consumption, the larger the negative effect on the treatment of depression. Although data are sparse, there is speculation that moderate alcohol use also may have a negative effect on the prognosis and course of dementing illnesses such as Alz-

heimer's disease. Moreover, alcohol use may elicit the onset of, or exacerbate preexisting, personality changes or behavioral disturbances in patients with dementia.

Screening and Diagnosis of Substance Use Problems

Potential Barriers to Screening and Diagnosis

As outlined previously, alcohol and drug problems are common in later life. However, substance misuse remains largely underrecognized and undertreated among older adults. It has been suggested that individuals older than 60 years be screened for alcohol and prescription drug use as part of their routine mental and physical health care (Blow 1998). Routine screening would enable the identification of not only those older adults who have problematic substance use but also those who are at risk for misusing drugs and alcohol (Table 14–2). Furthermore, proper screening helps determine whether additional assessment is needed. Nonetheless, various factors may interfere with screening and diagnostic processes.

At the patient level, confusion as to what constitutes a substance use problem and who might benefit from an intervention affects patients' behavior with regard to seeking assessment. Like providers, older adults may perceive physical symptoms (e.g., fatigue, sleep problems, anxiety, and confusion) as normative or attribute them to other medical illnesses. Older adults and their families also may not think that their substance use is problematic because of either denial or lack of knowledge about recommendations and guidelines for acceptable drinking and prescription and over-the-counter drug use levels. In addition to these factors, age- and substance-related declines in memory may contribute to underreporting of past and current alcohol or drug use. Despite these potential issues, research suggests that retrospective self-report is as reliable as a prospective diet record in identifying patterns of alcohol use (Werch 1989).

TABLE 14–2. Common signs and symptoms of potential substance misuse and abuse in older adults

Anxiety

Blackouts, dizziness

Depression, mood swings

Disorientation

Falls, bruises, and burns

Family problems

Financial problems

Headaches

Idiopathic seizures

Incontinence

Increased tolerance to alcohol or medications

Legal difficulties

Memory loss

New difficulties in decision making

Poor hygiene

Poor nutrition

Sleep problems

Social isolation

Source. Adapted from Barry KL, Blow FC, Oslin DW: "Substance Abuse in Older Adults: Review and Recommendations for Education and Practice in Medical Settings," in *Strategic Plan for Interdisciplinary Faculty Development: Arming the Nation's Health Professional Workforce for a New Approach to Substance Use Disorders.* Edited by Haack MR, Adger H. Providence, RI, Association for Medical Education and Research in Substance Abuse (AMERSA), September 2002, pp 105–131.

Assessing the Frequency and Quantity of Use

Retrospective accounts of daily use over some defined period (i.e., the timeline follow-back method) represent the most commonly used technique in treatment studies for addiction and have become the method of choice for such studies. Among older adults, 7-day timeline follow-back method assessments are highly correlated with reports from prospective diaries. Nevertheless, certain difficulties arise when using this method. First, the specific week of measurement under assessment may not be representative of the individual's usual drinking behavior. Second, although the timeline follow-back method closely matches prospective diary reports for nondrinkers or daily drinkers, it underestimates use for less frequent users of alcohol (Lemmens et al. 1992). General questions about the average, rather than daily, quantity and frequency of use over a specified time are least likely to match prospective diary reports and may underestimate the frequency of moderate drinking.

Standardized Screening Instruments

Brief, low-cost, convenient, standardized assessments that can be used to screen not only for frequency and quantity of alcohol use but also for drinking consequences and alcohol or medication interactions are essential in the success of efforts targeted toward prevention and early intervention for older adults at risk. As described earlier, screening should be a component of routine mental and physical health care and should be updated annually, before the older adult begins taking any new medications, or in response to problems that may be alcohol- or medication-related.

To complement questions assessing the quantity and frequency of use discussed in the previous subsection, the Short Michigan Alcoholism Screening Test–Geriatric Version (SMAST-G; Figure 14–1), the Alcohol Use Disorders Identification Test (AUDIT), and the CAGE questionnaire often are used to screen for at-risk substance use or misuse among older adults. The AUDIT and its abbreviated version, the AUDIT-C (Figure 14–2), are simple screening measures that capture the frequency of drinking and bingeing in the past year (Bush et al. 1998; Dawson et al. 2005). The AUDIT-C is scored on a scale of 0–12, with a score of 0 indicating no alcohol use during the preceding year. For older adults, a score of 3 or more reflects a positive screen and suggests the need for further evaluation. Generally, the higher the AUDIT-C score, the more likely it is that the individual's drinking is affecting his or her health and safety (Bush et al. 1998; Dawson et al. 2005).

In the past year:	Yes	No
1. When talking with others, do you ever underestimate how much you actually drink?	(1)	(0)
2. After a few drinks, have you sometimes not eaten or been able to skip a meal because you didn't feel hungry?	(1)	(0)
3. Does having a few drinks help decrease your shakiness or tremors?	(1)	(0)
4. Does alcohol sometimes make it hard for you to remember parts of the day or night?	(1)	(0)
5. Do you usually take a drink to relax or calm your nerves?	(1)	(0)
In the past year:		
6. Do you drink to take your mind off your problems?	(1)	(0)
7. Have you ever increased your drinking after experiencing a loss in your life?	(1)	(0)
8. Has a doctor or nurse ever said they were worried or concerned about your drinking?	(1)	(0)
9. Have you ever made rules to manage your drinking?	(1)	(0)
10. When you feel lonely, does having a drink help?	(1)	(0)
TOTAL SMAST-G SCORE (0–10)		

FIGURE 14–1. Short Michigan Alcohol Screening Test–Geriatric Version (SMAST-G).

Three or more positive responses is indicative of an alcohol abuse problem.

Source. Reprinted from the University of Michigan Alcohol Research Center. Copyright 1991 The Regents of the University of Michigan. Used with permission.

1. How often did you have a drink containing alcohol in the past year?

_____	Never	(0 points)
_____	Monthly or less	(1 point)
_____	Two to four times a month	(2 points)
_____	Two to three times per week	(3 points)
_____	Four or more times a week	(4 points)

If you answered "never," score questions 2 and 3 as zero.

2. How many drinks did you have on a typical day when you were drinking in the past year?

_____	1 or 2	(0 points)
_____	3 or 4	(1 point)
_____	5 or 6	(2 points)
_____	7 to 9	(3 points)
_____	10 or more	(4 points)

3. How often did you have six or more drinks on one occasion in the past year?

_____	Never	(0 points)
_____	Less than monthly	(1 point)
_____	Monthly	(2 points)
_____	Weekly	(3 points)
_____	Daily or almost daily	(4 points)

Possible range = 0–12. For older adults, a score of 3 or more is considered positive.

FIGURE 14–2. Alcohol Use Disorders Identification Test–C (AUDIT-C) alcohol screening.

Source. Adapted from Bush K, Kivlahan DR, McDonell MB, et al.: "The AUDIT Alcohol Consumption Questions (AUDIT-C): An Effective Brief Screening Test for Problem Drinking." *Archives of Internal Medicine* 158:1789–1795, 1998. Copyright 1998, American Medical Association. All rights reserved. Used with permission.

The CAGE questionnaire (Mayfield et al. 1974), however, is the most widely used alcohol screening test in clinical practice. A modified version of the original CAGE questionnaire asks only about recent problems, and the threshold is often reduced to one positive response as an indicator of problems in older individuals. This modified version of the CAGE has demonstrated high specificity for detecting alcohol abuse but relatively low sensitivity for alcohol dependence or problem drinking (Buchsbaum et al. 1992; Moore et al. 2002).

Following administration of a screening instrument, clinicians can ask follow-up questions about consequences, health risks, and social and family issues related to substance use. In accordance with DSM-IV-TR criteria, to assess dependence, questions should be asked about alcohol-related problems, a history of failed attempts to stop or to cut back, or withdrawal symptoms (e.g., anxiety, tremors, sleep disturbance). The use of a substance abuse assessment instrument such as DSM-IV-TR criteria can assist clinicians and researchers by providing a structured approach to assessment as well as a checklist of items that can be evaluated across older adults. Furthermore, such assessments can inform clinicians' decision making and help determine whether specialized alcohol treatment might be needed.

Use of Biological Markers for Screening

Biological markers of alcohol and drug use have proved to be less accepted in clinical practice but can be useful. Several laboratory values indicate recent use or abuse, including blood alcohol or acetate level, which is a metabolite of alcohol (Salaspuro 1994). Long-term markers of alcohol use include γ-glutamyl transferase (GGT), mean corpuscular volume, high-density lipoprotein level, and carbohydrate-deficient transferrin (Oslin et al. 1998b). Finally, urine drug screens are useful as both screening tools and confirmation of self-report when assessing prescription or over-the-counter medication and illicit drug abuse. Most drugs of abuse will remain detectable in a urine drug screen for 4 or more days, with some still detectable after several weeks.

Treatments for Substance Use Problems

Although numerous treatment options are available for substance use in later life, little formal research has been conducted to compare the relative efficacy of these various approaches among older adults. Nevertheless, results from naturalistic studies are promising: older individuals who engage in treatment not only have comparable or significantly better outcomes than their younger counterparts (Lemke and Moos 2003b; Oslin et al. 2002; Satre et al. 2003, 2004) but also are more likely to complete treatment than are younger patients (Schuckit and Pastor 1978; Wiens et al. 1982). Moreover, brief interventions and therapies have been shown to reduce drinking levels among older at-risk drinkers (F. Blow, "Brief Interventions in the Treatment of At-Risk Drinking in Older Adults," personal communication, 2003). Therefore, despite popular belief, older adults are quite receptive and responsive to treatment, especially in programs that offer age-appropriate care and have providers who are knowledgeable about aging issues.

Brief Interventions and Therapies

Low-intensity brief interventions or brief therapies are cost-effective and practical techniques that can be used in the initial treatment of at-risk and problem drinkers in a variety of clinical settings (Barry 1999). Brief interventions are time-limited and nonconfrontational in their approach. Given that these interventions are based on con-

cepts and techniques from the behavioral self-control literature, one of the hallmarks of brief interventions is to encourage individuals to change their behavior through motivational interviewing (Miller and Rollnick 1991). Randomized clinical trials of brief interventions for alcohol problems among older populations reveal that older adults can be engaged in brief intervention protocols and find the protocols acceptable. Results also point to a greater reduction in alcohol consumption among at-risk drinkers receiving interventions as compared with control groups. For example, in one randomized clinical study, older primary care patients randomly assigned to a brief intervention arm received two 10- to 15-minute physician counseling visits and two follow-up telephone calls from clinic staff that involved advice, education, and the creation of contracts (Fleming et al. 1999). Results from this study demonstrated that rates of alcohol use at 12-month follow-up were significantly lower for patients randomly assigned to the brief intervention arm relative to those in the control group. Likewise, older primary care patients randomly assigned to a single brief intervention session have been shown to have significantly greater reductions in alcohol consumption compared with usual care 1 year later (F. Blow, "Brief Interventions in the Treatment of At-Risk Drinking in Older Adults," personal communication, 2003).

Psychosocial Treatments

The literature on the efficacy of psychological therapies specifically for the treatment of substance abuse and dependence in older adulthood is sparse. In one study of older veterans with substance abuse problems, Schonfeld and Dupree (2000) showed that individuals who completed 16 weeks of a group intervention for relapse prevention were more likely to be abstinent at 6-month follow-up than noncompleters. Using cognitive-behavioral and self-management approaches, the group sessions included modules on coping with factors such as social problems, loneliness, depression, and anxiety and on dealing with high-risk situations for relapse. In yet another treatment study, three different manual-guided, individually delivered psychosocial treatments (cognitive-behavioral therapy, motivational enhancement therapy, and 12-Step facilitation) that spanned 12 weeks were found to be effective in reducing alcohol consumption among adults (7% of whom were age 60 years or older) with alcohol dependence 1 year posttreatment (Cooney et al. 1997).

Twelve-Step Programs

A large proportion of community-based and residential treatment programs incorporate the traditional 12-Step peer support model of recovery and rehabilitation. Participants share their experiences with one another and follow the 12 steps, which include admitting to one's addiction, recognizing the influence of a greater power as a source of strength, and acknowledging and atoning for past mistakes (Alcoholics Anonymous Services 2004).

Although self-help groups have been associated with positive outcomes for many individuals, findings regarding rates of group engagement and outcomes among older adults remain mixed. In their matched comparison of older versus younger and middle-aged adults who participated in age-integrated residential treatment, Lemke and Moos (2003a) found that older patients engaged in 12-Step programs as frequently as their younger and middle-aged counterparts when assessed at follow-up. Similarly, an investigation of patients who had com-

pleted an outpatient treatment program for chemical dependency yielded no age group differences in AA affiliation 5 years posttreatment (Satre et al. 2004). However, despite the fact that rates of attendance appeared to be comparable across age groups, the depth of involvement differed; older adults were less likely than middle-aged adults to self-identify as being a 12-Step group member and were less likely than younger and middle-aged adults to report calling a fellow group member for help. Comparable results were observed in examining 1-month postdischarge outcomes among alcohol-dependent patients admitted to a 12-Step residential rehabilitation program (Oslin et al. 2005). Although rates of postdischarge abstinence and AA attendance did not differ across middle-aged and older adults, older adults were significantly less likely to contact a sponsor. Furthermore, older adults were less likely than middle-aged adults to engage in formal aftercare (31.2% vs. 56.4%).

Taken together, these findings highlight the importance of more careful examination of factors that may be related to 12-Step program attendance, degree of engagement, and outcomes among older adults. These include but are not limited to perceived stigma, level of comfort regarding disclosure of personal information in group settings, degree to which age-relevant issues are addressed during group meetings, and logistical barriers such as lack of transportation and health problems that may preclude older adults from attending group sessions and engaging with sponsors (Oslin et al. 2005; Satre et al. 2004).

Pharmacotherapy

Until recently, the long-term treatment of alcohol dependence in older adults did not involve the use of pharmacological agents.

Although disulfiram was originally the only medication approved for the treatment of alcohol dependence, it was seldom used in older patients because of the potential for adverse effects. More recently, naltrexone has been shown to be effective among older adults. For example, results from a double-blind, placebo-controlled, randomized trial indicated that among older veterans ages 50–70, half as many naltrexone-treated subjects relapsed to significant drinking when compared with those who received placebo (Oslin et al. 1997a). Acamprosate has emerged as another promising agent in the treatment of alcohol dependence. Although the exact action of acamprosate is still unclear, it is believed to reduce glutamate response (Pelc et al. 1997). Unfortunately, no studies of the efficacy or safety of acamprosate among older patients have been conducted to date.

Detoxification and Withdrawal

When patients stop consuming substances or drastically cut down their consumption after heavy use, withdrawal symptoms are likely to occur. During hospitalizations, patients may be particularly vulnerable to alcohol or benzodiazepine withdrawal if the clinical team is unaware of problems with these substances. In light of the potential for life-threatening complications, clinicians caring for patients who abuse substances, particularly in settings in which withdrawal management or treatment is available, need to have a fundamental understanding of withdrawal symptoms and be able to provide detoxification management. The classic set of symptoms associated with alcohol withdrawal includes autonomic hyperactivity (increased pulse rate, increased blood

pressure, and increased temperature), restlessness, disturbed sleep, anxiety, nausea, and tremor. Severe withdrawal is marked by auditory, visual, or tactile hallucinations; delirium; seizures; and coma. It is important to recognize that among older patients, the duration of withdrawal symptoms is longer, and withdrawal has the potential to complicate other medical and psychiatric illnesses. Nonetheless, no evidence suggests that older patients are more prone to alcohol withdrawal or require longer treatment for withdrawal symptoms (Brower et al. 1994).

Moderators and Correlates of Treatment Response and Adherence

Some evidence indicates that certain factors may have an effect on the degree of treatment response and adherence among older adults receiving treatment. For example, age-specific treatment, or age matching, has been shown to improve treatment completion and to result in higher rates of attendance at group meetings when compared with mixed-age treatments. In one study of male veterans with alcohol problems who were randomly assigned after detoxification to either age-specific or standard mixed-age treatment, outcomes at 6 months and 1 year showed that patients assigned to the elder-specific program were 2.9 times more likely at 6 months and 2.1 times more likely at 1 year to report abstinence compared with patients receiving mixed-age group treatment (Kashner et al. 1992).

The type of treatment setting also may affect rates of adherence. In a study comparing engagement outcomes among older primary care patients referred to specialty mental health providers and those referred to an integrated care model using a brief intervention, 60.4% of at-risk drinkers attended at least one visit in the integrated care model (Bartels et al. 2004). In contrast, only 33% of the patients attended at least one visit to a specialty provider. It is important to note that these differences emerged despite efforts to address barriers to specialty care, such as copayments and insurance claims, and to ensure appointments within 2 weeks of patients being identified with at-risk drinking.

Medical and Psychiatric Comorbidity

The co-occurrence of problematic substance use and other medical and psychiatric conditions deserves special attention because such comorbidity may affect the course, treatment, and prognosis of both conditions. For example, in a review of 3,986 Veterans Affairs hospital patients between ages 60 and 69 presenting for alcohol treatment, the most common comorbid psychiatric disorder was an affective disorder (present in 21% of the patients) (Blow et al. 1992). Of these patients, 43% had major depression. Similarly, in a study of community-dwelling elderly, of the 4.5% of older adults who had a history of alcohol abuse, almost half had a comorbid diagnosis of depression or dysthymia (Blazer et al. 1987).

Comorbid symptoms of depression and alcohol misuse not only are common in late life but also may have a reciprocal effect on one another. Depressed individuals with alcoholism may have a more complicated clinical course of depression, marked by an increased risk of suicide and more social dysfunction, than nondepressed alcoholic

individuals (Conwell 1991; Cook et al. 1991; Waern 2003). In the same vein, alcohol use prior to late life has been shown to influence treatment of late-life depression; for example, a history of alcohol abuse is associated with a more severe and chronic course of depression (Cook et al. 1991).

Co-occurrence of alcohol use and dementing illnesses such as Alzheimer's disease is also a complex issue. Although Wernicke-Korsakoff syndrome is well defined and often caused by alcohol dependence, alcohol-related dementia may be difficult to differentiate from Alzheimer's disease because of a lack of well-specified diagnostic criteria. As a result, clinical diagnostic criteria for alcohol-related dementia have been proposed and validated in at least one trial examining a method for distinguishing alcohol-related dementia, including Wernicke-Korsakoff syndrome, from other types of dementia (Oslin and Cary 2003; Oslin et al. 1998a). Despite these diagnostic issues, it is generally agreed that alcohol abuse contributes to cognitive deficits in later life.

Sleep disorders and disturbances also frequently co-occur with excessive alcohol use. It is well established that alcohol causes changes in sleep patterns, such as decreased sleep latency, decreased stage 4 sleep, and precipitation or aggravation of sleep apnea (Wagman et al. 1977). Age-related changes in sleep patterns also occur with advancing age and include increased rapid eye movement (REM) episodes, a decrease in REM length and stage 3 and 4 sleep, and increased awakenings. Age-associated changes in sleep can be exacerbated by factors such as alcohol use and depression. For instance, in their study of younger subjects, Moeller et al. (1993) found that alcohol and depression had additive effects on sleep disturbances when occurring together. Furthermore, Wagman et al. (1977) reported that abstinent alcoholic individuals had poor sleep as a result of insomnia, frequent awakenings, and REM fragmentation. Nevertheless, after drinking alcohol, sleep periodicity normalized and REM sleep was temporarily suppressed, suggesting that alcohol use could be used to self-medicate for sleep disturbances.

Future Directions

Substance misuse among older adults represents a pressing public health issue, both now and for years to come. In light of changes in demographic and cohort trends, recent years have seen an increase in the number of older individuals who misuse or abuse alcohol and drugs. Moreover, there is a growing awareness that older adults often engage in at-risk or problem substance use. Nevertheless, individuals in need of treatment or at risk for future problems often go unidentified and untreated. Thus, research and clinical efforts aimed at improving screening efforts and identifying system, provider, and patient-level factors that may interfere with screening and referral processes for older individuals at risk are warranted. In this vein, a better understanding among clinicians and patients of recommended drinking levels and of the risks associated with moderate to heavy alcohol consumption is needed, particularly in light of the high prevalence of co-occurring medical and psychiatric problems in the older adult population. Clinicians should also ensure that screening becomes a part of routine practice when caring for their older patients.

Key Points

- Despite demographic and cohort trends that suggest rates of substance misuse among older adults are increasing, the misuse of alcohol and/or drugs among this group remains largely underrecognized and undertreated. Accordingly, substance misuse in later life has been referred to as an "invisible epidemic."

- Proper screening, diagnosis, and treatment of older adults with drug and/or alcohol problems require an understanding of both age-specific guidelines and the full range of substance use behavior seen among older adults.

- In light of physiological changes that accompany aging, it is recommended that adults age 65 years and older should consume no more than one standard drink per day.

- The use of multiple pharmaceutical drugs is prevalent in older adulthood, and thus the risk of misusing prescription and over-the-counter medications increases with age. Psychotherapeutic medications, in particular, should be closely monitored because they are subject to improper use and can lead to negative health outcomes and interactions, both used alone and in combination with other drugs and alcohol.

- Factors such as medical comorbidity, history of use, gender, and social and family environment are related to increased late-life vulnerability to substance misuse and the maintenance of problematic substance use patterns.

- Diagnostic criteria and symptoms for alcohol and drug misuse are not easily applied to older adults because they are often confounded with symptoms of comorbid medical illnesses. Thus, when diagnosing and treating symptoms in older adults, it is important that providers be able to distinguish between symptoms of substance misuse and those stemming from comorbid conditions.

- Routine screening allows for the identification of not only problematic and dependent drinkers but also older adults who are at risk for misusing drugs and alcohol. Proper screening also helps determine needs for additional assessment and/or intervention. Standardized brief, low-cost assessments can be used to assess the quantity and frequency of alcohol and drug use in clinical practice.

- Various treatments for substance misuse, such as brief interventions, psychotherapy, 12-Step programs, and pharmacotherapy, have been shown to be effective among older adults.

- Special attention should be paid to co-occurrence of problematic substance use and other medical and psychiatric conditions (e.g., depression, dementia, sleep disturbance) because such comorbidity may affect the course, treatment, and prognosis of both conditions.

References

Alcoholics Anonymous Services: Twelve Steps and Twelve Traditions. New York, Alcoholics Anonymous, 2004

American Psychiatric Association: Diagnostic and Statistical Manual of Mental Disorders, 4th Edition. Washington, DC, American Psychiatric Association, 1994

American Psychiatric Association: Diagnostic and Statistical Manual of Mental Disorders, 4th Edition, Text Revision. Washington, DC, American Psychiatric Association, 2000

Barry KL (Consensus Panel Chair): Brief Interventions and Brief Therapies for Substance Abuse. Treatment Improvement Protocol (TIP) Series 34 (DHHS SAMHSA Publ No SMA-99-3353). Rockville, MD, Center for Substance Abuse Treatment, 1999

Bartels S, Coakley E, Zubritsky C, et al: Improving access to geriatric mental health services: a randomized trial comparing treatment engagement with integrated versus enhanced referral care for depression, anxiety, and at-risk alcohol use. Am J Psychiatry 16:1455–1462, 2004

Blazer DG, Hughes DC, George LK: The epidemiology of depression in an elderly community population. Gerontologist 27:281–287, 1987

Blow FC (Consensus Panel Chair): Substance Abuse Among Older Adults. Treatment Improvement Series Protocol (TIP) Series No. 26. Center for Substance Abuse Treatment. Rockville, MD, U.S. Department of Health and Human Services, 1998

Blow F, Cook CL, Booth B, et al: Age-related psychiatric comorbidities and level of functioning in alcoholic veterans seeking outpatient treatment. Hosp Community Psychiatry 43:990–995, 1992

Brower KJ, Mudd S, Blow FC, et al: Severity and treatment of alcohol withdrawal in elderly versus younger patients. Alcohol Clin Exp Res 18:196–201, 1994

Buchsbaum DG, Buchanan R, Welsh J, et al: Screening for drinking disorders in the elderly using the CAGE questionnaire. J Am Geriatr Soc 40:662–665, 1992

Bush K, Kivlahan DR, McDonell MB, et al: The AUDIT alcohol consumption questions (AUDIT-C): an effective brief screening test for problem drinking. Ambulatory Care Quality Improvement Project (ACQUIP). Alcohol Use Disorders Identification Test. Arch Intern Med 158:1789–1795, 1998

Cawthon PM, Fink HA, Barrett-Connor E, et al: Alcohol use, physical performance, and functional limitations in older men. J Am Geriatr Soc 55:212–220, 2007

Chermack ST, Blow FC, Hill EM, et al: The relationship between alcohol symptoms and consumption among older drinkers. Alcohol Clin Exp Res 20:1153–1158, 1996

Closser MH, Blow FC: Special populations: women, ethnic minorities, and the elderly. Psychiatr Clin North Am 16:199–209, 1993

Conwell Y: Suicide in elderly patients, in Diagnosis and Treatment of Depression in Late Life. Edited by Schneider LS, Reynolds CF, Lebowitz BD, et al. Washington, DC, American Psychiatric Press, 1991, pp 397–418

Cook B, Winokur G, Garvey M, et al: Depression and previous alcoholism in the elderly. Br J Psychiatry 158:72–75, 1991

Cooney NL, DiClemente CC, Carbonari J, et al: Matching alcoholism treatments to client heterogeneity: Project MATCH posttreatment drinking outcomes. J Stud Alcohol 58:7–29, 1997

Dawson DA, Grant BF, Stinson FS, et al: Effectiveness of the derived Alcohol Use Disorders Identification Test (AUDIT-C) in screening for alcohol use disorders and risk drinking in the U.S. general population. Alcohol Clin Exp Res 29:844–854, 2005

Dufour MC, Archer L, Gordis E: Alcohol and the elderly. Clin Geriatr Med 8:127–141, 1992

Fleming MF, Manwell LB, Barry KL, et al: Brief physician advice for alcohol problems in older adults: a randomized community-based trial. J Fam Pract 48:378–384, 1999

Gambert S, Katsoyannis K: Alcohol-related medical disorders of older heavy drinkers, in Alcohol and Aging. Edited by Beresford T, Gomberg E. New York, Oxford University Press, 1995, pp 70–81

Gfroerer J, Penne M, Pemberton M, et al: Substance abuse treatment need among older adults in 2020: the impact of the aging baby-boom cohort. Drug Alcohol Depend 69:127–135, 2003

Golden AG, Preston RA, Barnett SD, et al: Inappropriate medication prescribing in homebound older adults. J Am Geriatr Soc 47:948–953, 1999

Grant BF, Dawson DA, Stinson FS, et al: The 12-month prevalence and trends in DSM-IV alcohol abuse and dependence: United States, 1991–1992 and 2001–2002. Drug Alcohol Depend 74:223–234, 2004

Holroyd S, Duryee J: Substance use disorders in a geriatric psychiatry outpatient clinic: prevalence and epidemiologic characteristics. J Nerv Ment Dis 185:627–632, 1997

Kashner TM, Rodell DI, Ogden SR, et al: Outcomes and costs of two VA inpatient treatment programs for older alcoholic patients. Hosp Community Psychiatry 43:985–989, 1992

Kirchner JE, Zubritsky C, Cody M, et al: Alcohol consumption among older adults in primary care. J Gen Intern Med 22:92–97, 2007

Klatsky AL, Armstrong A: Alcohol use, other traits and risk of unnatural death: a prospective study. Alcohol Clin Exp Res 17:1156–1162, 1993

Koenig HG, George LK, Schneider R: Mental health care for older adults in the year 2020: a dangerous and avoided topic. Gerontologist 34:674–679, 1994

Lang I, Wallace RB, Huppert FA, et al: Moderate alcohol consumption in older adults is associated with better cognition and well-being than abstinence. Age Ageing 36:256–261, 2007

Lassila HC, Stoehr GP, Ganguli M, et al: Use of prescription medications in an elderly rural population: the MoVIES project. Ann Pharmacother 30:589–595, 1996

Lemke S, Moos RH: Outcomes at 1 and 5 years for older patients with alcohol disorders. J Subst Abuse Treat 24:43–50, 2003a

Lemke S, Moos RH: Treatment and outcomes of older patients with alcohol use disorders in community residential programs. J Stud Alcohol 64:219–226, 2003b

Lemmens P, Tan ES, Knibbe RA: Measuring quantity and frequency of drinking in a general population survey: a comparison of five indices. J Stud Alcohol 53:476–486, 1992

Liberto JG, Oslin DW, Ruskin PE: Alcoholism in older persons: a review of the literature. Hosp Community Psychiatry 43:975–984, 1992

Mayfield D, McLeod G, Hall P: The CAGE questionnaire: validation of a new alcoholism instrument. Am J Psychiatry 131:1121–1123, 1974

Miller W, Rollnick S: Motivational Interviewing: Preparing People to Change Addictive Behavior. New York, Guilford, 1991

Moeller FG, Gillin JC, Irwin M, et al: A comparison of sleep EEGs in patients with primary major depression and major depression secondary to alcoholism. J Affect Disord 27:39–42, 1993

Montamat SC, Cusack B: Overcoming problems with polypharmacy and drug misuse in the elderly. Clin Geriatr Med 8:143–158, 1992

Moore AA, Hays RD, Reuben DB, et al: Using a criterion standard to validate the Alcohol-Related Problems Survey (ARPS): a screening measure to identify harmful and hazardous drinking in older persons. Aging (Milano) 12:221–227, 2000

Moore AA, Beck JC, Babor TF, et al: Beyond alcoholism: identifying older, at-risk drinkers in primary care. J Stud Alcohol 63:316–324, 2002

Moore AA, Gould R, Reuben DB, et al: Longitudinal patterns and predictors of alcohol consumption in the United States. Am J Public Health 95:458–465, 2005

Moore AA, Whiteman EJ, Ward KT: Risks of combined alcohol/medication use in older adults. Am J Geriatr Pharmacother 5:64–74, 2007

Moos RH, Schutte K, Brennan P, et al: Ten-year patterns of alcohol consumption and drinking problems among older women and men. Addiction 99:829–838, 2004

National Institute on Alcohol Abuse and Alcoholism: Diagnostic criteria for alcohol abuse. Alcohol Alert No. 30 (October) PH 359, 1995. Bethesda, MD, U.S. Department of Health and Human Services, Public Health Service, National Institutes of Health, 1995, pp 1–6

Oslin DW, Cary MS: Alcohol-related dementia: validation of diagnostic criteria. Am J Geriatr Psychiatry 11:441–447, 2003

Oslin D, Liberto JG, O'Brien J, et al: Naltrexone as an adjunctive treatment for older patients with alcohol dependence. Am J Geriatr Psychiatry 5:324–332, 1997a

Oslin D, Streim JE, Parmelee P, et al: Alcohol abuse: a source of reversible functional disability among residents of a VA nursing home. Int J Geriatr Psychiatry 12:825–832, 1997b

Oslin D, Atkinson RM, Smith DM, et al: Alcohol related dementia: proposed clinical criteria. Int J Geriatr Psychiatry 13:203–212, 1998a

Oslin DW, Pettinati HM, Luck G, et al: Clinical correlations with carbohydrate-deficient transferrin levels in women with alcoholism. Alcohol Clin Exp Res 22:1981–1985, 1998b

Oslin DW, Katz IR, Edell WS, et al: Effects of alcohol consumption on the treatment of depression among elderly patients. Am J Geriatr Psychiatry 8:215–220, 2000

Oslin DW, Pettinati HM, Volpicelli JR: Alcoholism treatment adherence: older age predicts better adherence and drinking outcomes. Am J Geriatr Psychiatry 10:740–747, 2002

Oslin DW, Slaymaker VJ, Blow FC, et al: Treatment outcomes for alcohol dependence among middle-aged and older adults. Addict Behav 30:1431–1436, 2005

Pelc I, Verbanck P, Le Bon O, et al: Efficacy and safety of acamprosate in the treatment of detoxified alcohol-dependent patients: a 90-day placebo-controlled dose-finding study. Br J Psychiatry 171:73–77, 1997

Poikolainen K: Epidemiologic assessment of population risks and benefits of alcohol use. Alcohol Alcohol Suppl 1:27–34, 1991

Rimm EB, Giovannucci EL, Willett WC, et al: Prospective study of alcohol consumption and risk of coronary disease in men. Lancet 338:464–468, 1991

Salaspuro M: Biological state markers of alcohol abuse. Alcohol Health Res World 18:131–135, 1994

Satre DD, Mertens JR, Arean PA, et al: Contrasting outcomes of older versus middle-aged and younger adult chemical dependency patients in a managed care program. J Stud Alcohol 64:520–530, 2003

Satre DD, Mertens JR, Arean PA, et al: Five-year alcohol and drug treatment outcomes of older adults versus middle-aged and younger adults in a managed care program. Addiction 99:1286–1297, 2004

Schonfeld L, Dupree LW: Cognitive-behavioral treatment of older veterans with substance abuse problems. J Geriatr Psychiatry Neurol 13:124–129, 2000

Schuckit M, Pastor P: The elderly as a unique population. Alcohol Clin Exp Res 2:31–38, 1978

Simoni-Wastila L, Yang HK: Psychoactive drug abuse in older adults. Am J Geriatr Pharmacother 4:380–394, 2006

Sorock GS, Chen LH, Gonzalgo SR, et al: Alcohol-drinking history and fatal injury in older adults. Alcohol 40:193–199, 2006

Stampfer MJ, Colditz GA, Willett WC, et al: A prospective study of moderate alcohol consumption and the risk of coronary disease and stroke in women. N Engl J Med 319:267–273, 1988

Stoehr GP, Ganguli M, Seaberg EC, et al: Over-the-counter medication use in an older rural community: the MoVIES project. J Am Geriatr Soc 45:158–165, 1997

Waern M: Alcohol dependence and misuse in elderly suicides. Alcohol Alcohol 38:249–254, 2003

Wagman AM, Allen RP, Upright D: Effects of alcohol consumption upon parameters of ultradian sleep rhythms in alcoholics. Adv Exp Med Biol 85A:601–616, 1977

Werch C: Quantity-frequency and diary measures of alcohol consumption for elderly drinkers. Int J Addict 24:859–865, 1989

Widlitz M, Marin D: Substance abuse in older adults: an overview. Geriatrics 57:29–34, 2002

Wiens AN, Menustik CE, Miller SI, et al: Medical-behavioral treatment for the older alcoholic patient. Am J Drug Alcohol Abuse 9:461–475, 1982

Wilsnack SC, Wilsnack RW: Drinking and problem drinking in U.S. women: patterns and recent trends. Recent Dev Alcohol 12:29–60, 1995

Suggested Readings

Blow FC (Consensus Panel Chair): Substance Abuse Among Older Adults. Treatment Improvement Series Protocol (TIP) Series No 26. Center for Substance Abuse Treatment. Rockville, MD, U.S. Department of Health and Human Services, 1998

Fleming MF, Manwell LB, Barry KL, et al: Brief physician advice for alcohol problems in older adults: a randomized community-based trial. J Fam Pract 48:378–384, 1999

Gfroerer J, Penne M, Pemberton M, et al: Substance abuse treatment need among older adults in 2020: the impact of the aging baby-boom cohort. Drug Alcohol Depend 69:127–135, 2003

Oslin D, Liberto JG, O'Brien J, et al: Naltrexone as an adjunctive treatment for older patients with alcohol dependence. Am J Geriatr Psychiatry 5:324–332, 1997

Satre DD, Mertens JR, Arean PA, et al: Five-year alcohol and drug treatment outcomes of older adults versus middle-aged and younger adults in a managed care program. Addiction 99:1286–1297, 2004

Schonfeld L, Dupree LW: Cognitive-behavioral treatment of older veterans with substance abuse problems. J Geriatr Psychiatry Neurol 13:124–129, 2000

Simoni-Wastila L, Yang HK: Psychoactive drug abuse in older adults. Am J Geriatr Pharmacother 4:380–394, 2006

Substance Abuse and Mental Health Services Administration: Results from the 2010 National Survey on Drug Use and Health: Summary of National Findings (NSDUH Series H-41, HHS Publication No. [SMA] 11-4658). Rockville, MD, Substance Abuse and Mental Health Services Administration, 2011

CHAPTER 15

AGITATION AND SUSPICIOUSNESS

HAROLD W. GOFORTH, M.D.
LISA P. GWYTHER, M.S.W.

Suspiciousness and Paranoia

Psychiatrists working with older adults frequently encounter suspicious or paranoid behaviors, especially in patients with agitation. In fact, such ideation is not uncommon in community populations of elderly adults. In a community study of elderly persons in San Francisco, California, 17% of the subjects reported that they were highly suspicious, and 13% reported delusions (Lowenthal and Berkman 1967). Another study that included elderly persons in both urban and rural areas of North Carolina found that 4% of older adults experienced a sense of persecution by those around them (Christenson and Blazer 1984). Perceptions of a hostile so-cial environment or ideas of persecution lead to greater stress, vigilance, and agitation among elderly persons, resulting in alienation from families and friends. Such individuals represent a challenge for clinicians who care for them.

Among suspicious or paranoid elderly individuals, one group has long been recognized, particularly in Europe. The term *late-life paraphrenia* has been used to identify psychosis that has a late age at onset and to distinguish late-onset psychosis from both chronic schizophrenia and dementia. Kraepelin used *paraphrenia* to classify a small group of patients who had paranoid delusions yet were able to maintain functioning in their social milieu for months or years. He observed that persons with paraphrenia were typically women, usually living alone.

Lisa Gwyther gratefully acknowledges support from the Joseph and Kathleen Bryan Alzheimer's Disease Research Center at Duke University Medical Center grant P30 AGO28377 from the National Institute on Aging.

Although current DSM diagnostic nomenclature would classify many of those individuals as having delusional disorder, this late-life syndrome may be more complex. Sometimes paranoid ideation is accompanied by hallucinations. In addition, patients with this condition may have comorbid sensory deficits, especially visual or hearing loss. Thus, although the condition may have features of delusional disorder, it may also have features and comorbidities that point to its being a different entity, perhaps along a continuum with schizophrenia. When the condition is accompanied by agitation, antipsychotics are usually the first-line treatment, although information is lacking on the effectiveness of this class of medications in delusional disorder. Caution with these medications is also warranted, given the increased sensitivity of elderly persons to antipsychotics (Soares and Gershon 1997).

Clearly, chronic paranoid schizophrenia persisting into late life is a major cause of suspiciousness and agitation in elderly persons. With accompanying functional decline and problematic behaviors occurring earlier in life in patients with schizophrenia, it is unusual for new cases of chronic schizophrenia to be diagnosed in elderly patients. Multimodal treatment—including antipsychotic medication, case management, and family education and involvement—is essential for ensuring adequate care. The occurrence of agitation in chronic paranoid schizophrenia patients is common and may indicate a need for an adjustment in antipsychotic dosing. However, new agitation arising in a previously stable older patient with schizophrenia may indicate another problem, and clinicians need to be particularly attuned to the possibility of an acute medical problem. The medical causes of agitation discussed later in this chapter for pa-

tients with dementia also may affect older patients with schizophrenia, who may require the same level of medical scrutiny.

Classic delusional disorder may occur at any age and is usually characterized by delusions centered on a single theme or series of connected themes. In elderly patients, delusions tend to be nonbizarre—for example, paranoid jealousy may be seen in individuals with a relatively intact premorbid personality (Yassa and Suranyi-Cadotte 1993). Agitation may become an issue when such individuals are confronted by family or clinicians about their delusion. Data are lacking on treatment for this disorder. Antipsychotics, particularly pimozide, have been reported to be helpful for the delusion (Opler and Feinberg 1991), but behavioral intervention and non-antipsychotic medication may be better choices for sporadic agitation that may arise.

Diagnostic Approach to Patients With New Onset of Suspiciousness and Paranoia

As with most mental disorders, a careful psychiatric evaluation and history are key components of the initial approach to the suspicious or paranoid patient. Interviews with family members may be necessary for establishing a diagnosis, particularly if delusions and agitation are present. Part of the task of the clinician is to determine whether the suspicious behavior may be warranted. Older individuals are occasionally abused or neglected; therefore, confronting family members about a patient's accusations of harm or neglect is often part of the assessment. If after such a confrontation the clinician is not convinced that the accusations are completely explained by the delusion, a social services agency or department should be requested to investigate further.

However, challenging the delusional patient usually is not recommended. It is important to seek an understanding of the patient's thought processes, so providing an atmosphere of acceptance (although not necessarily agreement) will allow the patient to express his or her beliefs and feelings. Reassurance should be provided in a manner conveying that although the clinician may not fully understand the whole situation, the goal is for the patient to feel better and more secure.

A laboratory workup is usually needed in new cases of paranoia to rule out an organic delusional syndrome. Blood chemistry, a complete blood count, and a thyroid profile should be obtained. If respiratory symptoms are present, a chest X ray may be needed. A computed tomography or magnetic resonance imaging brain scan may be indicated, especially if cognitive impairment or focal neurological findings are present. Because suspiciousness is often associated with sensory impairment, particularly visual and auditory deficits, audiometric and visual testing may identify potential areas for further intervention.

Treatment of paranoia may include antipsychotic medication, depending on the diagnosis, as discussed earlier in this chapter. (For a complete discussion of antipsychotics, please see Mulsant and Pollock, Chapter 16, "Psychopharmacology," in this volume.) Regardless of whether antipsychotics are prescribed, key components of management of paranoia include reassurance for the patient, education for the family, and careful monitoring for development of agitation.

Agitation in Elderly Persons

Behavioral manifestations of dementia are common (Lyketsos et al. 2000) and represent major predictors of caregiver depression, burden, and stress across cultures (Chen et al. 2000; Gallicchio et al. 2002; Teri 1997). Anxiety and agitation, the most commonly cited psychiatric manifestations of dementia, can be as disruptive and painful for the person with dementia as they are for family caregivers. Disruptive or resistive behaviors resulting from anxiety and agitation increase the risk of harm to the affected individual and others (Chow and MacLean 2001; Tractenberg et al. 2001), and caregivers frequently become frightened, upset, or simply exhausted by the demands of caring for a family member with agitation.

Nonpharmacological Approaches

Nonpharmacological strategies are recommended as first-line approaches for the noncognitive manifestations of dementia. These approaches can be taught effectively to family and nonprofessional caregivers (Belle et al. 2006; Cohen-Mansfield et al. 2007; Doody et al. 2001; Hepburn et al. 2007; Logsdon et al. 2007; Teri et al. 2005). Nonpharmacological approaches are most effective as adjuncts to pharmacotherapy, when pharmacotherapy is contraindicated, and when behaviors are manifested in response to unmet needs and environmental or interpersonal triggers.

These strategies focus on changing the patient's activity, routines, and/or human, physical, and social environment to provide reassurance, appropriate stimulation, and security. As the person with dementia becomes less adaptable to change, the human and physical environment must adapt to him or her. Behavioral approaches generally include person-specific problem solving, enriched cues, adapted work or expressive activities, exercise, communication strategies, and caregiver skills training.

Key Messages for Families About Agitation in Dementia

Families of persons with dementia should be told directly that anxiety, suspiciousness, and restless agitation are common symptoms of brain disorders, even in the context of excellent, well-intentioned family care. At the same time, it is helpful to suggest that disruptive behaviors have a person-specific situational context and meaning that may often, but not always, be understood. Agitated or even aggressive behavior is often beyond the person's control, intentionality, or even awareness.

Frequent or escalating agitation requires a prompt, multimodal response. Ignoring agitated or disruptive behaviors will not make them go away. Persons with dementia are most likely to be angry at what they perceive as an intolerable situation that no longer makes sense. For this reason, families are advised not to take attacks or accusations personally. Persons with dementia are more likely to take out their frustration on those closest to them while maintaining appropriate behavior in brief visits with others.

It is not helpful to exact promises from people with dementia to "try harder" or "never do that again." A corollary is that reasoning, arguing, coaxing, pleading, confronting, or punishing agitated persons may only escalate the distressing behavior. People with dementia are likely scared and overwhelmed by disorientation. They often forget appropriate public or private behavior. Agitation is frequently accompanied by a loss of impulse control, resulting in uncharacteristic cursing, insensitivity, tactlessness, or sexually inappropriate behavior. Despite their seeming insensitivity to others, people with

dementia are extremely sensitive to and will respond negatively to patronizing, angry, tense, or rushed nonverbal communication from family members.

Agitated persons with dementia generally respond well to calm, familiar settings with predictable routines and to requests tailored to their capacities, retained strengths, and energy levels. Although they may appear to do less as a result of apathy, they can become fatigued from just trying to make sense of what is expected. Late-day fatigue may explain some agitated behavior or exaggerated reactions to minor incidents associated with "sundowning" (patients' becoming more confused, agitated, or psychotic in the late afternoon or early evening). Furthermore, people with mild to moderate Alzheimer's disease may actively resist activities they perceive as too difficult or too demeaning to limit embarrassment or failure.

Questions to Guide Problem Solving for Agitation in Dementia

Consideration of the following nine questions can help to address caregivers' problems with an older adult's agitated behavior:

1. Which agitated, anxious, suspicious, or resistive behaviors are most disruptive to family life at this point?
2. Describe the behavior. Is it harmful or does it cause distress to the person with dementia or to others? Can the family change expectations or increase tolerance for this change in the person as they knew him or her?
3. Is there any pattern, trigger, or time of day that sets off the behavior (e.g., bathing, children's visits)?
4. Does anything happen afterward that makes it worse (e.g., caregiver anger or abandonment)?

5. Is the person uncomfortable (e.g., pain, hunger, constipation, full bladder, fatigue, infection, cold, fear, misperceived threats, difficult communication)?

6. Is the person looking for something familiar from the past (e.g., rummaging in drawers)?

7. Will a change in environment help (e.g., reduce number of people, stimuli, noise)?

8. Will use of familiar phrases calm or reassure the person (e.g., "I'll get right on it"; "Even the Lord rested on Sundays")?

9. Can routines be changed or adapted to prevent future occurrences of the behavior (e.g., exercising early in the day, bathing less frequently, avoiding rush-hour shopping)?

Common Strategies That Reduce Agitation

Nonpharmacological strategies for reducing agitation usually involve reassurance, redirection of the person's attention away from triggering contexts, or distraction with offers of person-specific pleasant events (going out for ice cream or a ride). Other strategies include breaking down complex tasks into one-step guided directions and allowing adequate rest or passive observation between stimulating activities. Environmental strategies include using labels, cues, or pictures; hazard-proofing the environment to reduce dangers of exploration or egress; removing guns or hazardous equipment; and using lighting or security objects to reduce nighttime confusion or daytime fear or uncertainty.

Communication Begins With Understanding

Families communicate effectively when they understand the experience of people with dementia. These excerpts from a Canadian support group of patients with early-stage dementias can offer guidance to family caregivers:

> Please don't correct me. Remember, my feelings are intact and I get hurt easily. Try to ignore offhand remarks that I wouldn't have made in the past. If you focus on my mistakes, it just makes me feel worse. I may say something that is real to me but not factual to you. It is not a lie. Don't argue—it won't solve anything. (Snyder 2001, p. 2)

Communication Strategies to Reduce Agitation

First, the clinician must get the person's attention and ensure that vision and hearing are "tuned up." The clinician should use eye contact, call the person by name in a clear adult tone, approach slowly from the side or front or crouch down at his or her level, and offer his or her hand, palm up. The clinician should listen but not feel compelled to talk constantly. Words are not as important as a calm tone, pleasant expression, and nondistracting environment (the television or radio should be turned off or down). Clinicians should use familiar words and speak in a normal tone and tempo but give the person time to process and respond. Words should be repeated exactly, if necessary. The clinician who is unsure of his or her meaning ("Am I getting closer to what you want?") should ask questions and be patient—repetition is reassuring.

If frustration mounts, the clinician should suggest a better time to talk or another topic. He or she should avoid ambiguous or vague expressions such as "Don't go there," "NOT," or "bottom line" and use concrete subjects, names, and references. The clinician should not test or ask if the patient remembers him or her. Positive statements such as "Let's go" should be used rather than "Do you want to go now?" The clinician should explain what happens next but wait until just before it will happen. He or she should demonstrate or model so that the patient can follow the clinician's lead. Complex multistep directions must be avoided. The clinician should use appropriate respectful humor or the patient's favorite phrases ("See ya later, alligator") and smile, nod, gesture, or touch gently when words fail.

Summary of Nonpharmacological Approaches

Families often want brief, concrete suggestions for dealing with agitation. The following format may be helpful (Alzheimer's Association 2010; Gwyther 2001):

- **DO**—slow down, soothe the person, or structure the situation. Reinforce positive adaptations that work for the person ("I depend on you for brute strength in carrying those grocery bags"). Be extra gracious and polite. Back off and ask permission. Repeatedly reassure. Use visual and verbal cues and add light. Offer guided choices between two options. Distract with a favorite snack or ask for help with an adult repetitive task. Increase time spent in pleasant activities like sitting in a porch glider at sunset. Offer security object, rest, or privacy after an upset. Limit caffeine and alcohol. Use comforting rituals like holding hands during grace or checking the bird feeder. Do for the person what he or she can no longer comfortably do on his or her own. Join the person in modified favorite activities—social, creative, or sports. Remove him or her from scary experiences like television shows that he or she believes are happening to him or her.
- **SAY**—May I help you? Do you have time to help me? Let's take a break—we have earned it. You're safe here. I will get right on it. Everything is under con-

trol. I apologize (even if you didn't do it!). I'm sorry you are upset. I know it's hard. We're in this together. I will make sure those men can't get in here.

Pharmacological and Medical Approaches

At times, agitation warrants pharmacological intervention, and the risks of persistent agitation versus the risks and benefits of treating the agitation must be weighed carefully. An accurate risk estimation of using antipsychotic agents in patients with dementia remains unclear, with some studies estimating up to a 3% risk of cerebrovascular events or death and other large population-based studies suggesting no increased risk at all (Herrmann and Lanctôt 2005; Kales et al. 2007; Layton et al. 2005; Raivio et al. 2007).

Most clinicians view agitation as a condition manifested by excessive verbal and/or motor behavior. It is distinguished from aggression, which can also be verbal (e.g., cursing or threats) or physical (e.g., hitting, kicking, shoving objects or people). Potential medical causes of agitation are shown in Table 15–1.

Agitation most commonly occurs in the context of delirium or dementia, and often these conditions coexist in elderly patients. Agitation also can be a feature of late-life depression. Acute, severe, or escalating agitation may require use of antipsychotics for adequate control. Benzodiazepines generally should be avoided in an agitated patient because of their high potential for worsening delirium except in cases of γ-aminobutyric acid (GABA)ergic withdrawal. Chronic treatment of agitation may require the clinician to consider other medications, including antidepressants and mood stabilizers. Choice of medication will depend on the setting and on the severity and chronicity of symptoms.

TABLE 15–1. Common medical causes of agitation in elderly persons

Medication

    Drug-drug interaction

    Accidental misuse

    Central nervous system–toxic side effect

    Systemic disturbance (e.g., medication-induced electrolyte imbalance)

Urinary tract infection

Poor nutrition, decreased oral intake of food and fluid

Respiratory infection

Recent stroke

Occult head trauma if patient fell recently

Pain

Constipation

Alcohol/substance withdrawal

Chronic obstructive pulmonary disease

Agitation in the Context of Delirium

Delirium is a common disorder, with an estimated prevalence of 15%–50% among hospitalized elderly patients (Inouye et al. 2007; Levkoff et al. 1991). Characterized by a disturbance of consciousness and a change in cognition, delirium typically has a rapid onset and runs a short course, although more recent data reflect the clinical observation that delirium may independently advance cognitive decline such that patients may not fully recover cognitive function as compared with their predelirium baseline (Bellelli et al. 2007; McCusker et al. 2001). DSM-IV-TR categorizes delirium by presumed etiology (including delirium secondary to a medical condition, substance intoxication, and substance withdrawal), mixed or multiple etiologies, and uncertain etiology (American Psychiatric Association 2000).

Delirium typically develops over hours to days and is provoked by certain medical illnesses, metabolic derangements, intoxications, and withdrawal states (Lipowski 1989). Confusion, clouding of sensorium or consciousness, and alterations in perception commonly occur, as do frankly psychotic symptoms. Marked disturbances of the sleep cycle contribute to delirium and are often present in these patients. Autonomic changes such as tachycardia and hypertension can also occur, particularly in delirium secondary to substance withdrawal. Patients who have hyperactive delirium show increased irritability and may be acutely sensitive to stimuli. Patients may experience profound shifts in mood and use rambling, illogical language while still having lucid intervals of relatively normal mental functioning. The duration of illness is largely controlled by the course of the underlying condition that provoked the delirious episode and, in susceptible individuals, may portend a permanent decline in mental functioning (Bellelli et al. 2007; McCusker et al. 2001). Hypoactive delirium is not generally accompanied by agitation and may mimic a depressive syndrome with accompanying fear. The need for treatment of hypoactive delirium with antipsychotics remains controversial, but its identification is important in that it is generally associated with higher mortality rates compared with nondelirious or hyperactively delirious subjects (Kiely et al. 2007).

Management of delirium is focused primarily on identifying and treating the underlying cause. Acute treatment of agitation generally requires the administration of intramuscular or intravenous antipsychotics, with the exception of delirium secondary to GABAergic withdrawal, in which case benzodiazepines become the treatment of choice. Oral administration of antipsychotics is frequently used in practice, and data regarding effective use are best for risperidone, quetiapine, and olanzapine (Breitbart et al. 2002; Han and Kim 2004; Pae et al. 2004; Rea et al. 2007; Sasaki et al. 2003).

Agitation in the Context of Dementia

Agitation is a frequent behavioral symptom in dementia, with 24% of caregivers in one survey reporting agitation and/or aggression (Lyketsos et al. 2000). Agitation occurs at various times of the day in about half of all patients with dementia (Little et al. 1995; Small et al. 1997). Behaviors associated with agitation in patients who have dementia include aggression, combativeness, disinhibition, wandering, and hyperactivity. As with all behavior problems, the first step in treatment is to identify potential precipitants. Evaluation should include assessment for common systemic causes (e.g., infection, dehydration, constipation, and other illnesses) as well as changes in medication or environment. Pharmacological Treatment

If environmental measures are insufficient to control a patient's agitated or aggressive behavior, medication is usually needed. Guidelines for pharmacological treatment of agitation in elderly patients with dementia have been developed (Alexopoulos et al. 1998). Antipsychotics are effective for controlling acute agitation, especially when psychotic features are present (Small et al. 1997), but care needs to be taken with these agents given the increased risk of extrapyramidal side effects in elderly patients. However, recent data regarding antipsychotics and increased cerebrovascular disease and mortality risks when used in demented populations are concerning and must be weighed carefully. Benzodiaz-

epines also can be used to treat anxiety or infrequent agitation, but they may be less effective than other agents for long-term treatment.

The anticonvulsants carbamazepine and divalproex sodium also have been noted to be effective in treating behavioral disturbances in dementia and have a side-effect profile distinct from that of antipsychotics. In a double-blind study, Tariot and colleagues (1998) found that compared with the placebo group, patients taking carbamazepine showed significant improvement in agitation and aggression. The drug was well tolerated in spite of its complex pharmacology. Divalproex also has been shown to be an effective treatment for agitation in dementia (Narayan and Nelson 1997). Both carbamazepine and divalproex have the ability to suppress blood cell lines, so periodic blood monitoring is required. Similarly, divalproex also has the capacity to induce liver dysfunction and pancreatitis, so periodic liver function testing should be performed for this agent as well—especially during initial dosing.

Other classes of drugs also can be useful for treating agitation. Antidepressants can be effective even in the absence of clear depressive symptoms. Acetylcholinesterase inhibitors have been shown to decrease agitation, possibly by stimulating attention and concentration (Levy et al. 1999). Similarly, memantine also has been shown to have some degree of favorable outcomes on functional measures and agitation at doses of 10–20 mg/day (Gauthier et al. 2008). The β-blocker propranolol hydrochloride inhibits impulsive behavior after frontal lobe injury and can be used to decrease agitation and aggressive behavior in dementia, but it may cause bradycardia and hypotension so should be used cautiously (Shankle et al. 1995).

The need for continued pharmacological treatment of agitation should be regularly reassessed. Generally, medication for agitation should not be viewed as long-term therapy because of the inherent risks associated with these agents. In one study, antipsychotic treatment was discontinued after agitation was successfully treated in nine patients with dementia (Borson and Raskind 1997), and eight did not need additional pharmacological treatment. After agitation is sufficiently controlled, trial reductions in the required dose of medication should be periodically attempted to minimize the need for polypharmacy and the incidence of adverse events.

However, some patients may require chronic medication treatment for agitation. In such cases, antidepressants, especially selective serotonin reuptake inhibitors, or anticonvulsants are emerging as the preferred treatments. Benzodiazepines and antipsychotics have obvious inherent risks when used chronically in elderly patients with dementia, and close monitoring for side effects (e.g., sedation and extrapyramidal side effects) is required. In the case of antipsychotics, agitated patients without an established psychotic illness should have clear documentation of previous failed trials of other medications or the presence of significantly agitated behavior that appears to represent a significant risk to the patient or others.

Key Points

- Agitation is a common and disabling nonspecific condition in elderly people.

- The causes of agitation include a wide differential that must be evaluated prior to treatment.

- A nonpharmacological approach should be a core component to address agitation.

- When the patient does not respond to nonpharmacological approaches, a wide range of pharmacological interventions can be attempted to provide effective intervention.

- If pharmacological means are used, they should not be continued indefinitely; rather, they should be reevaluated periodically and dosages tapered or eliminated if possible.

References

Alexopoulos GS, Silver JM, Kahn DA, et al (eds): Agitation in Older Persons With Dementia: A Postgraduate Medicine Special Report (The Expert Consensus Guideline Series). New York, McGraw-Hill, 1998

Alzheimer's Association: Behaviors: how to respond when dementia causes unpredictable behaviors. Chicago, IL, Alzheimer's Association, 2010. Available at: http://www.alz.org/national/documents/brochure_behaviors.pdf. Accessed November 2, 2011.

American Psychiatric Association: Diagnostic and Statistical Manual of Mental Disorders, 4th Edition, Text Revision. Washington, DC, American Psychiatric Association, 2000

Belle SH, Burgio L, Burns R, et al: Enhancing the quality of life of dementia caregivers from different ethnic and racial groups: a randomized, controlled trial. Ann Intern Med 145:727–738, 2006

Bellelli G, Frisoni GB, Turco R, et al: Delirium superimposed on dementia predicts 12-month survival in elderly patients discharged from a postacute rehabilitation facility. J Gerontol A Biol Sci Med Sci 62:1306–1309, 2007

Borson S, Raskind MA: Clinical features and pharmacologic treatment of behavioral symptoms of Alzheimer's disease. Neurology 48 (suppl 6):S17–S24, 1997

Breitbart W, Tremblay A, Gibson C: An open trial of olanzapine for the treatment of delirium in hospitalized cancer patients. Psychosomatics 43:175–182, 2002

Chen JC, Borson S, Scanlan JM: Stage-specific prevalence of behavioral symptoms in Alzheimer's disease in a multi-ethnic community sample. Am J Geriatr Psychiatry 8:123–133, 2000

Chow TW, MacLean CH: Quality indicators for dementia in vulnerable community-dwelling and hospitalized elders. Ann Intern Med 135:668–676, 2001

Christenson R, Blazer D: Epidemiology of persecutory ideation in an elderly population in the community. Am J Psychiatry 141:1088–1091, 1984

Cohen-Mansfield J, Libin A, Marx MS: Non-pharmacological treatment of agitation: a controlled trial of systematic individualized intervention. J Gerontol A Biol Sci Med Sci 62:908–916, 2007

Doody RS, Stevens JC, Beck C, et al: Practice parameter: management of dementia (an evidence-based review): report of the Quality Standards Subcommittee of the American Academy of Neurology. Neurology 56:1154–1166, 2001

Gallicchio L, Siddiqui N, Langenberg P, et al: Gender differences in burden and depression among informal caregivers of demented elders in the community. Int J Geriatr Psychiatry 17:154–163, 2002

Gauthier S, Loft H, Cummings J: Improvement in behavioural symptoms in patients with moderate to severe Alzheimer's disease by memantine: a pooled data analysis. Int J Geriatr Psychiatry 23:537–545, 2008

Gwyther L: Caring for People With Alzheimer's Disease: A Manual for Facility Staff. Washington, DC, American Health Care Association and Alzheimer's Association, 2001

Han CS, Kim YK: A double-blind trial of risperidone and haloperidol for the treatment of delirium. Psychosomatics 45:297–301, 2004

Hepburn K, Lewis M, Tomatore J, et al: The Savvy Caregiver Program: the effectiveness of a transportable dementia caregiver psychoeducational program. J Gerontol Nurs 33:30–36, 2007

Herrmann N, Lanctôt KL: Do atypical antipsychotics cause stroke? CNS Drugs 19:91–103, 2005

Inouye SK: Delirium in hospitalized older patients. Clin Geriatr Med 14:745–764, 1998

Inouye SK, Zhang Y, Jones RN, et al: Risk factors for delirium at discharge: development and validation of a predictive model. Arch Intern Med 167:1406–1413, 2007

Kales HC, Valenstein M, Kim HM, et al: Mortality risk in patients with dementia treated with antipsychotics versus other psychiatric medications. Am J Psychiatry 164:1568–1576, 2007

Kiely DK, Jones RN, Bergmann MA, et al: Association between psychomotor activity delirium subtypes and mortality among newly admitted post-acute facility patients. J Gerontol A Biol Sci Med Sci 62:174–179, 2007

Layton D, Harris S, Wilton LV, et al: Comparison of incidence rates of cerebrovascular accidents and transient ischaemic attacks in observational cohort studies of patients prescribed risperidone, quetiapine or olanzapine in general practice in England including patients with dementia. J Psychopharmacol 19:473–482, 2005

Levkoff S, Cleary P, Liptzin B, et al: Epidemiology of delirium: an overview of research issues and findings. Int Psychogeriatr 3:149–167, 1991

Levy ML, Cummings JL, Kahn-Rose R: Neuropsychiatric symptoms and cholinergic therapy for Alzheimer's disease. Gerontology 45 (suppl 1):15–22, 1999

Lipowski ZJ: Delirium in the elderly patient. N Engl J Med 320:578–582, 1989

Little JT, Satlin A, Sunderland T, et al: Sundown syndrome in severely demented patients with probable Alzheimer's disease. J Geriatr Psychiatry Neurol 8:103–106, 1995

Logsdon RG, McCurry SM, Teri L: Evidence-based psychological treatments for disruptive behaviors in individuals with dementia. Psychol Aging 22:28–36, 2007

Lowenthal MF, Berkman PL: Aging and Mental Disorders in San Francisco: A Social Psychiatry Study. San Francisco, CA, Jossey-Bass, 1967

Lyketsos CG, Steinberg M, Tschanz JT, et al: Mental and behavioral disturbances in dementia: findings from the Cache County Study on Memory in Aging. Am J Psychiatry 157:708–714, 2000

McCusker J, Cole M, Dendukuri N, et al: Delirium in older medical inpatients and subsequent cognitive and functional status: a prospective study. CMAJ 165:575–583, 2001

Narayan M, Nelson JC: Treatment of dementia with behavioral disturbance using divalproex or a combination of divalproex and a neuroleptic. J Clin Psychiatry 58:351–354, 1997

Opler LA, Feinberg SS: The role of pimozide in clinical psychiatry: a review. J Clin Psychiatry 52:221–233, 1991

Pae CU, Lee SJ, Lee CU, et al: A pilot trial of quetiapine for the treatment of patients with delirium. Hum Psychopharmacol 19:125–127, 2004

Raivio MM, Laurila JV, Strandberg TE, et al: Neither atypical nor conventional antipsychotics increase mortality or hospital admissions among elderly patients with dementia: a two-year prospective study. Am J Geriatr Psychiatry 15:416–424, 2007

Rea RS, Battistone S, Fong JJ, et al: Atypical antipsychotics versus haloperidol for treatment of delirium in acutely ill patients. Pharmacotherapy 27:588–594, 2007

Sasaki Y, Matsuyama T, Inoue S, et al: A prospective, open-label, flexible-dose study of quetiapine in the treatment of delirium. J Clin Psychiatry 64:1316–1321, 2003

Shankle WR, Nielson KA, Cotman CW: Low-dose propranolol reduces aggression and agitation resembling that associated with orbitofrontal dysfunction in elderly demented patients. Alzheimer Dis Assoc Disord 9:233–237, 1995

Small GW, Rabins PV, Barry PP, et al: Diagnosis and treatment of Alzheimer disease and related disorders: consensus statement of the American Association for Geriatric Psychiatry, the Alzheimer's Association, and the American Geriatrics Society. JAMA 278:1363–1371, 1997

Snyder L: Perspectives: A Newsletter for Individuals Diagnosed With Alzheimer's Disease. Alzheimer's Disease Research Center, University of California, San Diego, 2001, p 2

Soares JC, Gershon S: Therapeutic targets in late-life psychoses: review of concepts and critical issues. Schizophr Res 27:227–239, 1997

Tariot PN, Erb R, Podgorski CA, et al: Efficacy and tolerability of carbamazepine for agitation and aggression in dementia. Am J Psychiatry 155:54–61, 1998

Teri L: Behavior and caregiver burden: behavioral problems in patients with Alzheimer disease and its association with caregiver burden. Alzheimer Dis Assoc Disord 11 (suppl 4):S35–S38, 1997

Teri L, Huda P, Gibbons L, et al: STAR: a dementia-specific training program for staff in assisted living residences. Gerontologist 45:686–693, 2005

Tractenberg RE, Garmst A, Weiner MF, et al: Frequency of behavioral symptoms characterizes agitation in Alzheimer's disease. Int J Geriatr Psychiatry 16:886–891, 2001

Yassa R, Suranyi-Cadotte B: Clinical characteristics of late-onset schizophrenia and delusional disorder. Schizophr Bull 19:701–707, 1993

Suggested Readings

Caine ED: Clinical perspectives on atypical antipsychotics for treatment of agitation. J Clin Psychiatry 67 (suppl 10):22–31, 2006

Nassisi D, Korc B, Hahn S, et al: The evaluation and management of the acutely agitated elderly patient. Mt Sinai J Med 73:976–984, 2006

Roger KS: A literature review of palliative care, end of life, and dementia. Palliat Support Care 4:295–303, 2006

Spira AP, Edelstein BA: Behavioral interventions for agitation in older adults with dementia: an evaluative review. Int Psychogeriatr 18:195–225, 2006

Zuidema S, Koopmans R, Verhey F: Prevalence and predictors of neuropsychiatric symptoms in cognitively impaired nursing home patients. J Geriatr Psychiatry Neurol 20:41–49, 2007

PART IV

Treatment of Psychiatric Disorders in Late Life

CHAPTER 16

PSYCHOPHARMACOLOGY

BENOIT H. MULSANT, M.D.
BRUCE G. POLLOCK, M.D., PH.D.

Pharmacological intervention in late life requires special care. Elderly patients are more susceptible to drug-induced adverse events. Particularly troublesome among older persons are peripheral and central anticholinergic effects such as constipation, urinary retention, delirium, and cognitive dysfunction; antihistaminergic effects such as sedation; and antiadrenergic effects such as postural hypotension. Sedation and orthostatic hypotension not only interfere with basic activities but also pose a significant safety risk to elderly patients because they can lead to falls and fractures. Increased susceptibility to adverse effects in elders may be a result of the pharmacokinetic and pharmacodynamic changes associated with aging, such as diminished glomerular filtration, changes in the density and activity of target receptors, reduced liver size and hepatic blood flow, and de-

creased cardiac output (Pollock et al. 2009; Uchida et al. 2009) (Table 16–1).

Illnesses that affect many elderly persons (e.g., diabetes) further diminish the processing and removal of medications from the body. In addition, polypharmacy and the associated risk of drug interactions add another level of complexity to pharmacological treatment in older patients. Poor adherence to treatment regimens—which can be a result of impaired cognitive function, confusing drug regimens, or lack of motivation or insight associated with the psychiatric disorder being treated—is a significant obstacle to effective and safe pharmacological treatment. Finally, it should be appreciated that psychotropic medications are not as extensively studied in elders as in younger subjects or those without comorbid medical illness with respect to pharmacokinetic and dosing information (Pollock et al. 2009). For example,

TABLE 16–1. Physiological changes in elderly persons associated with altered pharmacokinetics

Organ system	Change	Pharmacokinetic consequence
Circulatory system	Decreased concentration of plasma albumin and increased α_1-acid glycoprotein	Increased or decreased free concentration of drugs in plasma
Gastrointestinal tract	Decreased intestinal and splanchnic blood flow	Decreased rate of drug absorption
Kidney	Decreased glomerular filtration rate	Decreased renal clearance of active metabolites
Liver	Decreased liver size; decreased hepatic blood flow; variable effects on cytochrome P450 isozyme activity	Decreased hepatic clearance
Muscle	Decreased lean body mass and increased adipose tissue	Altered volume of distribution of lipid-soluble drugs, leading to increased elimination half-life

Source.   Adapted from Pollock BG: "Psychotropic Drugs and the Aging Patient." *Geriatrics* 53 (suppl 1):S20–S24, 1998. Used with permission.

fewer than one-third of the package inserts for the drugs most commonly prescribed in elderly patients have specific dosing recommendations (Steinmetz et al. 2005). New methodologies such as population pharmacokinetics can help to address this lack of information about dosage and drug-drug interactions (Bigos et al. 2006; Jin et al. 2010). Nonetheless, even with currently available knowledge, medications cause considerable morbidity in elders. In a study by Laroche et al. (2007), 66% of the admissions to an acute geriatric medical unit were preceded by the prescription of at least one inappropriate medication; even among patients taking appropriate medications, the prevalence of adverse drug reactions was 16%.

Despite these challenges, psychiatric disorders can be treated successfully in late life with psychotropic drugs. In this chapter, we summarize relevant data published in scientific journals as of December 2010

on the efficacy, tolerability, and safety of the major psychotropic drugs.

Antidepressant Medications

Selective Serotonin Reuptake Inhibitors

Six selective serotonin reuptake inhibitors (SSRIs) are available in the United States (see Table 16–2). They are approved by the U.S. Food and Drug Administration (FDA) for the treatment of major depressive disorder (all except fluvoxamine) and several anxiety disorders (generalized anxiety disorder: escitalopram, paroxetine; obsessive-compulsive disorder: fluoxetine, fluvoxamine, paroxetine, sertraline; panic disorder: fluoxetine, paroxetine, sertraline; posttraumatic stress disorder: paroxetine, sertraline; and social anxiety disorder: paroxetine, sertraline) in adults. In older adults, SSRIs remain first-line antidepressants (Sonnenberg et al. 2008) because of this broad spectrum of action, high efficacy (Mukai and Tampi 2009; Pinquart et al. 2006), ease of use, good tolerability, and relative safety. More than 40 randomized controlled trials of SSRIs involving more than 6,000 geriatric patients with depression have been published (Table 16–2). However, as with most drugs, few clinical trials of SSRIs have been conducted under "real-life" geriatric situations (e.g., in long-term care facilities) or in very old patients. Overall, published trials support the efficacy and tolerability of SSRIs in older patients with major depression. These patients are at high risk for relapse and recurrence, and maintenance therapy with escitalopram or paroxetine has been shown to be effective in their prevention (Gorwood et al. 2007; Reynolds et al. 2006). Many open studies and some small controlled trials in special populations also have concluded that SSRIs are reasonably efficacious, safe, and well tolerated in older patients with mild cognitive impairment (Devanand et al. 2003; Reynolds et al. 2011), minor depression (Lavretsky et al. 2010; Rocca et al. 2005), schizophrenia (Kasckow et al. 2001), cardiovascular disease (Glassman et al. 2002; Serebruany et al. 2003), cerebrovascular disease (Y. Chen et al. 2007; Murray et al. 2005; Rampello et al. 2004; Rasmussen et al. 2003; Robinson et al. 2000, 2008), Parkinson's disease (Barone et al. 2006; Devos et al. 2008), or other medical conditions (Arranz and Ros 1997; Evans et al. 1997; Goodnick and Hernandez 2000; Karp et al. 2005; Lotrich et al. 2007; Trappler and Cohen 1998) and in family dementia caregivers with minor or major depression (Lavretsky et al. 2010).

Two published placebo-controlled trials of citalopram (Lenze et al. 2005) and escitalopram (Lenze et al. 2009) support the ef-ficacy of SSRIs in older patients with generalized anxiety disorders. The use of SSRIs to treat other anxiety disorders is based on small open trials (Flint 2005; Lenze et al. 2002; Sheikh et al. 2004b; Wylie et al. 2000) or extrapolation from studies in younger adults.

Some published studies—including two randomized controlled trials—suggest that SSRIs may be efficacious in the treatment of behavioral disturbances associated with dementia, including not only agitation and disinhibition but also delusions and hallucinations (Nyth and Gottfries 1990; Nyth et al. 1992; Pollock et al. 1997, 2002, 2007). Some older open studies and small single-site controlled trials also supported the use of SSRIs for the treatment of depression associated with Alzheimer's dementia (Katona et al. 1998; Lyketsos et al. 2003; Nyth and Gottfries 1990; Nyth et al. 1992; Olafsson et al. 1992; Petracca et al. 2001; Taragano et al. 1997). However, a larger multicenter trial failed to confirm these results: in this study, sertraline was not more efficacious and was less well tolerated than placebo for the treatment of depression in Alzheimer's disease (Rosenberg et al. 2010; Weintraub et al. 2010).

Some administrative or quasi-experimental geriatric data suggest that escitalopram may be more efficacious or better tolerated than other SSRIs (Wu et al. 2008a, 2008b). However, available data from head-to-head randomized comparisons support that all SSRIs currently available have similar efficacy and tolerability in the treatment of depression (see Table 16–2). Nevertheless, experts favor the use of citalopram, escitalopram, or sertraline over fluvoxamine, fluoxetine, or paroxetine (Alexopoulos et al. 2001; Mulsant et al. 2001a; Rajji et al. 2008) because of their favorable pharmacokinetic profiles (Table 16–3) and their lower poten-

TABLE 16–2. Summary of published randomized controlled trials of selective serotonin reuptake inhibitors for acute treatment of geriatric depression

	No. of published trials (cumulative no. of older participants)	Dosages studied (mg/day)	Comments
Citalopram	7[a] (N=1,343)	10–40	Citalopram was more efficacious than placebo in one of two trials and as efficacious as amitriptyline and venlafaxine. It was better tolerated than nortriptyline but associated with a lower remission rate. Several trials included patients with stroke and dementia.
Escitalopram	2[b] (N=781)	10–20	In one failed trial, escitalopram and fluoxetine were well tolerated but not superior to placebo. In another trial, escitalopram did not differ from placebo.
Fluoxetine	13[c] (N=2,092)	10–80	Fluoxetine was more efficacious than placebo in two of five trials and as efficacious as amitriptyline, doxepin, escitalopram, paroxetine, sertraline, trimipramine, and venlafaxine. In patients with dysthymic disorder, fluoxetine was marginally superior to placebo. In patients with dementia of the Alzheimer's type, fluoxetine did not differ from placebo.
Fluvoxamine	4[d] (N=278)	50–200	Fluvoxamine was more efficacious than placebo and as efficacious as dothiepin, imipramine, mianserin, and sertraline.
Paroxetine	9[e] (N=1,474)	10–60	Paroxetine was more efficacious than placebo and as efficacious as amitriptyline, bupropion, clomipramine, doxepin, fluoxetine, and imipramine. Paroxetine was less efficacious than venlafaxine in older patients (n=30) who had previously failed to respond to two other antidepressants. Mirtazapine was marginally superior to paroxetine. In very old long-term-care patients with minor depression, paroxetine was not more efficacious but was more cognitively toxic than placebo. One trial included patients with dementia.

TABLE 16–2. Summary of published randomized controlled trials of selective serotonin reuptake inhibitors for acute treatment of geriatric depression

	No. of published trials (cumulative no. of older participants)	Dosages studied (mg/day)	Comments
Sertraline	11[f] (N=1,948)	50–200	Sertraline was more efficacious than placebo and as efficacious as amitriptyline, fluoxetine, fluvoxamine, imipramine, nortriptyline, and venlafaxine. Greater cognitive improvement occurred with sertraline than with nortriptyline or fluoxetine. Some trials included long-term–care patients. In one small single-site trial, sertraline was more efficacious than placebo for the treatment of depression associated with Alzheimer's dementia. However, this finding was not replicated in a larger multicenter trial.

[a]Allard et al. 2004; Andersen et al. 1994; Kyle et al. 1998; Navarro et al. 2001; Nyth et al. 1992; Roose et al. 2004b; Rosenberg et al. 2007.

[b]Bose et al. 2008; Kasper et al. 2005.

[c]Altamura et al. 1989; Devanand et al. 2005; Doraiswamy et al. 2001; Evans et al. 1997; Feighner and Cohn 1985; Finkel et al. 1999; Kasper et al. 2005; Petracca et al. 2001; Schatzberg and Roose 2006; Schone and Ludwig 1993; Taragano et al. 1997; Tollefson et al. 1995; Wehmeier et al. 2005.

[d]Phanjoo et al. 1991; Rahman et al. 1991; Rossini et al. 2005; Wakelin 1986.

[e]Burrows et al. 2002; Dunner et al. 1992; Geretsegger et al. 1995; Guillibert et al. 1989; Katona et al. 1998; Mazeh et al. 2007; Mulsant et al. 2001b; Rapaport et al. 2003; Schatzberg et al. 2002; Schone and Ludwig 1993.

[f]Bondareff et al. 2000; Cohn et al. 1990; Doraiswamy et al. 2003; Finkel et al. 1999; Forlenza et al. 2001; Lyketsos et al. 2003; Newhouse et al. 2000; Oslin et al. 2000, 2003; Rosenberg et al. 2010; Rossini et al. 2005; Schneider et al. 2003; Sheikh et al. 2004a; Weintraub et al. 2010.

tial for clinically significant drug interactions (Table 16–4). Some data also suggest that they may be better tolerated (Cipriani et al. 2009) and more beneficial in terms of cognitive improvement (Burrows et al. 2002; Doraiswamy et al. 2003; Furlan et al. 2001; Jorge et al. 2010; Newhouse et al. 2000; Savaskan et al. 2008). However, some recent data suggest that citalopram—like other SSRIs—may have deleterious cognitive effects in some very old patients (Culang et al. 2009) and that those with executive dysfunction may not benefit from citalopram and other SSRIs (Sneed et al. 2010). Also, in August 2011, the FDA issued a warning recommending against the use of citalopram dosages greater than 40 mg/day in any person and greater than 20 mg/day in people older than 60 years, because of a risk of prolonged QTc and torsade de pointes (see footnote b in Table 16–3).

In older patients, SSRI starting dosages are typically half the minimal efficacious dosage (see Table 16–3), and the dosage is usually doubled after 1 week. All of the SSRIs can be administered in a single daily dose except for fluvoxamine, which should be given in two divided doses. Even though frail older patients typically tolerate these drugs relatively well (Oslin et al. 2000), some patients experience some gastrointestinal distress (e.g., nausea) during the first few days of treatment. Significant hyponatremia resulting from the syndrome of inappropriate secretion of antidiuretic hormone (SIADH) is a rare but potentially dangerous adverse effect that is observed almost exclusively in elderly patients (Fabian et al. 2004).

SSRIs may directly affect platelet activation (Pollock et al. 2000), and they are associated with a small increase in the risk of gastrointestinal or postsurgical bleeding (Dalton et al. 2006; Looper 2007). SSRIs act synergistically with other medications that increase the risk of gastrointestinal bleeding, such as nonsteroidal anti-inflammatory drugs (NSAIDs) and low-dose aspirin. Thus, SSRIs should be used cautiously in older patients taking these medications, and the prophylactic use of acid-suppressing agents should be considered in some high-risk patients (de Abajo and Garcia-Rodriguez 2008; Yuan et al. 2006).

SSRIs also can be associated with bradycardia and should be started with caution in patients with low heart rates (e.g., patients taking β-blockers). They rarely cause extrapyramidal symptoms (Mamo et al. 2000), and they are well tolerated by most patients with Parkinson's disease (P. Chen et al. 2007). The risk of falls and hip fracture does not differ among different classes of antidepressants (Liu et al. 1998), and there is concern that chronic use of SSRIs may contribute to the risk of fractures through their direct effects on bone metabolism (Diem et al. 2007; Richards et al. 2007).

A large pharmacoepidemiological study found that SSRIs in elders, compared with non-SSRI antidepressants, are associated with a greater risk for suicide during the first month of therapy (Juurlink et al. 2006). However, the absolute risk is low, which suggests that there may be a vulnerable subgroup at risk for an idiosyncratic response. A very large meta-analysis and controlled data available to the FDA indicated a substantial reduction in the risk for suicidal ideation in older individuals taking SSRIs compared with those taking placebo (Barbui et al. 2009; Friedman and Leon 2007; Nelson et al. 2007).

TABLE 16–3. Pharmacokinetic properties of selective serotonin reuptake inhibitors and serotonin-norepinephrine reuptake inhibitors

	Half-life (days), including active metabolites	Proportionality of dosage to plasma concentration	Risk of uncomfortable withdrawal symptoms	Efficacious dosage range in elderly (mg/day)[a]
Citalopram	1–3	Linear across therapeutic range	Low	20[b]
Desvenlafaxine	0.5	Linear up to 600 mg/day	High	50
Duloxetine	0.5	Linear across therapeutic range	Moderate	60–120
Escitalopram	1–2	Linear across therapeutic range	Low	10–20
Fluoxetine	7–10	Nonlinear at higher dosages	Very low	20–40
Fluvoxamine	0.5–1	Nonlinear at higher dosages	Moderate	50–300
Paroxetine	1	Nonlinear at higher dosages	Moderate	20–40
Sertraline	1–3	Linear across therapeutic range	Low	50–200
Venlafaxine XR	0.2	Linear across therapeutic range	High	75–300

Note. XR = extended release.

[a]Starting dosage is typically half of the lowest efficacious dosage; all the selective serotonin reuptake inhibitors can be administered in single daily doses except for fluvoxamine, which should be given in two divided doses.

[b]In August 2011, the U.S. Food and Drug Administration issued a drug safety communication stating the following: "20 mg per day is the maximum recommended dose for patients with hepatic impairment, who are greater than 60 years of age, who are CYP 2C19 poor metabolizers, or who are taking concomitant cimetidine (Tagamet), because these factors lead to increased blood levels of citalopram, increasing the risk of QT interval prolongation and Torsade de Pointes" (www.fda.gov/Drugs/DrugSafety/ucm269086.htm).

TABLE 16–4. Newer antidepressants' inhibition of cytochrome P450 (CYP) and potential for causing clinically significant drug-drug interactions

	CYP1A2	CYP2C9/ 2C19	CYP2D6	CYP3A4	Potential for causing clinically significant drug-drug interaction
Bupropion	0	0	++	0	Low
Citalopram	+	0	+	0	Low
Desvenlafaxine	0	0	+	0	Minimal
Duloxetine	0	0	++	+	Low
Escitalopram	+	0	+	0	Minimal
Fluoxetine	+	++	+++	++	High
Fluvoxamine	+++	+++	+	++	High
Mirtazapine	0	0	0	+	Low
Nefazodone	0	+	0	+++	High
Paroxetine	+	+	+++	+	Moderate
Sertraline	+	+	+	+	Low
Venlafaxine	0	0	0	0	Low

Note. 0=minimal or no inhibition; +=mild inhibition; ++=moderate inhibition; +++=strong inhibition.

Serotonin-Norepinephrine Reuptake Inhibitors

As of December 2010, three serotonin-norepinephrine reuptake inhibitors (SNRIs) are approved by the FDA for the treatment of major depressive disorder in adults: desvenlafaxine, duloxetine, and venlafaxine. Duloxetine and venlafaxine are also approved for the treatment of generalized anxiety disorder; duloxetine for diabetic peripheral neuropathic pain and fibromyalgia; and venlafaxine for panic disorder and social anxiety disorder. Because of their usually favorable side-effect profile in younger patients and their dual mechanism of action (Chalon et al. 2003; Harvey et al. 2000), SNRIs have become the preferred alternatives to SSRIs. Some meta-analyses have suggested that venlafaxine is associated with a higher rate of remission than are SSRIs in younger depressed patients (Shelton et al. 2005; Smith et al. 2002; Stahl et al. 2002; Thase et al. 2001, 2005a). However, several other meta-analyses and head-to-head trials have contradicted these results or challenged their clinical significance in both younger (Cipriani et al. 2009; Hansen et al. 2005; Kornstein et al. 2010a; Lam et al. 2010; Papakostas et al. 2007; Vis et al. 2005) and older patients (Mukai and Tampi 2009; Nelson et al. 2008; Rajji et al. 2008). Also, the risk-benefit ratio of SNRIs may be different in younger versus older individuals, which may change their relative desirability in the treatment of older patients (see below).

The efficacy, tolerability, and relative safety of SNRIs in the treatment of late-life depression are supported by 10 published controlled trials involving about 1,300 older patients (9 trials with venlafaxine and 1 with duloxetine; see Table 16–5). Two additional

TABLE 16–5. Summary of published randomized controlled trials of serotonin-norepinephrine reuptake inhibitors (desvenlafaxine, duloxetine, venlafaxine), bupropion, and mirtazapine for acute treatment of geriatric depression

	No. of published trials (cumulative no. of older participants)	Dosages studied (mg/day)	Comments
Bupropion	2[a] (N=163)	100–450	Bupropion was as efficacious as imipramine and paroxetine.
Desvenlafaxine	0	NA	No published geriatric randomized trials as of December 2010.
Duloxetine	1[b] (N=311)	20–60	Duloxetine was more efficacious and as well tolerated as placebo. Duloxetine also showed efficacy on pain and cognitive measures.
Mirtazapine	2[c] (N=370)	15–45	Mirtazapine was as efficacious as low-dose (total daily dose = 30–90 mg) amitriptyline and marginally superior to paroxetine.
Venlafaxine	9[d] (N=1,032)	50–300	Venlafaxine did not differ from placebo in one trial. Venlafaxine was as efficacious as citalopram, clomipramine, dothiepin, fluoxetine, nortriptyline, and sertraline and was more efficacious than paroxetine (in 30 older patients who had previously failed to respond to two other antidepressants) and trazodone. It was less well tolerated than placebo, fluoxetine, and sertraline; tolerated as well as citalopram and dothiepin; and better tolerated than clomipramine, nortriptyline, and trazodone.

Note.   NA=not applicable.
[a]Branconnier et al. 1983; Doraiswamy et al. 2001; Weihs et al. 2000.
[b]Raskin et al. 2007; Wohlreich et al. 2009.
[c]Hoyberg et al. 1996; Schatzberg et al. 2002.
[d]Allard et al. 2004; Gasto et al. 2003; Kok et al. 2007; Mahapatra and Hackett 1997; Mazeh et al. 2007; Oslin et al. 2003; Schatzberg and Roose 2006; Smeraldi et al. 1998; Trick et al. 2004.

analyses of geriatric data pooled from randomized placebo-controlled trials conducted in mixed-age adults support the efficacy of desvenlafaxine and duloxetine for late-life depression (Kornstein et al. 2010a; Nelson et al. 2005). In randomized comparisons of desvenlafaxine with escitalopram and placebo in perimenopausal and postmenopausal women ages 40–70 years with major depressive disorder, desvenlafaxine and escitalopram had similar efficacy and tolerability (Kornstein et al. 2010b; Soares et al. 2010). Additional data from open-label studies and case series support the efficacy of SNRIs in older patient populations, including patients with atypical depression (Roose et al. 2004a), treatment-resistant depression (Mazeh et al. 2007), dysthymic disorder (Devanand et al. 2004), poststroke depression (Dahmen et al. 1999), generalized anxiety disorder (Katz et al. 2002), chronic pain syndromes (Grothe et al. 2004), stress urinary incontinence (Mariappan et al. 2005), or pain symptoms associated with geriatric depression (Karp et al. 2010; Raskin et al. 2007; Wohlreich et al. 2009).

SNRIs do not inhibit significantly any of the major cytochrome P450 (CYP) isoenzymes, and thus they are unlikely to cause clinically significant drug-drug interactions (Oganesian et al. 2009) (see Table 16–4). However, venlafaxine and duloxetine are metabolized by CYP2D6, and their concentration can increase markedly in genetically poor metabolizers or in patients who are taking drugs that inhibit this isoenzyme (Whyte et al. 2006). The concentration of duloxetine also can be increased by drugs that inhibit CYP1A2. Dose adjustments of SNRIs are not recommended on the basis of age (see Table 16–3), but they should be used with caution in older patients with renal or liver disease (Dolder et al. 2010).

SNRIs inhibit the reuptake of serotonin. Thus, they share the side-effect profile of the SSRIs, including not only nausea, diarrhea, headaches, and excessive sweating but also sexual dysfunction (Montejo et al. 2001), SIADH and hyponatremia (Kirby et al. 2002), upper gastrointestinal tract bleeding (de Abajo and Garcia-Rodriguez 2008), serotonin syndrome (McCue and Joseph 2001; Perry 2000), and discontinuation symptoms (Montgomery et al. 2009). SNRIs are also associated with adverse effects that can be linked to their action on the adrenergic system, including dry mouth, constipation, urinary retention, increased ocular pressure, cardiovascular problems, and transient agitation (Aragona and Inghilleri 1998; Benazzi 1997; Dolder et al. 2010). These adverse effects appear to be dose-dependent (Clayton et al. 2009; Liebowitz et al. 2010; Thase 1998), and they are usually self-limiting. However, cardiovascular effects of SNRIs are of special concern in the elderly. SNRIs can cause not only some increase in blood pressure (Clayton et al. 2009; Thase 1998; Thase et al. 2005c; Zimmer et al. 1997) but also clinically significant orthostatic hypotension, syncope, electrocardiographic changes, arrhythmia, acute ischemia, and death in overdose (Clayton et al. 2009; Davidson et al. 2005; Johnson et al. 2006; Lessard et al. 1999; Reznik et al. 1999). At this time, we do not know whether the cardiovascular risks of the three SNRIs differ. However, venlafaxine has been used for the longest time, and the bulk of the relevant available data implicates venlafaxine. In the United Kingdom, the National Institute for Clinical Excellence has recommended that venlafaxine should not be prescribed to patients with preexisting heart disease, that an electrocardiogram should be obtained at baseline, and that blood pressure and cardiac functions should be monitored in those patients who are taking higher doses

(National Collaborating Centre for Mental Health 2004). Overall, duloxetine and venlafaxine may be less well tolerated than escitalopram and sertraline (Cipriani et al. 2009), and a randomized trial conducted under double-blind conditions in older nursing home residents found that venlafaxine was less well tolerated and less safe than sertraline without evidence for an increase in efficacy (Oslin et al. 2003).

In conclusion, it seems prudent not to use SNRIs as first-line agents in older patients but to reserve them for those whose symptoms do not respond to SSRIs (Alexopoulos et al. 2001; Cooper et al. 2011; Karp et al. 2008; Mulsant et al. 2001a; Whyte et al. 2004) or those who present with depression and chronic pain (Karp et al. 2010; Raskin et al. 2007; Wohlreich et al. 2009). This recommendation is congruent with the results from the Sequenced Treatment Alternatives to Relieve Depression study (STAR*D; Rush et al. 2006). In this large study, mixed-age patients who had failed a first-line SSRI had similar outcomes when the next treatment step was augmenting the SSRI with sustained-release bupropion or buspirone, switching to another SSRI, or switching to an agent from another class (i.e., bupropion or venlafaxine extended-release [XR]). The following steps included using a combination of venlafaxine XR and mirtazapine, with outcomes similar to those associated with switching to the monoamine oxidase inhibitor (MAOI) tranylcypromine (Rush et al. 2006).

Other Newer Antidepressants

Only limited controlled data support the efficacy and safety of bupropion or mirtazapine in older patients (see Table 16–5). Nevertheless, because of their usually favorable side-effect profiles and their different mechanisms of action, these two drugs are often used in older individuals whose symptoms do not respond to or who are unable to tolerate SSRIs (Alexopoulos et al. 2001).

Bupropion

Published data supporting the safety and efficacy of bupropion in geriatric depression are limited to two small controlled trials (see Table 16–5) and one small open study (Steffens et al. 2001). Expert consensus favors the use of bupropion—alone or as an augmentation agent—in older patients with depression whose symptoms have not responded to SSRIs or who cannot tolerate them (Alexopoulos et al. 2001). In particular, bupropion can be helpful for patients who complain of nausea, diarrhea, unbearable fatigue, or sexual dysfunction during SSRI treatment (Nieuwstraten and Dolovich 2001; Thase et al. 2005b). Although augmentation with bupropion has been reported to be helpful in patients who were partial responders to SSRIs or venlafaxine (Bodkin et al. 1997; Spier 1998), the safety of this combination in older patients has not been established (Joo et al. 2002). Controlled data on the use of bupropion in patients with heart disease (Kiev et al. 1994; Roose et al. 1991), in smokers (Tashkin et al. 2001), and in patients with neuropathic pain (Semenchuk et al. 2001) confirm clinical experience that bupropion is relatively well tolerated by medically ill patients. Bupropion is contraindicated in patients who have or are at risk for seizure disorders (e.g., poststroke patients). However, the sustained-release preparation of bupropion appears to be associated with a very low incidence of seizure, comparable to that of other antidepressants (Dunner et al. 1998).

Bupropion also has been associated with the onset of psychosis in case reports (Howard and Warnock 1999), and it is prudent to avoid this medication in psychotic patients or in agitated patients who are at risk for the development of psychotic symptoms. The propensity of bupropion to induce psychosis in patients at risk has been attributed to its action on dopaminergic neurotransmission (Howard and Warnock 1999). The same mechanism has been hypothesized to underlie the association of bupropion with gait disturbance and falls in some individuals (Joo et al. 2002; Szuba and Leuchter 1992).

Bupropion is a moderate inhibitor of CYP2D6 (Kotlyar et al. 2005). It appears to be metabolized by CYP2B6 (Hesse et al. 2004), and adverse effects of bupropion such as seizures or gait disturbance may be more likely in patients who take drugs that inhibit CYP2B6, such as fluoxetine or paroxetine (Joo et al. 2002).

Mirtazapine

The antidepressant activity of mirtazapine has been attributed to its blockade of α_2 autoreceptors, resulting in a direct enhancement of noradrenergic neurotransmission and an increase in the synaptic levels of serotonin (5-hydroxytryptamine [5-HT]), indirectly enhancing neurotransmission mediated by serotonin type 1A (5-HT_{1A}) receptors. In addition, like the antinausea drugs granisetron and ondansetron, mirtazapine inhibits the 5-HT_2 and 5-HT_3 receptors. Thus, mirtazapine could be particularly helpful for individuals who do not tolerate SSRIs because of sexual dysfunction (Gelenberg et al. 2000; Montejo et al. 2001), tremor (Pact and Giduz 1999), or severe nausea (Pedersen and Klysner 1997). In one case series, mirtazapine was used

successfully to treat depression in 19 mixed-age oncology patients who were receiving chemotherapy (Thompson 2000). It also has been combined with SSRIs (Pedersen and Klysner 1997). However, these combinations should be used cautiously because they have been associated with a serotonin syndrome in an older individuals (Benazzi 1998). The STAR*D study found that a combination of mirtazapine and venlafaxine XR had modest efficacy in patients with treatment-resistant depression, comparable to the efficacy of the MAOI tranylcypromine (Rush et al. 2006). However, only a few STAR*D participants were elderly, and the safety of this combination has not been established in older patients.

No published placebo-controlled trials and only two comparator-controlled trials of mirtazapine in geriatric depression have been done (see Table 16–5). Consistent with this paucity of controlled data, experts favor the use of mirtazapine as a third-line drug in older depressed patients who cannot tolerate or whose symptoms have not responded to SSRIs or venlafaxine (Alexopoulos et al. 2001). Mirtazapine also has been used to treat depression in frail nursing home patients (Roose et al. 2003) and in older patients with dementia (Raji and Brady 2001), but there are concerns about its effect on cognition. Mirtazapine has been shown to impair driving performance in two placebo- and active comparator–controlled trials in healthy volunteers (Ridout et al. 2003; Wingen et al. 2005) and to cause delirium in older patients with organic brain syndromes (Bailer et al. 2000). This deleterious effect on cognition is possibly a result of mirtazapine's antihistaminergic and sedative effects. Other adverse effects of mirtazapine include weight gain with lipid increase (Nicholas et al. 2003), hyponatremia (Cheah et al. 2008), and, very rarely, neutropenia or even agranulocytosis (Hutchison 2001).

Nefazodone

Given the absence of any controlled trials in geriatric depression, mediocre outcomes in an open study (Saiz-Ruiz et al. 2002), potentially problematic drug-drug interactions caused by its strong inhibition of CYP3A4 (see Table 16–4), and reports that the incidence of hepatic toxicity or even liver failure is 10- to 30-fold higher with nefazodone than with other antidepressants (Carvajal García-Pando et al. 2002), nefazodone should not be used in older patients.

Tricyclic Antidepressants and Monoamine Oxidase Inhibitors

As is the case in younger patients (Rush et al. 2006), tricyclic antidepressants (TCAs) and MAOIs have been relegated to third- and fourth-line drugs in the treatment of late-life depression because of their adverse effects and the special precautions that their use entails (Mottram et al. 2006; Mulsant et al. 2001a; Rajji et al. 2008; Wilson and Mottram 2004).

The tertiary-amine TCAs—amitriptyline, clomipramine, doxepin, and imipramine—can cause significant orthostatic hypotension and anticholinergic effects, including cognitive impairment, and they should be avoided in the elderly (Beers 1997). The secondary amines desipramine and nortriptyline are preferred in older patients. They have a lower propensity to cause orthostasis and falls, linear pharmacokinetics, and more modest anticholinergic effects (Chew et al. 2008). Their relatively

narrow therapeutic index (i.e., the plasma level range separating efficacy and toxicity) necessitates monitoring of plasma levels and electrocardiograms in older patients. A single dose is given at bedtime; 5–7 days after initiating desipramine at 50 mg or nortriptyline at 25 mg, plasma levels should be measured after 5–7 days and dosages adjusted linearly, targeting plasma levels of 200–400 ng/mL for desipramine and 50–150 ng/mL for nortriptyline. These narrow ranges ensure efficacy while decreasing risks of cardiac toxicity and other side effects. Like the tertiary-amine TCAs, desipramine and nortriptyline are type 1 antiarrhythmics: they have quinidine-like effects on cardiac conduction and should not be used in patients who have or are at risk for cardiac conduction defects (Roose et al. 1991). Most anticholinergic side effects of desipramine or nortriptyline (e.g., dry mouth, constipation) resolve with time or usually can be mitigated with symptomatic treatment (Rosen et al. 1993). However, TCAs have been associated with cognitive worsening (Reifler et al. 1989) or with less cognitive improvement than with sertraline (Bondareff et al. 2000; Doraiswamy et al. 2003) or other SSRIs.

Even though MAOIs have been found to be efficacious in older depressed patients (Georgotas et al. 1986), and they may have a special role in patients with atypical or treatment-resistant depression, these medications are now rarely used in older patients (Shulman et al. 2009). This is in large part because they can cause significant hypotension or life-threatening hypertensive or serotonergic crises as a result of dietary or drug interactions. When MAOIs are used in older patients whose symptoms have typically failed to respond to SSRIs, SNRIs, and TCAs, phenelzine is preferred to tranylcypromine because it has been more extensively studied in older patients (Georgotas et al. 1986). A typical starting dosage would be 15 mg/day, with a target dosage of 45–90 mg/day in three divided doses. Patients need to follow dietary restrictions (Shulman and Walker 2001) and to inform any health care providers (including pharmacists) that they are taking an MAOI. Another option is the selegiline transdermal patch. It was developed to deliver selegiline blood concentrations sufficient to inhibit monoamine oxidase–A (MAO-A) and MAO-B in the brain without inhibiting MAO-A in the gastrointestinal tract, thereby reducing the risk of hypertensive crisis (Nandagopal and DelBello 2009). No geriatric data are available, but dietary restrictions are not needed at the 6-mg/24-hour dose. However, they are recommended with higher doses (Robinson and Amsterdam 2008), and potentially lethal drug interactions remain a concern.

Psychostimulants

Even though psychostimulants are used in the treatment of late-life mood disorders by some clinicians, this practice has minimal empirical support. A few small double-blind trials suggested that methylphenidate is generally well tolerated and modestly efficacious for medically burdened elderly patients with depression (Satel and Nelson 1989; Wallace et al. 1995). Methylphenidate also has been used for the treatment of apathy and anergia associated with late-life depression or dementia (Herrmann et al. 2008). SSRIs inhibit dopamine release and may contribute to apathy and fatigue. A small study suggested that methylphenidate can be used to augment SSRIs in older depressed patients (Lavretsky et al. 2006). The wakefulness-promoting agent modafinil,

which appears to induce a calm alertness through nondopaminergic mechanisms, also may have utility when targeting apathy and fatigue in patients who are taking SSRIs (Dunlop et al. 2007; Fava et al. 2007), but geriatric data are currently nonexistent. Caution is advised regarding the possible exacerbation by methylphenidate and other psychostimulant agents of anxiety, psychosis, anorexia, or hypertension and potential interactions with warfarin. Experience with other dopaminergic medications—such as pergolide, piribedil, pramipexole, and ropinirole—in the elderly has been limited, but there have been several encouraging controlled trials in patients with Parkinson's disease and depression (Aiken 2007; Barone et al. 2006, 2010; Rektorova et al. 2003) and in cognitively impaired elders (Nagaraja and Jayashree 2001).

Antipsychotic Medications

As in other age groups, atypical antipsychotics are being prescribed in late life as first-line drugs for the treatment of psychotic symptoms of any etiology. Studies support the efficacy of these agents in the treatment of late-life schizophrenia and late-onset psychoses (Scott et al. 2011), but their role in the treatment of behavioral and psychological symptoms of dementia is being questioned (Ballard and Corbett 2010; Salzman et al. 2008; Siddiqi et al. 2007). A highly publicized report and an FDA warning have indicated a nearly twofold increase in the rate of deaths in older patients with behavioral and psychological symptoms of dementia treated with atypical antipsychotics when compared with placebo (Kuehn 2005; Schneider et al. 2005). These reports have led to a reexamination of the safety of both conventional and atypical antipsychotics in older patients. A series of studies emphasize their association with mortality (Ballard et al. 2009; Wang et al. 2005; Ray et al. 2009), stroke (Gill et al. 2005; Herrmann et al. 2004), severe hyperglycemia in patients with diabetes (Lipscombe et al. 2009), femur fractures (Liperoti et al. 2007), and venous thromboembolism (Kleijer et al. 2010). The relative safety of atypical compared with conventional antipsychotics remains unclear: atypical antipsychotics may cause fewer falls (Hien et al. 2005; Landi et al. 2005) and fewer extrapyramidal symptoms (Lee et al. 2004; Rochon et al. 2005; van Iersel et al. 2005), but they may cause more cerebrovascular events (Percudani et al. 2005), venous thromboembolism (Liperoti et al. 2005), and pancreatitis (Koller et al. 2003). Given the current uncertainty regarding the safety of antipsychotics—and, for most indications, the absence of consistent evidence supporting the efficacy or safety of drugs from alternative classes (Ballard and Corbett 2010; Sink et al. 2005)—clinicians need to consider the risk-benefit ratio for each individual patient (Gauthier et al. 2010; Rabins and Lyketsos 2005).

Risperidone

Of the atypical antipsychotics currently available in the United States, risperidone has the most published geriatric data for a variety of conditions (Schneider et al. 2005, 2006a; Sink et al. 2005). The efficacy and safety of risperidone in the treatment of behavioral and psychological symptoms of dementia have been reported in several randomized placebo-controlled trials (e.g., Brodaty et al. 2003; De Deyn et al. 1999, 2005b; Katz et al. 1999; Schneider et al. 2006a, 2006b; Sink et al. 2005); randomized comparisons with haloperidol (Chan

et al. 2001; De Deyn et al. 1999; Suh et al. 2004), promazine, and olanzapine (Gareri et al. 2004) or olanzapine (Fontaine et al. 2003; Mulsant et al. 2004); and many uncontrolled studies or large case series.

The efficacy and tolerability of risperidone in the treatment of late-life schizophrenia are supported by one randomized comparison with olanzapine (Harvey et al. 2003; Jeste et al. 2003) and one randomized open-label study involving crossover from a conventional antipsychotic to risperidone or olanzapine (Ritchie et al. 2003, 2006). The parallel study showed similar efficacy between olanzapine and risperidone but more weight gain and less cognitive improvement with olanzapine. In the crossover study, patients who were switched to olanzapine were more likely to complete the switching process and to show an improvement in psychological quality of life. The results from these two controlled trials are supported by a large body of uncontrolled data in older patients with schizophrenia and other psychotic disorders (e.g., Davidson et al. 2000; Madhusoodanan et al. 1999). In addition, an analysis of the patients with schizophrenia age 65 years and older ($N=57$) who participated in randomized studies of the long-acting injectable ("depot" or Risperdal Consta) risperidone concluded that it was well tolerated and produced significant symptomatic improvements (Lasser et al. 2004).

One randomized comparison with haloperidol (Han and Kim 2004) and some uncontrolled data (e.g., Mittal et al. 2004; Parellada et al. 2004) support the efficacy and tolerability of risperidone in the treatment of delirium. However, there have been several case reports of delirium induced by risperidone. One small randomized comparison with clozapine ($N=10$)

(Ellis et al. 2000) and several open trials of low-dose risperidone in the treatment of Parkinson's disease and drug-induced psychosis or Lewy body dementia have had inconsistent results, with clear worsening of parkinsonian symptoms occurring in some studies (e.g., Culo et al. 2010; Ellis et al. 2000; Leopold 2000). Thus, risperidone should be used with great caution in the treatment of these disorders (Parkinson Study Group 1999).

As with other atypical antipsychotics, the efficacy and tolerability of risperidone in younger patients with bipolar disorder (and possibly other mood disorders) (Andreescu et al. 2006) are well established. However, no efficacy data in older patients with bipolar disorder would favor the selection of a specific atypical antipsychotic for these patients. As a result, experts continue to favor the use of mood stabilizers as first-line agents except in the presence of severe mania or mania with psychosis, in which case they favor combining risperidone, olanzapine, or quetiapine with a mood stabilizer (Sajatovic et al. 2005b; Young et al. 2004).

Commonly reported side effects of risperidone include orthostatic hypotension (on initiation of treatment) and extrapyramidal symptoms that are dose-dependent (Katz et al. 1999). At a given dosage, concentrations of risperidone (and possibly those of its active metabolite paliperidone or 9-hydroxyrisperidone) seem to increase with age (Aichhorn et al. 2005). Therefore, typical dosages should be between 0.5 and 2.0 mg/day for older patients with dementia and lower than 4 mg/day for older patients without dementia. Of all the atypical antipsychotics, risperidone appears to be the most likely to be associated with hyperprolactinemia (Kinon et al. 2003). Risperi-

done causes only moderate electroencephalographic abnormalities (Centorrino et al. 2002), and it is rarely associated with cognitive impairment, probably because of its low affinity for muscarinic receptors (Chew et al. 2006; Harvey et al. 2003; Mulsant et al. 2004). Like other antipsychotics, risperidone can cause weight gain, diabetes, or dyslipidemia. It is more likely to do so than are aripiprazole and ziprasidone but less likely than are clozapine, olanzapine, and quetiapine (American Diabetes Association et al. 2004; Feldman et al. 2004; Zheng et al. 2009).

Paliperidone

Paliperidone is the active 9-hydroxy metabolite of risperidone, and therefore its pharmacological action, efficacy, and side effects should be very similar to those of risperidone. It is being marketed as a once-daily XR formulation that takes 24 hours to reach a maximum concentration. As a hydroxylated metabolite, paliperidone clearance is not affected by hepatic impairment or CYP2D6 metabolism, but it is affected by renal function. FDA approval was based on three 6-week trials that included a total of only 125 subjects who were age 65 years or older (e.g., Davidson et al. 2007; Kane et al. 2007). Limited available data indicate that paliperidone may be effective in the treatment of schizophrenia in the elderly (Madhusoodanan and Zaveri 2010). However, paliperidone has not yet been studied in patients with dementia, and doses remain speculative for this population.

Olanzapine

Next to risperidone, olanzapine has the greatest amount of published geriatric data. Its efficacy and tolerability in the treatment of behavioral and psychological symptoms of dementia have been reported in several randomized placebo-controlled trials (e.g., Clark et al. 2001; De Deyn et al. 2004; Schneider et al. 2006b; Street et al. 2000) and in randomized comparisons with haloperidol (Verhey et al. 2006), promazine and risperidone (Gareri et al. 2004), and risperidone (Fontaine et al. 2003; Mulsant et al. 2004). However, a meta-analysis of both published and nonpublished placebo-controlled trials of olanzapine in the treatment of behavioral and psychological symptoms of dementia concluded that "olanzapine was not associated with efficacy overall" (Schneider et al. 2006a, p. 205). Also, the study by Street and colleagues (2000) found an inverted dose-response relation (i.e., patients receiving 15 mg/day had worse outcomes than did patients receiving 5 mg/day), suggesting that higher dosages may be toxic in these patients (see discussion later in this subsection).

The efficacy and tolerability of olanzapine in the treatment of late-life schizophrenia have been confirmed in two randomized comparisons with haloperidol (Barak et al. 2002; Kennedy et al. 2003) and two randomized comparisons with risperidone (Harvey et al. 2003; Jeste et al. 2003; Ritchie et al. 2003, 2006).

In one randomized controlled trial in patients with delirium, olanzapine and haloperidol were found to have comparable efficacy (Skrobik et al. 2004). However, caution is needed when using olanzapine in patients with delirium because some controlled trials have reported some cognitive worsening in patients with dementia taking olanzapine (Kennedy et al. 2005; Mulsant et al. 2004), and several case reports of delirium induced by olanzapine have been published. Similarly, the need for caution

when olanzapine is used to treat psychosis in patients with Parkinson's disease or Lewy body dementia is reinforced by two comparative trials (Breier et al. 2002; Goetz et al. 2000) and several open trials or case series (e.g., Marsh et al. 2001; Molho and Factor 1999; Parkinson Study Group 1999; Walker et al. 1999) that have reported a significant worsening of motor symptoms in these patients.

The evidence supporting the efficacy and safety of olanzapine in younger patients with bipolar disorder and other mood disorders (Andreescu et al. 2006; Shelton et al. 2001; Thase 2002) is strong. However, there is a paucity of data relevant to older patients with mood disorders (Meyers et al. 2009; Sajatovic et al. 2005a, 2005b; Young et al. 2004). Similarly, very few geriatric data are available on the rapidly dissolving or the intramuscular preparations of olanzapine (Belgamwar and Fenton 2005).

On review of all evidence available in 2004, a consensus conference concluded that among the atypical antipsychotics, clozapine and olanzapine were associated with the highest risk for diabetes and caused the greatest amount of weight gain and dyslipidemia (American Diabetes Association et al. 2004). Limited geriatric data show a similar higher risk of metabolic problems in older patients (Feldman et al. 2004; Micca et al. 2006; Zheng et al. 2009). Other common side effects include sedation and gait disturbance. Extrapyramidal symptoms appear to be dose-dependent and are rare at the lower dosages typically used in older populations (5–10 mg/day). Olanzapine also has been associated with electroencephalographic abnormalities (Centorrino et al. 2002), and its strong blocking of the muscarinic receptor (Chew et al. 2005, 2006; Mulsant et al. 2003) (Table 16–6) may explain why it has been associated with the following effects: constipation in a large series of long-term care patients (Martin et al. 2003); decreased efficacy at higher doses in a randomized trial in older agitated or psychotic patients with dementia (Street et al. 2000); a differential cognitive effect from risperidone in randomized trials involving older patients with schizophrenia (Harvey et al. 2003) or dementia (Mulsant et al. 2004); worsening of cognition in a large placebo-controlled trial in older nonagitated, nonpsychotic patients with Alzheimer's disease (Kennedy et al. 2005); and frank delirium in some clinical cases. Patients who are older, female, or nonsmokers or who are taking a medication that inhibits CYP1A2 (e.g., fluvoxamine or ciprofloxacin) have higher concentrations of olanzapine and may be at higher risk for adverse effects (Gex-Fabry et al. 2003). Because of its adverse-effect profile, experts do not recommend olanzapine as a first-line antipsychotic in older patients at special risk for anticholinergic or metabolic adverse effects (Bell et al. 2010).

Quetiapine

Results of randomized placebo-controlled trials of quetiapine in older patients with behavioral and psychological symptoms of dementia—both published and unpublished—are inconclusive (Schneider et al. 2006a). For instance, in a large trial of 333 institutionalized participants, quetiapine, 200 mg/day (but not 100 mg/day), differed from placebo on global impressions and positive symptom ratings but not on the important primary outcome measures of agitation and psychosis (Zhong et al. 2007). However, several published but uncontrolled or unblinded studies in older patients with primary psychotic disorders (e.g., Madhusoodanan et al. 2000; Tariot et

al. 2000; Yang et al. 2005), dementia, or delirium (e.g., Kim et al. 2003; Pae et al. 2004; Sasaki et al. 2003) suggested that quetiapine may be effective for these disorders. The good tolerability of quetiapine observed clinically in patients at high risk for extrapyramidal symptoms suggests that quetiapine should be the first-line antipsychotic for older individuals with Parkinson's disease, dementia with Lewy body, or tardive dyskinesia (Fernandez et al. 2002; Poewe 2005). However, quetiapine was not found to be efficacious in such patients in two double-blind trials (Kurlan et al. 2007; Rabey et al. 2007).

Quetiapine is approved by the FDA for the treatment of acute mania and depression associated with bipolar disorder in adults. However, relevant geriatric published data are limited (Carta et al. 2007; Tadger et al. 2011). There have been several case reports of inappropriate antidiuretic and serotonin syndromes in these patients (e.g., Atalay et al. 2007; Kohen et al. 2007). Like other antipsychotics, quetiapine also can cause somnolence or dizziness (Jaskiw et al. 2004; Yang et al. 2005), but the incidence of these adverse effects can be minimized by a slower dose titration. The risk for weight gain, diabetes, or dyslipidemia associated with quetiapine appears similar to the risk associated with the use of risperidone but lower than the risk associated with the use of clozapine or olanzapine (American Diabetes Association et al. 2004; Feldman et al. 2004).

Clozapine

Clozapine is still considered the drug of choice for younger patients with treatment-refractory schizophrenia, and one small case series suggested that it can be similarly helpful in older patients for the treatment of

TABLE 16–6. Receptor blockade of atypical antipsychotics

	D_2	$5\text{-}HT_2$	M_1	α_1
Aripiprazole	★	++	0	+
Asenapine	+++	+++	0	+++
Clozapine	+	++	+++	+
Iloperidone	+++	++++	0	++++
Lurasidone	+++	++	0	++
Olanzapine	++	+++	++	+
Paliperidone	+++	+++	0	++
Quetiapine	+	++	+	+
Risperidone	+++	++++	0	+++
Ziprasidone	++	++	0	+

Note. Receptor types: α_1 = alpha-adrenergic type 1; D_2 = dopamine type 2; $5\text{-}HT_2$ = 5-hydroxy-tryptamine (serotonin) type 2; M_1 = muscarinic type 1.
0 = none; + = minimal; ++ = intermediate; +++ = high; ++++ = very high.
★High-affinity partial agonist.

primary psychotic disorders refractory to other treatments (Sajatovic et al. 1997). A randomized controlled trial comparing clozapine and chlorpromazine in older patients with schizophrenia (Howanitz et al. 1999) and one large case series (Barak et al. 1999) also supported the use of clozapine in moderate dosages (i.e., approximately 50–200 mg/day) in older patients with primary psychotic disorders. The strongest published geriatric studies of clozapine have been focused on the treatment of drug-induced psychosis in patients with Parkinson's disease (Ellis et al. 2000; Goetz et al. 2000; Parkinson Study Group 1999). The results of these studies suggest that clozapine at low dosages (12.5–50 mg/day) could be the preferred treatment for this condition (Parkinson Study Group 1999). However, the use of clozapine in older patients is severely limited because of its significant hematological, neurological, cognitive, metabolic, and cardiac adverse effects (Alvir et al. 1993; Centorrino et al. 2002;

Chew et al. 2006; Koller et al. 2001; O'Connor et al. 2010; Rajji et al. 2010).

Aripiprazole

Aripiprazole has partial dopamine type 2 (D_2) receptor agonist properties (i.e., in high dopaminergic states, it acts as an antagonist, and in low dopaminergic states, it acts as an agonist). This may explain why it is unlikely to cause extrapyramidal side effects or prolactin elevation (associated with osteoporosis), even at high D_2 receptor occupancy (Mamo et al. 2007). Aripiprazole has only moderate affinity to the adrenergic α_1 receptor and histamine H_1 receptor and negligible affinity to the muscarinic receptor (Chew et al. 2006). As a result, orthostatic hypotension and antihistaminergic and anticholinergic adverse effects are less likely to occur with aripiprazole than with other atypical agents. However, akathisia may be a common side effect in older patients (Coley et al. 2009; Sheffrin et al. 2009). Three randomized placebo-controlled trials of aripiprazole in older patients with behavioral and psychological symptoms of dementia have been published (De Deyn et al. 2005a; Mintzer et al. 2007; Streim et al. 2008), and a meta-analysis of these trials concluded that "efficacy on rating scales was observed by meta-analysis for aripiprazole" (Schneider et al. 2006a, p. 191).

Aripiprazole is approved by the FDA for the treatment of manic or mixed episodes associated with bipolar disorder and as an adjunctive treatment for major depressive disorder. Although no relevant controlled trials have been done in older patients, some prospective open studies (Sajatovic et al. 2008; Sheffrin et al. 2009) and analyses of pooled geriatric data have been published (Steffens et al. 2011; Suppes et al. 2008).

Ziprasidone

On the basis of ziprasidone's lower effect on glucose, lipids, and weight (American Diabetes Association et al. 2004) and its lack of affinity for the muscarinic receptor (see Table 16–6) (Chew et al. 2006) and thus its low potential to cause cognitive impairment, ziprasidone is an attractive medication for older patients with psychosis. However, geriatric data on the use of oral ziprasidone remain very limited (Berkowitz 2003; Wilner et al. 2000). Three published studies on the use of intramuscular ziprasidone found no adverse cardiovascular or electrocardiographic changes in a small number of older patients (Greco et al. 2005; Kohen et al. 2005; Rais et al. 2010). However, in the absence of systematic study, concern about the potential effects of ziprasidone on cardiac conduction persists, and ziprasidone should not be used in older patients with QTc prolongation or congestive heart failure.

Newer Atypical Antipsychotics

In 2009–2010, three other atypical antipsychotics were approved by the FDA for use in schizophrenia: asenapine, iloperidone, and lurasidone. However, at this time, the paucity of geriatric data for these medications precludes making recommendations for their use in older patients.

Mood Stabilizers

As a class, mood stabilizers are high-risk medications for older patients. There is a paucity of controlled studies and an abundance of concerns regarding their potential toxicity, problematic side effects, and drug interactions. Beyond their approved indications, anticonvulsants are also used in the management of agitation accompanying dementia. Currently, no consensus exists as to which drug should be preferred as a first-line mood stabilizer in older patients with bipolar disorder or secondary mania (Sajatovic et al. 2005b; Shulman 2010; Young et al. 2004).

Lithium

Lithium continues to be used in older patients for the treatment of bipolar disorder (Shulman 2010) or, less commonly, as an augmentation agent in treatment-resistant depression (Cooper et al. 2011; Flint and Rifat 2001; Ross 2008) and for the prevention of depressive relapse following electroconvulsive therapy (ECT) (Sackeim et al. 2001). Data from open and controlled trials suggest that lithium is efficacious in the acute treatment and prophylaxis of mania in older patients (Sajatovic et al. 2005a; Shulman 2010). However, age-related reductions in renal clearance and decreased total body water significantly affect the pharmacokinetics of lithium in older patients, increasing the risk of toxicity. Medical comorbidities common in late life—such as impaired renal function, hyponatremia, dehydration, and heart failure—exacerbate further the risk of toxicity (Sajatovic et al. 2006). Thiazide diuretics, angiotensin converting enzyme inhibitors, and NSAIDs may precipitate toxicity by further diminishing the renal clearance of lithium. Lithium toxicity can produce persistent central nervous system impairment or be fatal: it is a medical emergency that requires careful correction of fluid and electrolyte imbalances and that may require administration of mannitol (or even hemodialysis) to increase lithium excretion.

Older patients require lower lithium dosages than do younger patients to produce similar serum lithium levels, and their lithium levels, electrolytes, and thyrotropin concentrations should be monitored regularly. Also, older individuals are more sensitive to neurological side effects at lower lithium levels. This sensitivity may be a consequence of increased permeability of the blood-brain barrier and subtle changes in sodium-lithium countertransport, resulting in a higher ratio of brain-to-serum concentration than in younger patients (Forester et al. 2009). Lithium neurotoxicity may manifest as coarse tremor, slurred speech, ataxia, hyperreflexia, and muscle fasciculations. In vitro, lithium has moderate anticholinergic activity (Chew et al. 2008). This may explain why cognitive impairment has been observed with levels well below 1 mEq/L, and frank delirium has been reported with levels as low as 1.5 mEq/L (Sproule et al. 2000). Consequently, treatment in older patients may require lithium levels to be kept as low as 0.4–0.8 mEq/L. Despite its potential toxicity, lithium remains an important drug in the treatment of bipolar

disorder and treatment-resistant depression in late life because of its potential effect on suicidality and neuroprotective properties (Muller-Oerlinghausen and Lewitzka 2010; Shulman 2010).

Anticonvulsants

Anticonvulsants are used as alternatives to lithium in the treatment of bipolar disorder and as alternatives to antipsychotics for the management of agitation associated with dementia. There may be a subgroup of patients with bipolar disorder with dysphoria or rapid cycling who respond poorly to lithium but do well with anticonvulsants (Post et al. 1998).

Divalproex

Divalproex, a compound of sodium valproate and valproic acid in an enteric-coated form, is a broad-spectrum anticonvulsant approved by the FDA for the treatment of acute manic or mixed episodes associated with bipolar disorder, with or without psychotic features. It also may be efficacious in the treatment of bipolar depression (Bond et al. 2010). Small case series have suggested that divalproex is relatively well tolerated by older patients with bipolar disorder (Kando et al. 1996; Noaghiul et al. 1998) and those with agitation in the context of dementia. Nonetheless, in four negative placebo-controlled trials, valproate was not more effective than placebo in treating agitation of dementia (Sink et al. 2005; Tariot et al. 2005). Sedation, nausea, weight gain, and hand tremors are common dose-related side effects. Reversible thrombocytopenia can occur in as many as half of the elderly patients taking divalproex and may ensue at lower total drug levels than in younger patients (Fenn et al. 2006). Other dose-related adverse effects include reversible elevations in liver enzymes and transient elevations in blood ammonia levels. However, liver failure and pancreatitis are rare. Divalproex has other metabolic effects of concern to aging patients, such as increases in bone turnover and reductions of serum folate, with concomitant elevations in plasma homocysteine concentrations (Sato et al. 2001; Schwaninger et al. 1999).

The pharmacokinetics of valproate vary according to formulation, and valproic acid, divalproex sodium, and its XR preparation are not interchangeable. Valproate is metabolized principally by mitochondrial β-oxidation and secondarily by the cytochrome P450 system; typical half-lives are in the range of 5–16 hours and are not affected by aging alone. Concomitant administration of valproate will increase concentrations of carbamazepine, diazepam, lamotrigine, phenobarbital, and primidone. Conversely, concurrent administration of carbamazepine, lamotrigine, phenytoin, and topiramate may decrease levels of valproate. Fluoxetine and erythromycin may potentiate the effects of valproate. Changes in protein binding as a result of drug interactions are no longer considered clinically important beyond causing the misinterpretation of total (i.e., free and bound) drug levels (Benet and Hoener 2002). Because valproate binding to plasma proteins is generally reduced in elderly patients, use of free drug levels correlates better with adverse effects (Fenn et al. 2006).

Lamotrigine

Lamotrigine is approved by the FDA for the maintenance treatment of bipolar I disorder to prevent mood episodes (depressive, manic, or mixed episodes), and it is considered a first-line agent for the treatment of bipolar depression (Fenn et al. 2006). Pooled data from two randomized placebo-controlled trials in geriatric subjects support the efficacy of lamotrigine in preventing bipolar depression in older patients (Sajatovic et al. 2005a, 2007). Open studies and case reports suggest a possible role for lamotrigine in the treatment of bipolar depression, bipolar mania, and agitation associated with dementia (Sajatovic et al. 2007). In contrast with many other mood stabilizers and antidepressants, lamotrigine does not seem to be associated with weight gain or to cause significant drug interactions. Typically, it is well tolerated, but somnolence and rashes have been observed in older patients. Rashes are the most common reason for discontinuation, but their incidence is far less frequent than with carbamazepine (Fenn et al. 2006). Severe rashes, including Stevens-Johnson syndrome or toxic epidermal necrolysis, have been observed in about 0.3% of adult patients (Messenheimer 1998). At the first sign of rash or other evidence of hypersensitivity (e.g., fever, lymphadenopathy), lamotrigine should be discontinued, and the patient should be evaluated. The incidence of rashes can be reduced by using a low initial dose and a slow titration. Because valproate increases lamotrigine concentration, the initial and target doses need to be halved in patients who are receiving divalproex and the titration of lamotrigine slowed down. Conversely, carbamazepine approximately halves lamotrigine concentrations, and the initial dose needs to be doubled in patients who are receiving carbamazepine.

Carbamazepine and Oxcarbazepine

The XR formulation of carbamazepine is approved by the FDA for the acute treatment of manic and mixed episodes associated with bipolar disorder. In a placebo-controlled trial in 51 nursing home patients, carbamazepine also was shown to be efficacious in treating agitation and aggression associated with dementia (Tariot et al. 1998). Common side effects in older patients include sedation, nausea, dizziness, rash, ataxia, neutropenia, and hyponatremia. Older patients are also at risk for agranulocytosis, aplastic anemia, hepatitis, and problematic drug interactions (Fenn et al. 2006). Carbamazepine is primarily eliminated by CYP3A4, and its clearance is reduced with aging. Its interactions with other drugs are protean: carbamazepine concentrations are increased to potential toxicity by CYP3A4 inhibitors such as macrolide antibiotics, antifungals, and some antidepressants (see Table 16–4). CYP3A4 inducers—such as phenobarbital, phenytoin, and carbamazepine itself—lower the concentration of carbamazepine and the concentrations of many drugs metabolized by this isoenzyme, including lamotrigine, valproate, some antidepressants, and antipsychotics (Fenn et al. 2006). Oxcarbazepine, the 10-keto analog of carbamazepine, is a less potent CYP3A4 inducer and less likely to be involved in medication interactions. Although oxcarbazepine has been studied in a small number of younger bipolar patients, there is a paucity of data pertaining to older psychiatric patients (Sommer et al. 2007). Thus, its use cannot be recommended in these patients.

Gabapentin and Pregabalin

Although gabapentin has been used in bipolar disorder, trials have not borne out its effectiveness, and only small case series or case reports of its use in dementia are available (Sommer et al. 2007). Nonetheless, it has a generally favorable side-effect profile and modest anxiolytic and analgesic effects, particularly for neuropathic pain. Gabapentin does not bind to plasma proteins and is not metabolized, being eliminated by renal excretion. In patients with renal impairment, neurological adverse effects such as ataxia, involuntary movements, disorganized thinking, excitation, and extreme sedation have been noted. Even in the absence of renal dysfunction, elderly patients may be prone to excessive sedation. Therefore, in the elderly, initial dosages of 100 mg twice a day are more prudent than the 900 mg/day recommended as a starting dosage for younger patients with epilepsy. Pregabalin is a structural congener of gabapentin. It has an improved pharmacokinetic profile and may be helpful for neuropathic pain in elderly patients. No data pertaining to its use are available in older psychiatric patients.

Topiramate

Early reports of the efficacy of topiramate in younger patients with bipolar disorder have not been confirmed by subsequent studies (Sommer et al. 2007). In younger patients, topiramate is one of the few psychotropic medications that has been associated with weight loss. However, it also has been associated with cognitive impairment that can be severe enough to interfere with functioning. Also, because of the paucity of data pertaining to use of topiramate in older psychiatric patients (Sommer et al. 2007), it cannot be recommended in these patients.

Anxiolytics and Sedative-Hypnotics

Social isolation, financial concerns, and declining intellectual and physical function may predispose elderly patients to anxiety. New-onset anxiety is a frequent accompaniment of physical illness, depression, or medication side effects. The SSRIs and

SNRIs have displaced benzodiazepines as first-line pharmacotherapy for anxiety in late life, whereas benzodiazepine receptor agonist hypnotics (i.e., eszopiclone, zaleplon, zolpidem) and the intermediate half-life benzodiazepine lorazepam have become the most commonly used hypnotics.

Benzodiazepines and Benzodiazepine Receptor Agonists

Detrimental effects of benzodiazepines in elderly patients frequently outweigh any short-term symptomatic relief that they may provide. Even single small doses of diazepam, nitrazepam, and temazepam cause significant impairment in memory and psychomotor performance in older subjects (Nikaido et al. 1990; Pomara et al. 1989). Even benzodiazepines with shorter half-lives increase the risk of falls and hip fractures in frail elderly patients (Ray et al. 2000). Benzodiazepine receptor agonists also have been associated with falls and hip fractures (Wang et al. 2001) or cognitive impairment and traffic accidents (Glass et al. 2005; Gustavsen et al. 2008; Leufkens et al. 2009).

Nevertheless, adjunctive treatment with a sedative-hypnotic may be indicated for a few weeks in the treatment of anxiety or depression-related sleep disturbance when the primary pharmacotherapy is an antidepressant. Relative contraindications include heavy snoring (because it suggests sleep apnea), dementia (because such patients are at increased risk for daytime confusion, impairment in activities of daily living, and daytime sleepiness), and the use of other sedating medications or alcohol. Benzodiazepines with long half-lives (clorazepate, chlordiazepoxide, clonazepam, diazepam,

flurazepam, halazepam, and quazepam) should be avoided (Fick et al. 2003; Hemmelgarn et al. 1997). Also, several drugs with shorter half-lives (i.e., alprazolam, triazolam, midazolam, eszopiclone, zaleplon, and zolpidem) undergo phase 1 hepatic metabolism by CYP3A4 that is subject to specific interactions and age-associated decline (Freudenreich and Menza 2000; Greenblatt et al. 1991). Sedatives with very short half-lives also may increase the likelihood that confused elderly patients will awake in the middle of the night to stagger off to the bathroom. Lorazepam and oxazepam do not undergo phase 1 hepatic metabolism, have no active metabolites, have acceptable half-lives that do not increase with age, and are not subject to drug interactions. Lorazepam is available in appropriately small doses (0.5-mg pills) and is well absorbed intramuscularly. It is preferred for inducing sleep because oxazepam has a relatively slow and erratic absorption.

Buspirone

The anxiolytic buspirone, a partial 5-HT$_{1A}$ agonist, is rarely used. Nevertheless, it may be beneficial for some patients with generalized anxiety disorder or as an augmentation agent in treatment-resistant depression (Trivedi et al. 2006). It appears to be well tolerated by elderly patients without the sedation or addiction liability of the benzodiazepines (Steinberg 1994). Thus, it may be helpful for some older patients prone to falls, confusion, or chronic lung disease. Nonetheless, buspirone may take several weeks to exert an anxiolytic effect, has no cross-tolerance with benzodiazepines, and may cause dizziness, headache, or nervousness (Strand et al. 1990). It is of limited use for panic or obsessive-compulsive disorders. The pharmacokinetics of buspirone are not affected by age or gender, but coadministration with verapamil, diltiazem, erythromycin, or itraconazole will substantially increase buspirone concentrations, and its combination with serotonergic medications may result in the serotonin syndrome (Mahmood and Sahajwalla 1999).

Cognitive Enhancers

Cholinesterase Inhibitors

Four of the five drugs currently approved by the FDA for the symptomatic improvement of Alzheimer's disease—tacrine, donepezil, galantamine, and rivastigmine—are cholinesterase inhibitors (Table 16–7). The use of tacrine is no longer recommended because of its potential hepatotoxic effects. The principal adverse effects of cholinesterase inhibitors are concentration dependent and result from their peripheral cholinergic actions. With these adverse effects in mind, clinicians should be aware of these medications' specific pathways of elimination and the potential for pharmacokinetic drug interactions with CYP2D6 or CYP3A4 inhibitors and CYP3A4 inducers when prescribing donepezil and galantamine (Pilotto et al. 2009; Seritan 2008). Rivastigmine is affected by renal function, and FDA warnings have emphasized the need for careful dosage titration (and retitration if restarting) to prevent severe vomiting (Birks et al. 2009). Drugs with potent anticholinergic effects directly antagonize cholinesterase inhibitors (Chew et al. 2008; Modi et al. 2009) and should be avoided in patients with dementia.

Cognitive enhancers produce modest improvements in cognition and function in patients with Alzheimer's disease (Hansen et al. 2008), including those with severe Alzheimer's disease (Winblad et al. 2006). A modest benefit of uncertain clinical significance is also observed in vascular dementia (Kavirajan and Schneider 2007). They may also have a role in the management of other dementias, such as Lewy body dementia (Gustavsson et al. 2009) or dementia with Parkinson's disease, mild cognitive impairment (Diniz et al. 2009; Doody et al. 2009), cognitive impairment associated with late-life depression (Reynolds et al. 2011), or behavioral and psychological symptoms of dementia (Gauthier et al. 2010; Rodda et al. 2009; Sink et al. 2005), but more research is needed.

A rapid symptomatic deterioration may occur when these drugs are discontinued, and no evidence suggests that they alter the underlying neuropathology of Alzheimer's disease or its eventual progression. Before initiating anticholinesterase therapy, it is imperative that unnecessary anticholinergic medications be discontinued (Lu and Tune 2003; Modi et al. 2009). In patients with diminished cognitive reserve, even small anticholinergic effects can substantially impair cognition (Mulsant et al. 2003; Nebes et al. 2005). Adverse effects including nausea, diarrhea, weight loss, bradycardia, syncope, and nightmares are associated with all three cholinesterase inhibitors and may lead to discontinuation (see Table 16–7; Gill et al. 2009; Hernandez et al. 2009; Park-Wyllie et al. 2009); gastrointestinal adverse effects may be less frequent with donepezil (Mayeux 2010).

NMDA Receptor Antagonist

The *N*-methyl-D-aspartate (NMDA) receptor antagonist memantine is approved by the FDA for the treatment of moderate to severe Alzheimer's disease. As an uncompetitive antagonist with moderate affinity

TABLE 16–7. Cholinesterase inhibitors

	Clearance	Dosing	Significant adverse effects	Pharmacodynamics
Donepezil	Half-life = 70–80 hours; CYP3A4, CYP2D6	5–10 mg/day in one dose; start at 5 mg at bedtime	Mild nausea, diarrhea, bradycardia	Reversible acetylcholinesterase inhibition
Galantamine, galantamine ER	Half-life = 7 hours; CYP2D6, CYP3A4	8–24 mg/day divided into two doses; start at 8 mg/day twice daily	Moderate nausea, vomiting, diarrhea, anorexia, tremor, insomnia	Reversible acetylcholinesterase inhibition; nicotinic modulation may increase acetylcholine release
Rivastigmine, rivastigmine patch	Half-life = 1.25 hours; Renal	6–12 mg/day divided into two doses; start at 1.5 mg twice daily. For patch, start at 4.6 mg/day and increase after 4 weeks to 9.5 mg/day. Retitrate if drug is stopped.	Severe nausea, vomiting, anorexia, weight loss, sweating, dizziness	Pseudoirreversible acetylcholinesterase inhibition; also butylcholinesterase inhibition

Note. CYP = cytochrome P450; ER = extended release.

for NMDA receptors, memantine may attenuate neurotoxicity without interfering with glutamate's normal physiological actions. In placebo-controlled clinical trials in patients with Alzheimer's disease, memantine was associated with a modest delay in deterioration of cognition and activities of daily living when given either alone (Reisberg et al. 2003) or in combination with donepezil (Tariot et al. 2004). Memantine also may have a role in the treatment of Parkinson's disease dementia and Lewy body dementia (Aarsland et al. 2009). It is well tolerated, although it may cause confusion in some patients (Kavirajan 2009). Memantine does not appear to be implicated in drug-drug interactions, but it is excreted by the kidneys, and its dosage needs to be reduced in patients with significant impairment in renal function.

Key Points

- Psychiatric disorders can be successfully treated in late life with psychotropic drugs, but pharmacological intervention requires special care because the elderly are more susceptible to drug-induced adverse events.

Antidepressants

- Selective serotonin reuptake inhibitors (SSRIs) remain first-line drugs for treating late-life depression because of their efficacy for both depressive and anxiety syndromes, ease of use, and overall safety and good tolerability. All available SSRIs have similar efficacy and tolerability; however, in late life, experts favor the use of citalopram, escitalopram, or sertraline because of their favorable pharmacokinetic profiles. SSRIs can cause the syndrome of inappropriate secretion of antidiuretic hormone; act synergistically with other medications that increase the risk of gastrointestinal bleeding, such as nonsteroidal anti-inflammatory drugs; and be associated with bradycardia.

- Serotonin-norepinephrine reuptake inhibitors (SNRIs) are the preferred alternatives in older patients whose symptoms do not respond to SSRIs. Bupropion and mirtazapine can be useful in older patients who do not tolerate SSRIs or SNRIs.

- Secondary amine tricyclic antidepressants and monoamine oxidase inhibitors continue to have a role in the management of treatment-resistant depression.

Antipsychotics

- For the treatment of psychotic symptoms of any etiology in late life, atypical antipsychotics are first-line drugs. Evidence supports their efficacy in the treatment of schizophrenia, behavioral and psychological symptoms of dementia, or delirium in older patients. However, significant questions remain regarding their tolerability and safety in older patients. They have been associated with a nearly twofold increase in the rate of deaths in older patients with behavioral and psychological symptoms of dementia. The selection of a specific drug to treat a specific patient should be guided by the strength of the available evidence relevant to the disorder being treated and, in the absence of such evidence, by the differing side-effect profiles of the drugs currently available.

Cognitive Enhancers

- The cognitive enhancers that are currently available have been shown in controlled trials to result in modest improvements in cognition and function. Before initiating anticholinesterase therapy, it is imperative that unnecessary anticholinergic medications be discontinued.

Other Psychotropic Medications

- The efficacy and safety of lithium and divalproex are supported only by open and naturalistic data at present. Both can cause significant adverse effects and require close monitoring. Minimal geriatric data are available for carbamazepine or lamotrigine.

- Detrimental effects of the benzodiazepines in elderly patients frequently outweigh any short-term symptomatic relief that they may provide.

References

Aarsland D, Ballard C, Walker Z, et al: Memantine in patients with Parkinson's disease dementia or dementia with Lewy bodies: a double-blind, placebo-controlled, multicentre trial. Lancet Neurol 8:613–618, 2009

Aichhorn W, Weiss U, Marksteiner J, et al: Influence of age and gender on risperidone plasma concentrations. J Psychopharmacol 19:395–401, 2005

Aiken CB: Pramipexole in psychiatry: a systematic review of the literature. J Clin Psychiatry 68:1230–1236, 2007

Alexopoulos GS, Katz IR, Reynolds CF 3rd, et al: Pharmacotherapy of depression in older patients: a summary of the expert consensus guidelines. J Psychiatr Pract 7:361–376, 2001

Allard P, Gram L, Timdahl K, et al: Efficacy and tolerability of venlafaxine in geriatric outpatients with major depression: a double-blind, randomised 6-month comparative study. Int J Geriatr Psychiatry 19:1123–1130, 2004

Altamura AC, De Novellis F, Guercetti G, et al: Fluoxetine compared with amitriptyline in elderly depression: a controlled clinical trial. Int J Clin Pharmacol Res 9:391–396, 1989

Alvir JJ, Lieberman JA, Safferman AZ, et al: Clozapine-induced agranulocytosis: incidence and risk factors in the United States. N Engl J Med 329:162–167, 1993

American Diabetes Association, American Psychiatric Association, American Association of Clinical Endocrinologists, et al: Consensus development conference on antipsychotic drugs and obesity and diabetes. Diabetes Care 27:596–601, 2004

Andersen G, Vestergaard K, Lauritzen L: Effective treatment of poststroke depression with the selective serotonin reuptake inhibitor citalopram. Stroke 25:1099–1104, 1994

Andreescu C, Mulsant BH, Rothschild AJ, et al: Pharmacotherapy of major depression with psychotic features: what is the evidence? Psychiatr Ann 35:31–38, 2006

Aragona M, Inghilleri M: Increased ocular pressure in two patients with narrow angle glaucoma treated with venlafaxine. Clin Neuropharmacol 21:130–131, 1998

Arranz FJ, Ros S: Effects of comorbidity and polypharmacy on the clinical usefulness of sertraline in elderly depressed patients: an open multicentre study. J Affect Disord 46:285–291, 1997

Atalay A, Turhan N, Aki OE: A challenging case of syndrome of inappropriate secretion of antidiuretic hormone in an elderly patient secondary to quetiapine. South Med J 100:832–833, 2007

Bailer U, Fischer P, Kufferle B, et al: Occurrence of mirtazapine-induced delirium in organic brain disorder. Int Clin Psychopharmacol 15:239–243, 2000

Ballard C, Corbett A: Management of neuropsychiatric symptoms in people with dementia. CNS Drugs 24:729–739, 2010

Ballard C, Hanney ML, Theodoulou M, et al: The Dementia Antipsychotic Withdrawal Trial (DART-AD): long-term follow-up of a randomised placebo-controlled trial. Lancet Neurol 8:151–157, 2009

Barak Y, Wittenberg N, Naor S, et al: Clozapine in elderly psychiatric patients: tolerability, safety, and efficacy. Compr Psychiatry 40:320–325, 1999

Barak Y, Shamir E, Zemishlani H, et al: Olanzapine vs. haloperidol in the treatment of elderly chronic schizophrenia patients. Prog Neuropsychopharmacol Biol Psychiatry 26:1199–1202, 2002

Barbui C, Esposito E, Cipriani A: Selective serotonin reuptake inhibitors and risk of suicide: a systematic review of observational studies. CMAJ 180:291–297, 2009

Barone P, Scarzella L, Marconi R, et al: Pramipexole versus sertraline in the treatment of depression in Parkinson's disease: a national multicenter parallel-group randomized study. J Neurol 253:601–607, 2006

Barone P, Poewe W, Albrecht S, et al: Pramipexole for the treatment of depressive symptoms in patients with Parkinson's disease: a randomised, double-blind, placebo-controlled trial. Lancet Neurol 9:573–580, 2010

Beers MH: Explicit criteria for determining potentially inappropriate medication use by the elderly. Arch Intern Med 157:1531–1536, 1997

Belgamwar RB, Fenton M: Olanzapine IM or velotab for acutely disturbed/agitated people with suspected serious mental illnesses. Cochrane Database of Systematic Reviews 2005, Issue 2. Art. No.: CD003729. DOI: 10.1002/14651858.CD003729.pub2.

Bell JS, Taipale HT, Soini H, et al: Sedative load among long-term care facility residents with and without dementia: a cross-sectional study. Clin Drug Investig 30:63–70, 2010

Benazzi F: Urinary retention with venlafaxine-haloperidol combination. Pharmacopsychiatry 30:27, 1997

Benazzi F: Serotonin syndrome with mirtazapine-fluoxetine combination. Int J Geriatr Psychiatry 13:495–496, 1998

Benet LZ, Hoener B: Changes in plasma protein binding have little clinical relevance. Clin Pharmacol Ther 71:115–121, 2002

Berkowitz A: Ziprasidone for dementia in elderly patients: case review. J Psychiatr Pract 9:469–473, 2003

Bigos KL, Bies RR, Pollock BG: Population pharmacokinetics in geriatric psychiatry. Am J Geriatr Psychiatry 14:993–1003, 2006

Birks J, Grimley Evans J, Iakovidou V, et al: Rivastigmine for Alzheimer's disease. Cochrane Database of Systematic Reviews 2009, Issue 2. Art. No.: CD001191. DOI: 10.1002/14651858.CD001191.pub2.

Bodkin JA, Lasser RA, Wines JD Jr, et al: Combining serotonin reuptake inhibitors and bupropion in partial responders to antidepressant monotherapy. J Clin Psychiatry 58:137–145, 1997

Bond DJ, Lam RW, Yatham LN: Divalproex sodium versus placebo in the treatment of acute bipolar depression: a systematic review and meta-analysis. J Affect Disord 124:228–234, 2010

Bondareff W, Alpert M, Friedhoff AJ, et al: Comparison of sertraline and nortriptyline in the treatment of major depressive disorder in late life. Am J Psychiatry 157:729–736, 2000

Bose A, Li D, Ghandi C: Escitalopram in the acute treatment of depressed patients aged 60 years and older. Am J Geriatr Psychiatry 16:14–20, 2008

Branconnier RJ, Cole JO, Ghazvinian S, et al: Clinical pharmacology of bupropion and imipramine in elderly depressives. J Clin Psychiatry 44 (5 pt 2):130–133, 1983

Breier A, Sutton VK, Feldman PD, et al: Olanzapine in the treatment of dopamimetic-induced psychosis in patients with Parkinson's disease. Biol Psychiatry 52:438–445, 2002

Brodaty H, Ames D, Snowdon J, et al: A randomized placebo-controlled trial of risperidone for the treatment of aggression, agitation, and psychosis of dementia. J Clin Psychiatry 64:134–143, 2003

Burrows AB, Salzman C, Satlin A, et al: A randomized, placebo-controlled trial of paroxetine in nursing home residents with non-major depression. Depress Anxiety 15:102–110, 2002

Carta MG, Zairo F, Mellino G, et al: Add-on quetiapine in the treatment of major depressive disorder in elderly patients with cerebrovascular damage. Clin Pract Epidemiol Ment Health 3:28, 2007

Carvajal García-Pando A, García del Pozo J, Sánchez AS, et al: Hepatotoxicity associated with the new antidepressants. J Clin Psychiatry 63:135–137, 2002

Centorrino F, Price BH, Tuttle M, et al: EEG abnormalities during treatment with typical and atypical antipsychotics. Am J Psychiatry 159:109–115, 2002

Chalon SA, Granier LA, Vandenhende FR, et al: Duloxetine increases serotonin and norepinephrine availability in healthy subjects: a double-blind, controlled study. Neuropsychopharmacology 28:1685–1693, 2003

Chan WC, Lam LC, Choy CN, et al: A double-blind randomised comparison of risperidone and haloperidol in the treatment of behavioural and psychological symptoms in Chinese dementia patients. Int J Geriatr Psychiatry 16:1156–1162, 2001

Cheah CY, Ladhams B, Fegan PG: Mirtazapine associated with profound hyponatremia: two case reports. Am J Geriatr Pharmacother 6:91–95, 2008

Chen P, Kales HC, Weintraub D, et al: Antidepressant treatment of veterans with Parkinson's disease and depression: analysis of a national sample. J Geriatr Psychiatry Neurol 20:161–165, 2007

Chen Y, Patel NC, Guo JJ, et al: Antidepressant prophylaxis for poststroke depression: a meta-analysis. Int Clin Psychopharmacol 22:159–166, 2007

Chew ML, Mulsant BH, Rosen J, et al: Serum anticholinergic activity and cognition in patients with moderate to severe dementia. Am J Geriatr Psychiatry 13:535–538, 2005

Chew ML, Mulsant BH, Pollock BG, et al: A model of anticholinergic activity of atypical antipsychotic medications. Schizophr Res 88:63–72, 2006

Chew ML, Mulsant BH, Pollock BG, et al: Anticholinergic activity of 107 medications commonly used by older adults. J Am Geriatr Soc 56:1333–1341, 2008

Cipriani A, Furukawa TA, Salanti G, et al: Comparative efficacy and acceptability of 12 new-generation antidepressants: a multiple-treatments meta-analysis. Lancet 373:746–758, 2009

Clark WS, Street JS, Feldman PD, et al: The effects of olanzapine in reducing the emergence of psychosis among nursing home patients with Alzheimer's disease. J Clin Psychiatry 62:34–40, 2001

Clayton AH, Kornstein SG, Rosas G, et al: An integrated analysis of the safety and tolerability of desvenlafaxine compared with placebo in the treatment of major depressive disorder. CNS Spectrums 14:183–195, 2009

Cohn CK, Shrivastava R, Mendels J, et al: Double-blind, multicenter comparison of sertraline and amitriptyline in elderly depressed patients. J Clin Psychiatry 51 (suppl B):28–33, 1990

Coley KC, Scipio TM, Ruby C, et al: Aripiprazole prescribing patterns and side effects in elderly psychiatric inpatients. J Psychiatr Pract 15:150–153, 2009

Cooper C, Katona C, Lyketsos K, et al: A systematic review of treatments for refractory depression in older people. Am J Geriatr Psychiatry 168:681–688, 2011

Culang ME, Sneed JR, Keilp JG, et al: Change in cognitive functioning following acute antidepressant treatment in late-life depression. Am J Geriatr Psychiatry 17:881–888, 2009

Culo S, Mulsant BH, Rosen J, et al: Treating neuropsychiatric symptoms in dementia with Lewy bodies: a randomized controlled trial. Alzheimer Dis Assoc Disord 24:360–364, 2010

Dahmen N, Marx J, Hopf HC, et al: Therapy of early poststroke depression with venlafaxine: safety, tolerability, and efficacy as determined in an open, uncontrolled clinical trial. Stroke 30:691–692, 1999

Dalton SO, Sorensen HT, Johansen C: SSRIs and upper gastrointestinal bleeding: what is known and how should it influence prescribing? CNS Drugs 20:143–151, 2006

Davidson J, Watkins L, Owens M, et al: Effects of paroxetine and venlafaxine XR on heart rate variability in depression. J Clin Psychopharmacol 25:480–484, 2005

Davidson M, Harvey PD, Vervarcke J, et al: A long-term, multicenter, open-label study of risperidone in elderly patients with psychosis. On behalf of the Risperidone Working Group. Int J Geriatr Psychiatry 15:506–514, 2000

Davidson M, Emsley R, Kramer M, et al: Efficacy, safety and early response of paliperidone extended-release tablets (paliperidone ER): results of a 6-week, randomized, placebo-controlled study. Schizophr Res 93:117–130, 2007

de Abajo FJ, Garcia-Rodriguez LA: Risk of upper gastrointestinal tract bleeding associated with selective serotonin reuptake inhibitors and venlafaxine therapy: interaction with nonsteroidal anti-inflammatory drugs and effect of acid-suppressing agents. Arch Gen Psychiatry 65:795–803, 2008

De Deyn PP, Rabheru K, Rasmussen A, et al: A randomized trial of risperidone, placebo, and haloperidol for behavioral symptoms of dementia. Neurology 53:946–955, 1999

De Deyn PP, Carrasco MM, Deberdt W, et al: Olanzapine versus placebo in the treatment of psychosis with or without associated behavioral disturbances in patients with Alzheimer's disease. Int J Geriatr Psychiatry 19:115–126, 2004

De Deyn PP, Jeste DV, Swanik R, et al: Aripiprazole for the treatment of psychosis in patients with Alzheimer's disease: a randomized placebo-controlled study. J Clin Psychopharmacol 25:463–467, 2005a

De Deyn PP, Katz IR, Brodaty H, et al: Management of agitation, aggression, and psychosis associated with dementia: a pooled analysis including three randomized, placebo-controlled double-blind trials in nursing home residents treated with risperidone. Clin Neurol Neurosurg 107:497–508, 2005b

Devanand DP, Pelton GH, Marston K, et al: Sertraline treatment of elderly patients with depression and cognitive impairment. Int J Geriatr Psychiatry 18:123–130, 2003

Devanand DP, Juszczak N, Nobler MS, et al: An open treatment trial of venlafaxine for elderly patients with dysthymic disorder. J Geriatr Psychiatry Neurol 17:219–224, 2004

Devanand DP, Nobler MS, Cheng J, et al: Randomized, double-blind, placebo-controlled trial of fluoxetine treatment for elderly patients with dysthymic disorder. Am J Geriatr Psychiatry 13:59–68, 2005

Devos D, Dujardin K, Poirot I, et al: Comparison of desipramine and citalopram treatments for depression in Parkinson's disease: a double-blind, randomized, placebo-controlled study. Mov Disord 23:850–857, 2008

Diem SJ, Blackwell TL, Stone KL, et al: Use of antidepressants and rates of hip bone loss in older women: the study of osteoporotic fractures. Arch Intern Med 167:1240–1245, 2007

Diniz BS, Pinto JA Jr, Gonzaga ML, et al: To treat or not to treat? A meta-analysis of the use of cholinesterase inhibitors in mild cognitive impairment for delaying progression to Alzheimer's disease. Eur Arch Psychiatry Clin Neurosci 259:248–256, 2009

Dolder C, Nelson M, Stump A: Pharmacological and clinical profile of newer antidepressants: implications for the treatment of elderly patients. Drugs Aging 27:625–640, 2010

Doody RS, Ferris SH, Salloway S, et al: Donepezil treatment of patients with MCI: a 48-week randomized, placebo-controlled trial. Neurology 72:1555–1561, 2009

Doraiswamy PM, Khan ZM, Donahue RM, et al: Quality of life in geriatric depression: a comparison of remitters, partial responders, and nonresponders. Am J Geriatr Psychiatry 9:423–428, 2001

Doraiswamy PM, Krishnan KR, Oxman T, et al: Does antidepressant therapy improve cognition in elderly depressed patients? J Gerontol A Biol Sci Med Sci 58:M1137–M1144, 2003

Dunlop BW, Crits-Christoph P, Evans DL, et al: Coadministration of modafinil and a selective serotonin reuptake inhibitor from the initiation of treatment of major depressive disorder with fatigue and sleepiness: a double-blind, placebo-controlled study. J Clin Psychopharmacol 27:614–619, 2007

Dunner DL, Cohn JB, Walshe TD, et al: Two combined, multicenter double-blind studies of paroxetine and doxepin in geriatric patients with major depression. J Clin Psychiatry 53 (suppl):57–60, 1992

Dunner DL, Zisook S, Billow AA, et al: A prospective safety surveillance study for bupropion sustained-release in the treatment of depression. J Clin Psychiatry 59:366–373, 1998

Ellis T, Cudkowicz ME, Sexton PM, et al: Clozapine and risperidone treatment of psychosis in Parkinson's disease. J Neuropsychiatry Clin Neurosci 12:364–369, 2000

Evans M, Hammond M, Wilson K, et al: Treatment of depression in the elderly: effect of physical illness on response. Int J Geriatr Psychiatry 12:1189–1194, 1997

Fabian TJ, Amico JA, Kroboth PD, et al: Paroxetine-induced hyponatremia in older adults: a 12-week prospective study. Arch Intern Med 164:327–332, 2004

Fava M, Thase ME, DeBattista C, et al: Modafinil augmentation of selective serotonin reuptake inhibitor therapy in MDD partial responders with persistent fatigue and sleepiness. Ann Clin Psychiatry 19:153–159, 2007

Feighner JP, Cohn JB: Double-blind comparative trials of fluoxetine and doxepin in geriatric patients with major depressive disorder. J Clin Psychiatry 46 (3 pt 2):20–25, 1985

Feldman PD, Hay LK, Deberdt W, et al: Retrospective cohort study of diabetes mellitus and antipsychotic treatment in a geriatric population in the United States. J Am Med Dir Assoc 5:38–46, 2004

Fenn HH, Sommer BR, Ketter TA, et al: Safety and tolerability of mood-stabilising anticonvulsants in the elderly. Expert Opin Drug Saf 5:401–416, 2006

Fernandez HH, Trieschmann ME, Burke MA, et al: Quetiapine for psychosis in Parkinson's disease versus dementia with Lewy bodies. J Clin Psychiatry 63:513–515, 2002

Fick DM, Cooper JW, Wade WE, et al: Updating the Beers criteria for potentially inappropriate medication use in older adults: results of a US consensus panel of experts. Arch Intern Med. 163:2716–2724, 2003

Finkel SI, Richter EM, Clary CM, et al: Comparative efficacy of sertraline vs. fluoxetine in patients age 70 or over with major depression. Am J Geriatr Psychiatry 7:221–227, 1999

Flint AJ: Generalised anxiety disorder in elderly patients: epidemiology, diagnosis and treatment options. Drugs Aging 22:101–114, 2005

Flint AJ, Rifat SL: Nonresponse to first-line pharmacotherapy may predict relapse and recurrence of remitted geriatric depression. Depress Anxiety 13:125–131, 2001

Fontaine CS, Hynan LS, Koch K, et al: A double-blind comparison of olanzapine versus risperidone in the acute treatment of dementia-related behavioral disturbances in extended care facilities. J Clin Psychiatry 64:726–730, 2003

Forester BP, Streeter CC, Berlow YA, et al: Brain lithium levels and effects on cognition and mood in geriatric bipolar disorder: a lithium-7 magnetic resonance spectroscopy study. Am J Geriatr Psychiatry 17:13–23, 2009

Forlenza OV, Almeida OP, Stoppe A Jr, et al: Antidepressant efficacy and safety of low-dose sertraline and standard-dose imipramine for the treatment of depression in older adults: results from a double-blind, randomized, controlled clinical trial. Int Psychogeriatr 13:75–84, 2001

Freudenreich O, Menza M: Zolpidem-related delirium: a case report. J Clin Psychiatry 61:449–450, 2000

Friedman RA, Leon AC: Expanding the black box: depression, antidepressants, and the risk of suicide. N Engl J Med 356:2343–2346, 2007

Furlan PM, Kallan MJ, Ten Have T, et al: Cognitive and psychomotor effects of paroxetine and sertraline on healthy elderly volunteers. Am J Geriatr Psychiatry 9:429–438, 2001

Gareri P, Cotroneo A, Lacava R, et al: Comparison of the efficacy of new and conventional antipsychotic drugs in the treatment of behavioral and psychological symptoms of dementia (BPSD). Arch Gerontol Geriatr Suppl 9:207–215, 2004

Gasto C, Navarro V, Marcos T, et al: Single-blind comparison of venlafaxine and nortriptyline in elderly major depression. J Clin Psychopharmacol 23:21–26, 2003

Gauthier S, Cummings J, Ballard C, et al: Management of behavioral problems in Alzheimer's disease. Int Psychogeriatr 22:346–372, 2010

Gelenberg AJ, Laukes C, McGahuey C, et al: Mirtazapine substitution in SSRI-induced sexual dysfunction. J Clin Psychiatry 61:356–360, 2000

Georgotas A, McCue RE, Hapworth W, et al: Comparative efficacy and safety of MAOIs versus TCAs in treating depression in the elderly. Biol Psychiatry 21:1155–1166, 1986

Geretsegger C, Stuppaeck CH, Mair M, et al: Multicenter double blind study of paroxetine and amitriptyline in elderly depressed inpatients. Psychopharmacology (Berl) 119:277–281, 1995

Gex-Fabry M, Balant-Gorgia AE, Balant LP: Therapeutic drug monitoring of olanzapine: the combined effect of age, gender, smoking, and comedication. Ther Drug Monit 25:46–53, 2003

Gill SS, Rochon PA, Herrmann N, et al: Atypical antipsychotic drugs and risk of ischaemic stroke: population based retrospective cohort study. BMJ 330:445, 2005

Gill SS, Anderson GM, Fischer HD, et al: Syncope and its consequences in patients with dementia receiving cholinesterase inhibitors: a population-based cohort study. Arch Int Med 169:867–873, 2009

Glass J, Lanctot KL, Herrmann N, et al: Sedative hypnotics in older people with insomnia: meta-analysis of risks and benefits. BMJ 331(7526):1169, 2005

Glassman AH, O'Connor CM, Califf RM, et al: Sertraline treatment of major depression in patients with acute MI or unstable angina [published erratum appears in JAMA 288:1720, 2002]. JAMA 288:701–709, 2002

Goetz CG, Blasucci LM, Leurgans S, et al: Olanzapine and clozapine: comparative effects on motor function in hallucinating PD patients. Neurology 55:789–794, 2000

Goodnick PJ, Hernandez M: Treatment of depression in comorbid medical illness. Expert Opin Pharmacother 1:1367–1384, 2000

Gorwood P, Weiller E, Lemming O, et al: Escitalopram prevents relapse in older patients with major depressive disorder. Am J Geriatr Psychiatry 15:581–593, 2007

Greco KE, Tune LE, Brown FW, et al: A retrospective study of the safety of intramuscular ziprasidone in agitated elderly patients. J Clin Psychiatry 66:928–929, 2005

Greenblatt DJ, Harmatz JS, Shapiro L, et al: Sensitivity to triazolam in the elderly. N Engl J Med 324:1691–1698, 1991

Grothe DR, Scheckner B, Albano D: Treatment of pain syndromes with venlafaxine. Pharmacotherapy 24:621–629, 2004

Guillibert E, Pelicier Y, Archambault JC, et al: A double-blind, multicentre study of paroxetine versus clomipramine in depressed elderly patients. Acta Psychiatr Scand Suppl 350:132–134, 1989

Gustavsen I, Bramness JG, Skurtveit S, et al: Road traffic accident risk related to prescriptions of the hypnotics zopiclone, zolpidem, flunitrazepam and nitrazepam. Sleep Med 9:818–822, 2008

Gustavsson A, Van Der Putt R, Jonsson L, et al: Economic evaluation of cholinesterase inhibitor therapy for dementia: comparison of Alzheimer's disease and dementia with Lewy bodies. Int J Geriatr Psychiatry 24:1072–1078, 2009

Han CS, Kim YK: A double-blind trial of risperidone and haloperidol for the treatment of delirium. Psychosomatics 45:297–301, 2004

Hansen RA, Gartlehner G, Lohr KN, et al: Efficacy and safety of second-generation antidepressants in the treatment of major depressive disorder. Ann Intern Med 143:415–426, 2005

Hansen RA, Gartlehner G, Webb AP, et al: Efficacy and safety of donepezil, galantamine, and rivastigmine for the treatment of Alzheimer's disease: a systematic review and meta-analysis. Clin Interv Aging 3:211–225, 2008

Harvey AT, Rudolph RL, Preskorn SH: Evidence of the dual mechanisms of action of venlafaxine. Arch Gen Psychiatry 57:503–509, 2000

Harvey PD, Napolitano JA, Mao L, et al: Comparative effects of risperidone and olanzapine on cognition in elderly patients with schizophrenia or schizoaffective disorder. Int J Geriatr Psychiatry 18:820–829, 2003

Hemmelgarn B, Suissa S, Huang A, et al: Benzodiazepine use and the risk of motor vehicle crash in the elderly. JAMA 278:27–31, 1997

Hernandez RK, Farwell W, Cantor MD, et al: Cholinesterase inhibitors and incidence of bradycardia in patients with dementia in the Veterans Affairs New England Healthcare System. J Am Geriatr Soc 57:1997–2003, 2009

Herrmann N, Mamdani M, Lanctot KL: Atypical antipsychotics and risk of cerebrovascular accidents. Am J Psychiatry 161:1113–1115, 2004

Herrmann N, Rothenburg LS, Black SE, et al: Methylphenidate for the treatment of apathy in Alzheimer disease: prediction of response using dextroamphetamine challenge. J Clin Psychopharmacol 28:296–301, 2008

Hesse LM, He P, Krishnaswamy S, et al: Pharmacogenetic determinants of interindividual variability in bupropion hydroxylation by cytochrome P450 2B6 in human liver microsomes. Pharmacogenetics 14:225–238, 2004

Hien le TT, Cumming RG, Cameron ID, et al: Atypical antipsychotic medications and risk of falls in residents of aged care facilities. J Am Geriatr Soc 53:1290–1295, 2005

Howanitz E, Pardo M, Smelson DA, et al: The efficacy and safety of clozapine versus chlorpromazine in geriatric schizophrenia. J Clin Psychiatry 60:41–44, 1999

Howard WT, Warnock JK: Bupropion-induced psychosis. Am J Psychiatry 156:2017–2018, 1999

Hoyberg OJ, Maragakis B, Mullin J, et al: A double-blind multicentre comparison of mirtazapine and amitriptyline in elderly depressed patients. Acta Psychiatr Scand 93:184–190, 1996

Hutchison LC: Mirtazapine and bone marrow suppression: a case report. J Am Geriatr Soc 49:1129–1130, 2001

Jaskiw GE, Thyrum PT, Fuller MA, et al: Pharmacokinetics of quetiapine in elderly patients with selected psychotic disorders. Clin Pharmacokinet 43:1025–1035, 2004

Jeste DV, Barak Y, Madhusoodanan S, et al: International multisite double-blind trial of the atypical antipsychotics risperidone and olanzapine in 175 elderly patients with chronic schizophrenia. Am J Geriatr Psychiatry 11:638–647, 2003

Jin Y, Pollock BG, Frank E, et al: Effect of age, weight and CYP2C19 genotype on escitalopram exposure. J Clin Pharmacol 50:62–72, 2010

Johnson EM, Whyte E, Mulsant BH, et al: Cardiovascular changes associated with venlafaxine in the treatment of late life depression. Am J Geriatr Psychiatry 14:796–802, 2006

Joo JH, Lenze EJ, Mulsant BH, et al: Risk factors for falls during treatment of late-life depression. J Clin Psychiatry 63:936–941, 2002

Jorge RE, Acion L, Moser D, et al: Escitalopram and enhancement of cognitive recovery following stroke. Arch Gen Psychiatry 67:187–196, 2010

Juurlink DN, Mamdani MM, Kopp A, et al: The risk of suicide with selective serotonin reuptake inhibitors in the elderly. Am J Psychiatry 163:813–821, 2006

Kando JC, Tohen M, Castillo J, et al: The use of valproate in an elderly population with affective symptoms. J Clin Psychiatry 57:238–240, 1996

Kane J, Canas F, Kramer M, et al: Treatment of schizophrenia with paliperidone extended-release tablets: a 6-week placebo-controlled trial. Schizophr Res 90:147–161, 2007

Karp JF, Weiner D, Seligman K, et al: Body pain and treatment response in late-life depression. Am J Geriatr Psychiatry 13:188–194, 2005

Karp JF, Whyte EM, Lenze EJ, et al: Rescue pharmacotherapy with duloxetine for selective serotonin reuptake inhibitor nonresponders in late-life depression: outcome and tolerability. J Clin Psychiatry 69:457–463, 2008

Karp JF, Weiner DK, Dew MA, et al: Duloxetine and care management treatment of older adults with comorbid major depressive disorder and chronic low back pain: results of an open-label pilot study. Int J Geriatr Psychiatry 25:633–642, 2010

Kasckow JW, Mohamed S, Thallasinos A, et al: Citalopram augmentation of antipsychotic treatment in older schizophrenia patients. Int J Geriatr Psychiatry 16:1163–1167, 2001

Kasper S, de Swart H, Andersen HF: Escitalopram in the treatment of depressed elderly patients. Am J Geriatr Psychiatry 13:884–891, 2005

Katona CLE, Hunter BN, Bray J: A double-blind comparison of the efficacy and safety of paroxetine and imipramine in the treatment of depression with dementia. Int J Geriatr Psychiatry 13:100–108, 1998

Katz IR, Jeste DV, Mintzer JE, et al: Comparison of risperidone and placebo for psychosis and behavioral disturbances associated with dementia: a randomized, double-blind trial. Risperidone Study Group. J Clin Psychiatry 60:107–115, 1999

Katz IR, Reynolds CF 3rd, Alexopoulos GS, et al: Venlafaxine ER as a treatment for generalized anxiety disorder in older adults: pooled analysis of five randomized placebo-controlled clinical trials. J Am Geriatr Soc 50:18–25, 2002

Kavirajan H: Memantine: a comprehensive review of safety and efficacy. Expert Opin Drug Saf 8:89–109, 2009

Kavirajan H, Schneider LS: Efficacy and adverse effects of cholinesterase inhibitors and memantine in vascular dementia: a meta-analysis of randomised controlled trials. Lancet Neurology 6:782–792, 2007

Kennedy JS, Jeste D, Kaiser CJ, et al: Olanzapine vs. haloperidol in geriatric schizophrenia: analysis of data from a double-blind controlled trial. Int J Geriatr Psychiatry 18:1013–1020, 2003

Kennedy J, Deberdt W, Siegal A, et al: Olanzapine does not enhance cognition in non-agitated and non-psychotic patients with mild to moderate Alzheimer's dementia. Int J Geriatr Psychiatry 20:1020–1027, 2005

Kiev A, Masco HL, Wenger TL, et al: The cardiovascular effects of bupropion and nortriptyline in depressed outpatients. Ann Clin Psychiatry 6:107–115, 1994

Kim KY, Bader GM, Kotlyar V, et al: Treatment of delirium in older adults with quetiapine. J Geriatr Psychiatry Neurol 16:29–31, 2003

Kinon BJ, Stauffer VL, McGuire HC, et al: The effects of antipsychotic drug treatment on prolactin concentrations in elderly patients. J Am Med Dir Assoc 4:189–194, 2003

Kirby D, Harrigan S, Ames D: Hyponatraemia in elderly psychiatric patients treated with selective serotonin reuptake inhibitors and venlafaxine: a retrospective controlled study in an inpatient unit. Int J Geriatr Psychiatry 17:231–237, 2002

Kleijer BC, Heerdink ER, Egberts TC, et al: Antipsychotic drug use and the risk of venous thromboembolism in elderly patients. J Clin Psychopharmacol 30:526–530, 2010

Kohen I, Preval H, Southard R, et al: Naturalistic study of intramuscular ziprasidone versus conventional agents in agitated elderly patients: retrospective findings from a psychiatric emergency service. Am J Geriatr Pharmacother 3:240–245, 2005

Kohen I, Gordon ML, Manu P: Serotonin syndrome in elderly patients treated for psychotic depression with atypical antipsychotics and antidepressants: two case reports. CNS Spectr 12:596–598, 2007

Kok RM, Nolen WA, Heeren TJ: Venlafaxine versus nortriptyline in the treatment of elderly depressed inpatients: a randomised, double-blind, controlled trial. Int J Geriatr Psychiatry 22:1247–1254, 2007

Koller E, Schneider B, Bennett K, et al: Clozapine-associated diabetes. Am J Med 111:716–723, 2001

Koller EA, Cross JT, Doraiswamy PM, et al: Pancreatitis associated with atypical antipsychotics: from the Food and Drug Administration's MedWatch surveillance system and published reports. Pharmacotherapy 23:1123–1130, 2003

Kornstein SG, Clayton AH, Soares CN, et al: Analysis by age and sex of efficacy data from placebo-controlled trials of desvenlafaxine in outpatients with major depressive disorder. J Clin Psychopharmacol 30:294–299, 2010a

Kornstein SG, Jiang Q, Reddy S, et al: Short-term efficacy and safety of desvenlafaxine in a randomized, placebo-controlled study of perimenopausal and postmenopausal women with major depressive disorder. J Clin Psychiatry 71:1088–1096, 2010b

Kotlyar M, Brauer LH, Tracy TS, et al: Inhibition of CYP2D6 activity by bupropion. J Clin Psychopharmacol 25:226–229, 2005

Kuehn BM: FDA warns antipsychotic drugs may be risky for elderly. JAMA 293:2462, 2005

Kurlan R, Cummings J, Raman R, et al: Quetiapine for agitation or psychosis in patients with dementia and parkinsonism. Neurology 68:1356–1363, 2007

Kyle CJ, Petersen HE, Overo KF: Comparison of the tolerability and efficacy of citalopram and amitriptyline in elderly depressed patients treated in general practice. Depress Anxiety 8:147–153, 1998

Lam RW, Lonn SL, Despiegel N: Escitalopram versus serotonin noradrenaline reuptake inhibitors as second step treatment for patients with major depressive disorder: a pooled analysis. Int Clin Psychopharmacol 25:199–203, 2010

Landi F, Onder G, Cesari M, et al: Psychotropic medications and risk for falls among community-dwelling frail older people: an observational study. J Gerontol A Biol Sci Med Sci 60:622–626, 2005

Laroche ML, Charmes JP, Nouaille Y, et al: Is inappropriate medication use a major cause of adverse drug reactions in the elderly? Br J Clin Pharmacol 63:177–186, 2007

Lasser RA, Bossie CA, Zhu Y, et al: Efficacy and safety of long-acting risperidone in elderly patients with schizophrenia and schizoaffective disorder. Int J Geriatr Psychiatry 19:898–905, 2004

Lavretsky H, Park S, Siddarth P, et al: Methylphenidate-enhanced antidepressant response to citalopram in the elderly: a double-blind, placebo-controlled pilot trial. Am J Geriatr Psychiatry 142:181–185, 2006

Lavretsky H, Siddarth P, Irwin MR: Improving depression and enhancing resilience in family dementia caregivers: a pilot randomized placebo-controlled trial of escitalopram. Am J Geriatr Psychiatry 18:154–162, 2010

Lee PE, Gill SS, Freedman M, et al: Atypical antipsychotic drugs in the treatment of behavioural and psychological symptoms of dementia: systematic review. BMJ 329:75, 2004

Lenze EJ, Mulsant BH, Shear MK, et al: Anxiety symptoms in elderly patients with depression: what is the best approach to treatment? Drugs Aging 19:753–760, 2002

Lenze EJ, Mulsant BH, Shear MK, et al: Efficacy and tolerability of citalopram in the treatment of late-life anxiety disorders: results from an 8-week randomized, placebo-controlled trial. Am J Psychiatry 162:146–150, 2005

Lenze EJ, Rollman BL, Shear MK, et al: Escitalopram for older adults with generalized anxiety disorder: a randomized controlled trial. JAMA 301:295–303, 2009

Leopold NA: Risperidone treatment of drug-related psychosis in patients with parkinsonism. Mov Disord 15:301–304, 2000

Lessard E, Yessine MA, Hamelin BA, et al: Influence of CYP2D6 activity on the disposition and cardiovascular toxicity of the antidepressant agent venlafaxine in humans. Pharmacogenetics 9:435–443, 1999

Leufkens TR, Lund JS, Vermeeren A: Highway driving performance and cognitive functioning the morning after bedtime and middle-of-the-night use of gaboxadol, zopiclone and zolpidem. J Sleep Res 18:387–396, 2009

Liebowitz MR, Tourian KA: Efficacy, safety, and tolerability of desvenlafaxine 50 mg/d for the treatment of major depressive disorder: a systematic review of clinical trials. Prim Care Companion J Clin Psychiatry 12(3), 2010

Liperoti R, Pedone C, Lapane KL, et al: Venous thromboembolism among elderly patients treated with atypical and conventional antipsychotic agents. Arch Intern Med 165:2677–2682, 2005

Liperoti R, Onder G, Lapane KL, et al: Conventional or atypical antipsychotics and the risk of femur fracture among elderly patients: results of a case-control study. J Clin Psychiatry 68:929–934, 2007

Lipscombe LL, Levesque L, Gruneir A, et al: Antipsychotic drugs and hyperglycemia in older patients with diabetes. Arch Intern Med 169:1282–1289, 2009

Liu B, Anderson G, Mittmann N, et al: Use of selective serotonin reuptake inhibitors or tricyclic antidepressants and risk of hip fractures in elderly people. Lancet 351:1303–1307, 1998

Looper KJ: Potential medical and surgical complications of serotonergic antidepressants. Psychosomatics 48:1–9, 2007

Lotrich FE, Rabinovitz F, Gironda P, et al: Depression following pegylated interferon-alpha: characteristics and vulnerability. J Psychosom Res 63:131–135, 2007

Lu CJ, Tune LE: Chronic exposure to anticholinergic medications adversely affects the course of Alzheimer disease. Am J Geriatr Psychiatry 14:458–461, 2003

Lyketsos CG, DelCampo L, Steinberg M, et al: Treating depression in Alzheimer disease: efficacy and safety of sertraline therapy, and the benefits of depression reduction: the DIADS. Arch Gen Psychiatry 60:737–746, 2003

Madhusoodanan S, Zaveri D: Paliperidone use in the elderly. Curr Drug Saf 5:149–152, 2010

Madhusoodanan S, Suresh P, Brenner R, et al: Experience with the atypical antipsychotics—risperidone and olanzapine in the elderly. Ann Clin Psychiatry 11:113–118, 1999

Madhusoodanan S, Brenner R, Alcantra A: Clinical experience with quetiapine in elderly patients with psychotic disorders. J Geriatr Psychiatry Neurol 13:28–32, 2000

Mahapatra SN, Hackett D: A randomised, double-blind, parallel-group comparison of venlafaxine and dothiepin in geriatric patients with major depression. Int J Clin Pract 51:209–213, 1997

Mahmood I, Sahajwalla C: Clinical pharmacokinetics and pharmacodynamics of buspirone, an anxiolytic drug. Clin Pharmacokinet 36:277–287, 1999

Mamo DC, Sweet RA, Mulsant BH, et al: The effect of nortriptyline and paroxetine on extrapyramidal signs and symptoms: a prospective double-blind study in depressed elderly patients. Am J Geriatr Psychiatry 8:226–231, 2000

Mamo D, Graff A, Mizrahi R, et al: Differential effects of aripiprazole on D2, 5-HT2, and 5-HT1A receptor occupancy in patients with schizophrenia: a triple tracer PET study. Am J Psychiatry 164:1411–1417, 2007

Mariappan P, Alhasso AA, Grant A, et al: Serotonin and noradrenaline reuptake inhibitors (SNRI) for stress urinary incontinence in adults. Cochrane Database of Systematic Reviews 2005, Issue 3. Art. No.: CD004742. DOI: 10.1002/14651858.CD004742.pub2.

Marsh L, Lyketsos C, Reich SG: Olanzapine for the treatment of psychosis in patients with Parkinson's disease and dementia. Psychosomatics 42:477–481, 2001

Martin H, Slyk MP, Deymann S, et al: Safety profile assessment of risperidone and olanzapine in long-term care patients with dementia. J Am Med Dir Assoc 4:183–188, 2003

Mayeux R: Early Alzheimer's disease. N Engl J Med 362:2194–2201, 2010

Mazeh D, Shahal B, Aviv A, et al: A randomized, single-blind, comparison of venlafaxine with paroxetine in elderly patients suffering from resistant depression. Int Clin Psychopharmacol 22:371–375, 2007

McCue RE, Joseph M: Venlafaxine- and trazodone-induced serotonin syndrome. Am J Psychiatry 158:2088–2089, 2001

Messenheimer JA: Rash in adult and pediatric patients treated with lamotrigine. Can J Neurol Sci 25:S14–S18, 1998

Meyers BS, Flint AJ, Rothschild AJ, et al: A double-blind randomized controlled trial of olanzapine plus sertraline versus olanzapine plus placebo for psychotic depression—the STOP-PD Study. Arch Gen Psychiatry 66:838–847, 2009

Micca JL, Hoffmann VP, Lipkovich I, et al: Retrospective analysis of diabetes risk in elderly patients with dementia in olanzapine clinical trials. Am J Geriatr Psychiatry 14:62–70, 2006

Mintzer JE, Tune LE, Breder CD, et al: Aripiprazole for the treatment of psychoses in institutionalized patients with Alzheimer dementia: a multicenter, randomized, double-blind, placebo-controlled assessment of three fixed doses. Am J Geriatr Psychiatry 15:918–931, 2007

Mittal D, Jimerson NA, Neely EP, et al: Risperidone in the treatment of delirium: results from a prospective open-label trial. J Clin Psychiatry 65:662–667, 2004

Modi A, Weiner M, Craig BA, et al: Concomitant use of anticholinergics with acetylcholinesterase inhibitors in Medicaid recipients with dementia and residing in nursing homes. J Am Geriatr Soc 57:1238–1244, 2009

Molho ES, Factor SA: Worsening of motor features of parkinsonism with olanzapine. Mov Disord 14:1014–1016, 1999

Montejo AL, Llorca G, Izquierdo JA, et al: Incidence of sexual dysfunction associated with antidepressant agents: a prospective multicenter study of 1022 outpatients. Spanish Working Group for the Study of Psychotropic-Related Sexual Dysfunction. J Clin Psychiatry 62 (suppl 3):10–21, 2001

Montgomery SA, Fava M, Padmanabhan SK, et al: Discontinuation symptoms and taper/poststudy-emergent adverse events with desvenlafaxine treatment for major depressive disorder. Int Clin Psychopharmacol 24:296–305, 2009

Mottram PG, Wilson K, Strobl JJ: Antidepressants for depressed elderly. Cochrane Database of Systematic Reviews 2006, Issue 1. Art. No.: CD003491. DOI: 10.1002/14651858.CD003491.pub2.

Mukai Y, Tampi RR: Treatment of depression in the elderly: a review of the recent literature on the efficacy of single- versus dual-action antidepressants. Clin Ther 31:945–961, 2009

Muller-Oerlinghausen B, Lewitzka U: Lithium reduces pathological aggression and suicidality: a mini-review. Neuropsychobiology 62:43–49, 2010

Mulsant BH, Alexopoulos GS, Reynolds CF 3rd, et al: Pharmacological treatment of depression in older primary care patients: the PROSPECT algorithm. Int J Geriatr Psychiatry 16:585–592, 2001a

Mulsant BH, Pollock BG, Nebes R, et al: A twelve-week, double-blind, randomized comparison of nortriptyline and paroxetine in older depressed inpatients and outpatients. Am J Geriatr Psychiatry 9:406–414, 2001b

Mulsant BH, Pollock BG, Kirshner M, et al: Serum anticholinergic activity in a community-based sample of older adults: relationship with cognitive performance. Arch Gen Psychiatry 60:198–203, 2003

Mulsant BH, Gharabawi GM, Bossie CA, et al: Correlates of anticholinergic activity in patients with dementia and psychosis treated with risperidone or olanzapine. J Clin Psychiatry 65:1708–1714, 2004

Murray V, von Arbin M, Bartfai A, et al: Double-blind comparison of sertraline and placebo in stroke patients with minor depression and less severe major depression. J Clin Psychiatry 66:708–716, 2005

Nagaraja D, Jayashree S: Randomized study of the dopamine receptor agonist piribedil in the treatment of mild cognitive impairment. Am J Psychiatry 158:1517–1519, 2001

Nandagopal JJ, DelBello MP: Selegiline transdermal system: a novel treatment option for major depressive disorder. Expert Opin Pharmacother 10:1665–1673, 2009

National Collaborating Centre for Mental Health: Management of Depression in Primary and Secondary Care (Clinical Guideline 23). London, National Institute for Clinical Excellence, 2004

Navarro V, Gasto C, Torres X, et al: Citalopram versus nortriptyline in late-life depression: a 12-week randomized single-blind study. Acta Psychiatr Scand 103:435–440, 2001

Nebes RD, Pollock BG, Meltzer CC, et al: Cognitive effects of serum anticholinergic activity and white matter hyperintensities. Neurology 65:1487–1489, 2005

Nelson JC, Wohlreich MM, Mallinckrodt CH, et al: Duloxetine for the treatment of major depressive disorder in older patients. Am J Geriatr Psychiatry 13:227–235, 2005

Nelson JC, Delucchi K, Schneider L: Suicidal thinking and behavior during treatment with sertraline in late-life depression. Am J Geriatr Psychiatry 15:573–580, 2007

Nelson JC, Delucchi K, Schneider LS: Efficacy of second generation antidepressants in late-life depression: a meta-analysis of the evidence. Am J Geriatr Psychiatry 16:558–567, 2008

Newhouse PA, Krishnan KR, Doraiswamy PM, et al: A double-blind comparison of sertraline and fluoxetine in depressed elderly outpatients. J Clin Psychiatry 61:559–568, 2000

Nicholas LM, Ford AL, Esposito SM, et al: The effects of mirtazapine on plasma lipid profiles in healthy subjects. J Clin Psychiatry 64:883–889, 2003

Nieuwstraten CE, Dolovich LR: Bupropion versus selective serotonin-reuptake inhibitors for treatment of depression. Ann Pharmacother 35:1608–1613, 2001

Nikaido AM, Ellinwood EH Jr, Heatherly DG, et al: Age-related increase in CNS sensitivity to benzodiazepines as assessed by task difficulty. Psychopharmacology 100:90–97, 1990

Noaghiul S, Narayan M, Nelson JC: Divalproex treatment of mania in elderly patients. Am J Geriatr Psychiatry 6:257–262, 1998

Nyth AL, Gottfries CG: The clinical efficacy of citalopram in treatment of emotional disturbances in dementia disorders: a Nordic multicentre study. Br J Psychiatry 157:894–901, 1990

Nyth AL, Gottfries CG, Lyby K, et al: A controlled multicenter clinical study of citalopram and placebo in elderly depressed patients with and without concomitant dementia. Acta Psychiatr Scand 86:138–145, 1992

O'Connor DW, Sierakowski C, Chin LF, et al: The safety and tolerability of clozapine in aged patients: a retrospective clinical file review. World J Biol Psychiatry 11:788–791, 2010

Oganesian A, Shilling AD, Young-Sciame R, et al: Desvenlafaxine and venlafaxine exert minimal in vitro inhibition of human cytochrome p450 and p-glycoprotein activities. Psychopharmacol Bull 42:47–63, 2009

Olafsson K, Jorgensen S, Jensen HV, et al: Fluvoxamine in the treatment of demented elderly patients: a double-blind, placebo-controlled study. Acta Psychiatr Scand 85:453–456, 1992

Oslin DW, Streim JE, Katz IR, et al: Heuristic comparison of sertraline with nortriptyline for the treatment of depression in frail elderly patients. Am J Geriatr Psychiatry 8:141–149, 2000

Oslin DW, Ten Have TR, Streim JE, et al: Probing the safety of medications in the frail elderly: evidence from a randomized clinical trial of sertraline and venlafaxine in depressed nursing home residents. J Clin Psychiatry 64:875–882, 2003

Pact V, Giduz T: Mirtazapine treats resting tremor, essential tremor, and levodopa-induced dyskinesias. Neurology 53:1154, 1999

Pae CU, Lee SJ, Lee CU, et al: A pilot trial of quetiapine for the treatment of patients with delirium. Hum Psychopharmacol 19:125–127, 2004

Papakostas GI, Thase ME, Fava M, et al: Are antidepressant drugs that combine serotonergic and noradrenergic mechanisms of action more effective than the selective serotonin reuptake inhibitors in treating major depressive disorder? A meta-analysis of studies of newer agents. Biol Psychiatry 62:1217–1227, 2007

Parellada E, Baeza I, de Pablo J, et al: Risperidone in the treatment of patients with delirium. J Clin Psychiatry 65:348–353, 2004

Park-Wyllie LY, Mamdani MM, Li P, et al: Cholinesterase inhibitors and hospitalization for bradycardia: a population-based study. PLoS Med 6(9):e1000157, 2009

Parkinson Study Group: Low-dose clozapine for the treatment of drug-induced psychosis in Parkinson's disease. N Engl J Med 340:757–763, 1999

Pedersen L, Klysner R: Antagonism of selective serotonin reuptake inhibitor-induced nausea by mirtazapine. Int Clin Psychopharmacol 12:59–60, 1997

Percudani M, Barbui C, Fortino I, et al: Second-generation antipsychotics and risk of cerebrovascular accidents in the elderly. J Clin Psychopharmacol 25:468–470, 2005

Perry NK: Venlafaxine-induced serotonin syndrome with relapse following amitriptyline. Postgrad Med J 76:254–256, 2000

Petracca GM, Chemerinski E, Starkstein SE: A double-blind, placebo-controlled study of fluoxetine in depressed patients with Alzheimer's disease. Int Psychogeriatr 13:233–240, 2001

Phanjoo AL, Wonnacott S, Hodgson A: Double-blind comparative multicentre study of fluvoxamine and mianserin in the treatment of major depressive episode in elderly people. Acta Psychiatr Scand 83:476–479, 1991

Pilotto A, Franceschi M, D'Onofrio G, et al: Effect of a CYP2D6 polymorphism on the efficacy of donepezil in patients with Alzheimer disease. Neurology 73:761–767, 2009

Pinquart M, Duberstein PR, Lyness JM: Treatments for later-life depressive conditions: a meta-analytic comparison of pharmacotherapy and psychotherapy. Am J Psychiatry 163:1493–1501, 2006

Poewe W: Treatment of dementia with Lewy bodies and Parkinson's disease dementia. Mov Disord 20 (suppl 12):S77–S82, 2005

Pollock BG, Mulsant BH, Sweet R, et al: An open pilot study of citalopram for behavioral disturbances of dementia. Am J Geriatr Psychiatry 5:70–78, 1997

Pollock BG, Laghrissi-Thode F, Wagner WR: Evaluation of platelet activation in depressed patients with ischemic heart disease after paroxetine or nortriptyline treatment. J Clin Psychopharmacol 20:137–140, 2000

Pollock BG, Mulsant BH, Rosen J, et al: Comparison of citalopram, perphenazine, and placebo for the acute treatment of psychosis and behavioral disturbances in hospitalized, demented patients. Am J Psychiatry 159:460–465, 2002

Pollock BG, Mulsant BH, Rosen J, et al: A double-blind comparison of citalopram and risperidone for the treatment of behavioral and psychotic symptoms associated with dementia. Am J Geriatr Psychiatry 15:942–952, 2007

Pollock BG, Forsyth CE, Bies RR: The critical role of clinical pharmacology in geriatric psychopharmacology. Clin Pharmacol Ther 85:89–93, 2009

Pomara N, Deptula D, Medel M, et al: Effects of diazepam on recall memory: relationship to aging, dose, and duration of treatment. Psychopharmacol Bull 25:144–148, 1989

Post RM, Frye MA, Denicoff KD, et al: Beyond lithium in the treatment of bipolar illness. Neuropsychopharmacology 19:206–219, 1998

Rabey JM, Prokhorov T, Miniovitz A, et al: Effect of quetiapine in psychotic Parkinson's disease patients: a double-blind labeled study of 3 months' duration. Mov Disord 22:313–318, 2007

Rabins PV, Lyketsos CG: Antipsychotic drugs in dementia: what should be made of the risks? JAMA 294:1963–1965, 2005

Rahman MK, Akhtar MJ, Savla NC, et al: A double-blind, randomised comparison of fluvoxamine with dothiepin in the treatment of depression in elderly patients. Br J Clin Pract 45:255–258, 1991

Rais AR, Williams K, Rais T, et al: Use of intramuscular ziprasidone for the control of acute psychosis or agitation in an inpatient geriatric population: an open-label study. Psychiatry (Edgmont) 7:17–24, 2010

Raji MA, Brady SR: Mirtazapine for treatment of depression and comorbidities in Alzheimer disease. Ann Pharmacother 35:1024–1027, 2001

Rajji TK, Mulsant BH, Lotrich FE, et al: Use of antidepressants in late-life depression. Drugs Aging 25:841–853, 2008

Rajji TK, Uchida H, Ismail Z, et al: Clozapine and global cognition in schizophrenia. J Clin Psychopharmacol 30:431–436, 2010

Rampello L, Chiechio S, Nicoletti G, et al: Prediction of the response to citalopram and reboxetine in post-stroke depressed patients. Psychopharmacology (Berl) 173:73–78, 2004

Rapaport MH, Schneider LS, Dunner DL, et al: Efficacy of controlled-release paroxetine in the treatment of late-life depression. J Clin Psychiatry 64:1065–1074, 2003

Raskin J, Wiltse CG, Siegal A, et al: Efficacy of duloxetine on cognition, depression, and pain in elderly patients with major depressive disorder: an 8-week, double-blind, placebo-controlled trial. Am J Psychiatry 164:900–909, 2007

Rasmussen A, Lunde M, Poulsen DL, et al: A double-blind, placebo-controlled study of sertraline in the prevention of depression in stroke patients. Psychosomatics 44:216–221, 2003

Ray WA, Thapa PB, Gideon P: Benzodiazepines and the risk of falls in nursing home residents. J Am Geriatr Soc 48:682–685, 2000

Ray WA, Chung CP, Murray KT, et al: Atypical antipsychotic drugs and the risk of sudden cardiac death. N Engl J Med 360:225–235, 2009

Reifler BV, Teri L, Raskind M: Double-blind trial of imipramine in Alzheimer's disease in patients with and without depression. Am J Psychiatry 146:45–49, 1989

Reisberg B, Doody R, Stöffler A, et al: Memantine in moderate-to-severe Alzheimer's disease. N Engl J Med 348:1333–1341, 2003

Rektorova I, Rektor I, Bares M, et al: Pramipexole and pergolide in the treatment of depression in Parkinson's disease: a national multicentre prospective randomized study. Eur J Neurol 10:399–406, 2003

Reynolds CF, Dew MA, Pollock BG, et al: Maintenance treatment of major depression in old age. N Engl J Med 354:1130–1138, 2006

Reynolds CF 3rd, Butters MA, Lopez O, et al: Maintenance treatment of depression in old age: a randomized, double-blind, placebo-controlled evaluation of the efficacy and safety of donepezil combined with antidepressant pharmacotherapy. Arch Gen Psychiatry 68:51–60, 2011

Reznik I, Rosen Y, Rosen B: An acute ischaemic event associated with the use of venlafaxine: a case report and proposed pathophysiological mechanisms. J Psychopharmacol 13:193–195, 1999

Richards JB, Papaioannou A, Adachi JD for the Canadian Multicentre Osteoporosis Study Research Group: Effect of selective serotonin reuptake inhibitors on the risk of fracture. Arch Intern Med 167:188–194, 2007

Ridout F, Meadows R, Johnsen S, et al: A placebo controlled investigation into the effects of paroxetine and mirtazapine on measures related to car driving performance. Hum Psychopharmacol 18:261–269, 2003

Ritchie CW, Chiu E, Harrigan S, et al: The impact upon extrapyramidal side effects, clinical symptoms and quality of life of a switch from conventional to atypical antipsychotics (risperidone or olanzapine) in elderly patients with schizophrenia. Int J Geriatr Psychiatry 18:432–440, 2003

Ritchie CW, Chiu E, Harrigan S, et al: A comparison of the efficacy and safety of olanzapine and risperidone in the treatment of elderly patients with schizophrenia: an open study of six months duration. Int J Geriatr Psychiatry 21:171–179, 2006

Robinson DS, Amsterdam JD: The selegiline transdermal system in major depressive disorder: a systematic review of safety and tolerability. J Affect Disord 105:15–23, 2008

Robinson R, Schultz S, Castillo C, et al: Nortriptyline versus fluoxetine in the treatment of depression and in short-term recovery after stroke: a placebo-controlled, double-blind study. Am J Psychiatry 157:351–359, 2000

Robinson RG, Jorge RE, Moser DJ, et al: Escitalopram and problem-solving therapy for prevention of poststroke depression: a randomized controlled trial. JAMA 299:2391–2400, 2008

Rocca P, Calvarese P, Faggiano F, et al: Citalopram versus sertraline in late-life nonmajor clinically significant depression: a 1-year follow-up clinical trial. J Clin Psychiatry 66:360–369, 2005

Rochon PA, Stukel TA, Sykora K, et al: Atypical antipsychotics and parkinsonism. Arch Intern Med 165:1882–1888, 2005

Rodda J, Morgan S, Walker Z: Are cholinesterase inhibitors effective in the management of the behavioral and psychological symptoms of dementia in Alzheimer's disease? A systematic review of randomized, placebo-controlled trials of donepezil, rivastigmine and galantamine. Int Psychogeriatr 21:813–824, 2009

Roose SP, Dalack GW, Glassman AH, et al: Cardiovascular effects of bupropion in depressed patients with heart disease. Am J Psychiatry 148:512–516, 1991

Roose SP, Nelson JC, Salzman C, et al: Open-label study of mirtazapine orally disintegrating tablets in depressed patients in the nursing home. Mirtazapine in the Nursing Home Study Group. Curr Med Res Opin 19:737–746, 2003

Roose SP, Miyazaki M, Devanand D, et al: An open trial of venlafaxine for the treatment of late-life atypical depression. Int J Geriatr Psychiatry 19:989–994, 2004a

Roose SP, Sackeim HA, Krishnan KR, et al: Antidepressant pharmacotherapy in the treatment of depression in the very old: a randomized, placebo-controlled trial. Am J Psychiatry 161:2050–2059, 2004b

Rosen J, Sweet R, Pollock BG, et al: Nortriptyline in the hospitalized elderly: tolerance and side effect reduction. Psychopharmacol Bull 29:327–331, 1993

Rosenberg C, Lauritzen L, Brix J, et al: Citalopram versus amitriptyline in elderly depressed patients with or without mild cognitive dysfunction: a Danish multicentre trial in general practice. Psychopharmacol Bull 40:63–73, 2007

Rosenberg PB, Drye LT, Martin BK, et al: Sertraline for the treatment of depression in Alzheimer disease. Am J Geriatr Psychiatry 18:136–145, 2010

Ross J: Discontinuation of lithium augmentation in geriatric patients with unipolar depression: a systematic review. Can J Psychiatry 53:117–120, 2008

Rossini D, Serretti A, Franchini L, et al: Sertraline versus fluvoxamine in the treatment of elderly patients with major depression: a double-blind, randomized trial. J Clin Psychopharmacol 25:471–475, 2005

Rush AJ, Trivedi MH, Wisniewski SR, et al: Acute and longer-term outcomes in depressed outpatients requiring one or several treatment steps: a STAR*D report. Am J Psychiatry 163:1905–1917, 2006

Sackeim HA, Haskett RF, Mulsant BH, et al: Continuation pharmacotherapy in the prevention of relapse following electroconvulsive therapy: a randomized controlled trial. JAMA 285:1299–1307, 2001

Saiz-Ruiz J, Ibanez A, Diaz-Marsa M, et al: Nefazodone in the treatment of elderly patients with depressive disorders: a prospective, observational study. CNS Drugs 16:635–643, 2002

Sajatovic M, Jaskiw G, Konicki PE, et al: Outcome of clozapine therapy for elderly patients with refractory primary psychosis. Int J Geriatr Psychiatry 12:553–558, 1997

Sajatovic M, Gyulai L, Calabrese JR, et al: Maintenance treatment outcomes in older patients with bipolar I disorder. Am J Geriatr Psychiatry 13:305–311, 2005a

Sajatovic M, Madhusoodanan S, Coconcea N: Managing bipolar disorder in the elderly: defining the role of the newer agents. Drugs Aging 22:39–54, 2005b

Sajatovic M, Blow FC, Ignacio RV: Psychiatric comorbidity in older adults with bipolar disorder. Int J Geriatr Psychiatry 21:582–587, 2006

Sajatovic M, Ramsay E, Nanry K, et al: Lamotrigine therapy in elderly patients with epilepsy, bipolar disorder or dementia. Int J Geriatr Psychiatry 22:945–950, 2007

Sajatovic M, Coconcea N, Ignacio RV, et al: Aripiprazole therapy in 20 older adults with bipolar disorder: a 12-week, open-label trial. J Clin Psychiatry 69:41–46, 2008

Salzman C, Jeste DV, Meyer RE, et al: Elderly patients with dementia-related symptoms of severe agitation and aggression: consensus statement on treatment options, clinical trials methodology, and policy. J Clin Psychiatry 69:889–898, 2008

Sasaki Y, Matsuyama T, Inoue S, et al: A prospective, open-label, flexible-dose study of quetiapine in the treatment of delirium. J Clin Psychiatry 64:1316–1321, 2003

Satel SL, Nelson JC: Stimulants in the treatment of depression: a critical overview. J Clin Psychiatry 50:241–249, 1989

Sato Y, Kondo I, Ishida S, et al: Decreased bone mass and increased bone turnover with valproate therapy in adults with epilepsy. Neurology 57:445–449, 2001

Savaskan E, Muller SE, Bohringer A, et al: Antidepressive therapy with escitalopram improves mood, cognitive symptoms, and identity memory for angry faces in elderly depressed patients. Int J Neuropsychopharmacol 11:381–388, 2008

Schatzberg A, Roose S: A double-blind, placebo-controlled study of venlafaxine and fluoxetine in geriatric outpatients with major depression. Am J Geriatr Psychiatry 14:361–370, 2006

Schatzberg AF, Kremer C, Rodrigues HE, et al: Double-blind, randomized comparison of mirtazapine and paroxetine in elderly depressed patients. Am J Geriatr Psychiatry 10:541–550, 2002

Schneider LS, Nelson JC, Clary CM, et al: An 8-week multicenter, parallel-group, double-blind, placebo-controlled study of sertraline in elderly outpatients with major depression. Am J Psychiatry 160:1277–1285, 2003

Schneider LS, Dagerman KS, Insel P: Risk of death with atypical antipsychotic drug treatment for dementia: meta-analysis of randomized placebo-controlled trials. JAMA 294:1934–1943, 2005

Schneider LS, Dagerman K, Insel PS: Efficacy and adverse effects of atypical antipsychotics for dementia: meta-analysis of randomized placebo-controlled trials. Am J Geriatr Psychiatry 14:191–210, 2006a

Schneider LS, Tariot PN, Dagerman KS, et al: Effectiveness of atypical antipsychotic drugs in patients with Alzheimer's disease. N Engl J Med 355:1525–1538, 2006b

Schone W, Ludwig M: A double-blind study of paroxetine compared with fluoxetine in geriatric patients with major depression. J Clin Psychopharmacol 13 (6 suppl 2):34S–39S, 1993

Schwaninger M, Ringleb P, Winter R, et al: Elevated plasma concentrations of homocysteine in antiepileptic drug treatment. Epilepsia 40:345–350, 1999

Scott J, Greenwald BS, Kramer E, et al: Atypical (second generation) antipsychotic treatment response in very late-onset schizophrenia-like psychosis. Int Psychogeriatr 23:742–748, 2011

Semenchuk MR, Sherman S, Davis B: Double-blind, randomized trial of bupropion SR for the treatment of neuropathic pain. Neurology 57:1583–1588, 2001

Serebruany VL, Glassman AH, Malinin AI, et al: Platelet/endothelial biomarkers in depressed patients treated with the selective serotonin reuptake inhibitor sertraline after acute coronary events: the Sertraline AntiDepressant Heart Attack Randomized Trial (SADHART) Platelet Substudy. Circulation 108:939–944, 2003

Seritan AL: Prevent drug-drug interactions with cholinesterase inhibitors: avoid adverse events when prescribing medications for patients with dementia. Curr Psychiatry 7:57–67, 2008

Sheffrin M, Driscoll HC, Lenze EJ, et al: Pilot study of augmentation with aripiprazole for incomplete response in late-life depression: getting to remission. J Clin Psychiatry 70:208–213, 2009

Sheikh JI, Cassidy EL, Doraiswamy PM, et al: Efficacy, safety, and tolerability of sertraline in patients with late-life depression and comorbid medical illness. J Am Geriatr Soc 52:86–92, 2004a

Sheikh JI, Lauderdale SA, Cassidy EL: Efficacy of sertraline for panic disorder in older adults: a preliminary open-label trial. Am J Geriatr Psychiatry 12:230, 2004b

Shelton C, Entsuah R, Padmanabhan SK, et al: Venlafaxine XR demonstrates higher rates of sustained remission compared to fluoxetine, paroxetine or placebo. Int Clin Psychopharmacol 20:233–238, 2005

Shelton RC, Tollefson GD, Tohen M, et al: A novel augmentation strategy for treating resistant major depression. Am J Psychiatry 158:131–134, 2001

Shulman KI: Lithium for older adults with bipolar disorder: should it still be considered a first-line agent? Drugs Aging 27:607–615, 2010

Shulman KI, Walker SE: A reevaluation of dietary restrictions for irreversible monoamine oxidase inhibitors. Psychiatr Ann 31:378–384, 2001

Shulman KI, Fischer HD, Herrmann N, et al: Current prescription patterns and safety profile of irreversible monoamine oxidase inhibitors: a population-based cohort study of older adults. J Clin Psychiatry 70:1681–1686, 2009

Siddiqi N, Holt R, Britton AM, et al: Interventions for preventing delirium in hospitalised patients. Cochrane Database of Systematic Reviews 2007, Issue 2. Art. No.: CD005563. DOI: 10.1002/14651858.CD005563.pub2.

Sink KM, Holden KF, Yaffe K: Pharmacological treatment of neuropsychiatric symptoms of dementia: a review of the evidence. JAMA 293:596–608, 2005

Skrobik YK, Bergeron N, Dumont M, et al: Olanzapine vs. haloperidol: treating delirium in a critical care setting. Intensive Care Med 30:444–449, 2004

Smeraldi E, Rizzo F, Crespi G: Double-blind, randomized study of venlafaxine, clomipramine and trazodone in geriatric patients with major depression. Primary Care Psychiatry 4:189–195, 1998

Smith D, Dempster C, Glanville J, et al: Efficacy and tolerability of venlafaxine compared with selective serotonin reuptake inhibitors and other antidepressants: a meta-analysis. Br J Psychiatry 180:396–404, 2002

Sneed JR, Culang ME, Keilp JG, et al: Antidepressant medication and executive dysfunction: a deleterious interaction in late-life depression. Am J Geriatr Psychiatry 18:128–135, 2010

Soares CN, Thase ME, Clayton A, et al: Desvenlafaxine and escitalopram for the treatment of postmenopausal women with major depressive disorder. Menopause 17:700–711, 2010

Sommer BR, Fenn HH, Ketter TA: Safety and efficacy of anticonvulsants in elderly patients with psychiatric disorders: oxcarbazepine, topiramate and gabapentin. Expert Opin Drug Saf 6:133–145, 2007

Sonnenberg CM, Deeg DJ, Comijs HC, et al: Trends in antidepressant use in the older population: results from the LASA-study over a period of 10 years. J Affect Disord 111:299–305, 2008

Spier SA: Use of bupropion with SRIs and venlafaxine. Depress Anxiety 7:73–75, 1998

Sproule BA, Hardy BG, Shulman KI: Differential pharmacokinetics of lithium in elderly patients. Drugs Aging 16:165–177, 2000

Stahl SM, Entsuah R, Rudolph RL: Comparative efficacy between venlafaxine and SSRIs: a pooled analysis of patients with depression. Biol Psychiatry 52:1166–1174, 2002

Steffens DC, Doraiswamy PM, McQuoid DR: Bupropion SR in the naturalistic treatment of elderly patients with major depression. Int J Geriatr Psychiatry 16:862–865, 2001

Steffens DC, Nelson JC, Eudicone JM, et al: Efficacy and safety of adjunctive aripiprazole in major depressive disorder in older patients; a pooled subpopulation analysis. Int J Geriatr Psychiatry 26:564–572, 2011

Steinberg JR: Anxiety in elderly patients: a comparison of azapirones and benzodiazepines. Drugs Aging 5:335–345, 1994

Steinmetz K, Coley K, Pollock BG: Assessment of the quantity and quality of geriatric information in the drug label for commonly prescribed drugs in the elderly. J Am Geriatr Soc 53:891–894, 2005

Strand M, Hetta J, Rosen A, et al: A double-blind controlled trial in primary care patients with generalized anxiety: a comparison between buspirone and oxazepam. J Clin Psychiatry 51(suppl):40–45, 1990

Street JS, Clark WS, Gannon KS, et al: Olanzapine treatment of psychotic and behavioral symptoms in patients with Alzheimer disease in nursing care facilities: a double-blind, randomized, placebo-controlled trial. The HGEU Study Group. Arch Gen Psychiatry 57:968–976, 2000

Streim JE, Porsteinsson AP, Breder CD, et al: A randomized, double-blind, placebo-controlled study of aripiprazole for the treatment of psychosis in nursing home patients with Alzheimer disease. Am J Geriatr Psychiatry 16:537–550, 2008

Suh GH, Son HG, Ju YS, et al: A randomized, double-blind, crossover comparison of risperidone and haloperidol in Korean dementia patients with behavioral disturbances. Am J Geriatr Psychiatry 12:509–516, 2004

Suppes T, Eudicone J, McQuade R, et al: Efficacy and safety of aripiprazole in subpopulations with acute manic or mixed episodes of bipolar I disorder. J Affect Disord 107:145–154, 2008

Szuba MP, Leuchter AF: Falling backward in two elderly patients taking bupropion. J Clin Psychiatry 53:157–159, 1992

Tadger S, Paleacu D, Barak Y: Quetiapine augmentation of antidepressant treatment in elderly patients suffering from depressive symptoms: a retrospective chart review. Arch Gerontol Geriatr 53:104–105, 2011

Taragano FE, Lyketsos CG, Mangone CA, et al: A double-blind, randomized, fixed-dose trial of fluoxetine vs. amitriptyline in the treatment of major depression complicating Alzheimer's disease. Psychosomatics 38:246–252, 1997

Tariot PN, Erb R, Podgorski CA, et al: Efficacy and tolerability of carbamazepine for agitation and aggression in dementia. Am J Psychiatry 155:54–61, 1998

Tariot PN, Salzman C, Yeung PP, et al: Long-term use of quetiapine in elderly patients with psychotic disorders. Clin Ther 22:1068–1084, 2000

Tariot PN, Farlow MR, Grossberg GT, et al: Memantine treatment in patients with moderate to severe Alzheimer disease already receiving donepezil: a randomized controlled trial. JAMA 291:317–324, 2004

Tariot PN, Raman R, Jakimovich L, et al: Divalproex sodium in nursing home residents with possible or probable Alzheimer disease complicated by agitation: a randomized, controlled trial. Am J Geriatr Psychiatry 13:942–949, 2005

Tashkin D, Kanner R, Bailey W, et al: Smoking cessation in patients with chronic obstructive pulmonary disease: a double-blind, placebo-controlled, randomised trial. Lancet 357:1571–1575, 2001

Thase ME: Effects of venlafaxine on blood pressure: a meta-analysis of original data from 3744 depressed patients. J Clin Psychiatry 59:502–508, 1998

Thase ME: What role do atypical antipsychotic drugs have in treatment-resistant depression? J Clin Psychiatry 63:95–103, 2002

Thase ME, Entsuah AR, Rudolph RL: Remission rates during treatment with venlafaxine or selective serotonin reuptake inhibitors. Br J Psychiatry 178:234–241, 2001

Thase ME, Entsuah R, Cantillon M, et al: Relative antidepressant efficacy of venlafaxine and SSRIs: sex-age interactions. J Womens Health 14:609–616, 2005a

Thase ME, Haight BR, Richard N, et al: Remission rates following antidepressant therapy with bupropion or selective serotonin reuptake inhibitors: a meta-analysis of original data from 7 randomized controlled trials. J Clin Psychiatry 66:974–981, 2005b

Thase ME, Tran PV, Wiltse C, et al: Cardiovascular profile of duloxetine, a dual re-uptake inhibitor of serotonin and norepinephrine. J Clin Psychopharmacol 25:132–140, 2005c

Thompson DS: Mirtazapine for the treatment of depression and nausea in breast and gynecological oncology. Psychosomatics 41:356–359, 2000

Tollefson GD, Bosomworth JC, Heiligenstein JH, et al: A double-blind, placebo-controlled clinical trial of fluoxetine in geriatric patients with major depression. The Fluoxetine Collaborative Study Group. Int Psychogeriatr 7:89–104, 1995

Trappler B, Cohen CI: Use of SSRIs in "very old" depressed nursing home residents. Am J Geriatr Psychiatry 6:83–89, 1998

Trick L, Stanley N, Rigney U, et al: A double-blind, randomized, 26-week study comparing the cognitive and psychomotor effects and efficacy of 75 mg (37.5 mg b.i.d.) venlafaxine and 75 mg (25 mg mane, 50 mg nocte) dothiepin in elderly patients with moderate major depression being treated in general practice. J Psychopharmacol 18:205–214, 2004

Trivedi MH, Fava M, Wisniewski SR, et al: Medication augmentation after the failure of SSRIs for depression. N Engl J Med 354:1243–1252, 2006

Uchida H, Mamo DC, Mulsant BH, et al: Increased antipsychotic sensitivity in elderly patients: evidence and mechanisms. J Clin Psychiatry 70:397–405, 2009

U.S. Food and Drug Administration: FDA Drug Safety Communication: Abnormal heart rhythms associated with high doses of Celexa (citalopram hydrobromide). August 24, 2011. Available at: http://www.fda.gov/Drugs/DrugSafety/ucm269086.htm. Accessed October 11, 2011.

van Iersel MB, Zuidema SU, Koopmans RT, et al: Antipsychotics for behavioral and psychological problems in elderly people with dementia: a systematic review of adverse events. Drugs Aging 22:845–858, 2005

Verhey FR, Verkaaik M, Lousberg R: Olanzapine versus haloperidol in the treatment of agitation in elderly patients with dementia: results of a randomized controlled double-blind trial. Dement Geriatr Cogn Disord 21:1–8, 2006

Vis PM, van Baardewijk M, Einarson TR: Duloxetine and venlafaxine-XR in the treatment of major depressive disorder: a meta-analysis of randomized clinical trials. Ann Pharmacother 39:1798–1807, 2005

Wakelin JS: Fluvoxamine in the treatment of the older depressed patient: double-blind, placebo-controlled data. Int Clin Psychopharmacol 1:221–230, 1986

Walker Z, Grace J, Overshot R, et al: Olanzapine in dementia with Lewy bodies: a clinical study. Int J Geriatr Psychiatry 14:459–466, 1999

Wallace AE, Kofoed LL, West AN: Double-blind placebo-controlled trial of methylphenidate in older, depressed, medically ill patients. Am J Psychiatry 152:929–931, 1995

Wang PS, Bohn RL, Glynn RJ, et al: Zolpidem use and hip fractures in older people. J Am Geriatr Soc 49:1685–1690, 2001

Wang PS, Schneeweiss S, Avorn J, et al: Risk of death in elderly users of conventional vs. atypical antipsychotic medications. N Engl J Med 353:2335–2341, 2005

Wehmeier PM, Kluge M, Maras A, et al: Fluoxetine versus trimipramine in the treatment of depression in geriatric patients. Pharmacopsychiatry 38:13–16, 2005

Weihs KL, Settle EC Jr, Batey SR, et al: Bupropion sustained release versus paroxetine for the treatment of depression in the elderly. J Clin Psychiatry 61:196–202, 2000

Weintraub D, Rosenberg PB, Drye LT, et al: Sertraline for the treatment of depression in Alzheimer disease: week-24 outcomes. Am J Geriatr Psychiatry 18:332–340, 2010

Whyte EM, Basinski J, Farhi P, et al: Geriatric depression treatment in nonresponders to selective serotonin reuptake inhibitors. J Clin Psychiatry 65:1634–1641, 2004

Whyte E, Romkes M, Mulsant BH, et al: CYP 2D6 genotype and venlafaxine-XR concentrations in depressed elderly. Int J Geriatr Psychiatry 21:1–8, 2006

Wilner KD, Tensfeldt TG, Baris B, et al: Single- and multiple-dose pharmacokinetics of ziprasidone in healthy young and elderly volunteers. Br J Clin Pharmacol 49 (suppl 1):15S–20S, 2000

Wilson K, Mottram P: A comparison of side effects of selective serotonin reuptake inhibitors and tricyclic antidepressants in older depressed patients: a meta-analysis. Int J Geriatr Psychiatry 19:754–762, 2004

Winblad B, Kilander L, Eriksson S, et al: Donepezil in patients with severe Alzheimer's disease: double-blind, parallel-group, placebo-controlled study. Lancet 367(9516):1057–1065, 2006

Wingen M, Bothmer J, Langer S, et al: Actual driving performance and psychomotor function in healthy subjects after acute and subchronic treatment with escitalopram, mirtazapine, and placebo: a crossover trial. J Clin Psychiatry 66:436–443, 2005

Wohlreich MM, Sullivan MD, Mallinckrodt CH, et al: Duloxetine for the treatment of recurrent major depressive disorder in elderly patients: treatment outcomes in patients with comorbid arthritis. Psychosomatics 50:402–412, 2009

Wu E, Greenberg P, Yang E, et al: Comparison of treatment persistence, hospital utilization and costs among major depressive disorder geriatric patients treated with escitalopram versus other SSRI/SNRI antidepressants. Curr Med Res Opin 24:2805–2813, 2008a

Wu E, Greenberg PE, Yang E, et al: Comparison of escitalopram versus citalopram for the treatment of major depressive disorder in a geriatric population. Curr Med Res Opin 24:2587–2595, 2008b

Wylie ME, Miller MD, Shear MK, et al: Fluvoxamine pharmacotherapy of anxiety disorders in late life: preliminary open-trial data. J Geriatr Psychiatry Neurol 13:43–48, 2000

Yang CH, Tsai SJ, Hwang JP: The efficacy and safety of quetiapine for treatment of geriatric psychosis. J Psychopharmacol 19:661–666, 2005

Young RC, Gyulai L, Mulsant BH, et al: Pharmacotherapy of bipolar disorder in old age: review and recommendations. Am J Geriatr Psychiatry 12:342–357, 2004

Yuan Y, Tsoi K, Hunt RH: Selective serotonin reuptake inhibitors and risk of upper GI bleeding: confusion or confounding? Am J Med 119:719–727, 2006

Zheng L, Mack WJ, Dagerman KS, et al: Metabolic changes associated with second-generation antipsychotic use in Alzheimer's disease patients: the CATIE-AD study. Am J Psychiatry 166:583–590, 2009

Zhong KX, Tariot PN, Mintzer J, et al: Quetiapine to treat agitation in dementia: a randomized, double-blind, placebo-controlled study. Curr Alzheimer Res 4:81–93, 2007

Zimmer B, Kant R, Zeiler D, et al: Antidepressant efficacy and cardiovascular safety of venlafaxine in young vs. old patients with comorbid medical disorders. Int J Psychiatry Med 27:353–364, 1997

Suggested Readings

Alexopoulos GS, Katz IR, Reynolds CF 3rd, et al: Pharmacotherapy of depression in older patients: a summary of the expert consensus guidelines. J Psychiatr Pract 7:361–376, 2001

Gauthier S, Cummings J, Ballard C, et al: Management of behavioral problems in Alzheimer's disease. Int Psychogeriatr 22:346–372, 2010

Pinquart M, Duberstein PR, Lyness JM: Treatments for later-life depressive conditions: a meta-analytic comparison of pharmaco-therapy and psychotherapy. Am J Psychiatry 163:1493–1501, 2006

Rabins PV, Lyketsos CG: Antipsychotic drugs in dementia: what should be made of the risks? JAMA 294:1963–1965, 2005

Schneider LS, Dagerman KS, Insel P: Efficacy and adverse effects of atypical antipsychotics for dementia: meta-analysis of randomized placebo-controlled trials. Am J Geriatr Psychiatry 14:191–210, 2006

Sink KM, Holden KF, Yaffe K: Pharmacological treatment of neuropsychiatric symptoms of dementia: a review of the evidence. JAMA 293:596–608, 2005

Young RC, Gyulai L, Mulsant BH, et al: Pharmacotherapy of bipolar disorder in old age: review and recommendations. Am J Geriatr Psychiatry 12:342–357, 2004

CHAPTER 17

ELECTROCONVULSIVE THERAPY

RICHARD D. WEINER, M.D., PH.D.
ANDREW D. KRYSTAL, M.D., M.S.

Electroconvulsive therapy (ECT) involves the electrical induction of a series of seizures as a treatment for mental disorders—most notably, major depression. In this chapter, we review ECT's history,; indications, and risks; the evaluation of patients for ECT; ECT technique; the use of ECT to alleviate episodes of illness; post-ECT course patient management; and the future of ECT. The primary focus of this chapter is on the use of ECT in the elderly.

History

The first use of ECT was in Italy in 1937, by Ugo Cerletti and Lucio Bini (Endler 1988; Shorter and Healey 2007). ECT was first used to treat schizophrenia; however, clinicians soon realized that its highest ther-

apeutic potency was in treating mood disorders. Although psychopharmacological agents obviated the need for ECT in many cases, beginning in the late 1950s, trials indicate that ECT remains the most rapid and effective means to induce remission of depression (UK ECT Review Group 2003).

In the early days of ECT, medical comorbidity common in older adults led to fears about the use of ECT in this population. As ECT methodology became more refined, its use with older adults steadily increased. ECT use rose from 4.2 per 10,000 to 5.1 per 10,000 among Medicare recipients between 1987 and 1992 (Rosenbach et al. 1997). There has been speculation about the reasons for the growing use of ECT among older individuals. Possible contributing factors include that depression tends to be relatively more severe and more resistant to medication in older adults, who are also more likely to be intolerant of medications. Thus, the available evidence indicates that ECT is likely used because it is safe, it works well, and it works rapidly (Stek et al. 2003).

Indications for Electroconvulsive Therapy

Diagnostic Indications

The most common diagnostic indication for ECT is major depression (American Psychiatric Association 2001). A significant body of literature not only supports the efficacy of ECT for major depression but also suggests that it is the most rapid and effective treatment for this condition (Husain et al. 2004; Stek et al. 2003). This literature includes a series of randomized, double-blind, placebo-controlled studies and meta-analytical studies comparing the efficacy of ECT with that of antidepressant medication (UK ECT Review Group 2003).

Regarding subtypes of depression, ECT appears to be effective in treating both melancholic and severe nonmelancholic depression, as well as bipolar and unipolar major depression (Weiner and Krystal 2001). In addition, it may be particularly effective in treating psychotic major depression (Petrides et al. 2001).

Although ECT is used more frequently for major depression than for other illnesses, evidence suggests that ECT has efficacy in several other mental disorders. A series of reports suggested that ECT has efficacy in the treatment of acute mania (Mukherjee et al. 1994). In this regard, ECT has been reported to achieve a response rate as high as 80%, to have efficacy equal to that of lith-

ium, and to have an advantage over lithium in patients not responding to lithium or antipsychotic medication. ECT also appears to have efficacy in schizophrenia (Tharyan and Adams 2005). Following the development of antipsychotic medications in the late 1950s, the use of ECT as a treatment for schizophrenia gradually declined. Regardless, several studies have suggested that antipsychotic medications and ECT have comparable efficacy and that the combination of antipsychotic medications and ECT may have greater efficacy than either ECT or medications alone (Tharyan and Adams 2005). The presence of affective symptoms appears to increase the likelihood of response to ECT in individuals with schizophrenia. Thus, individuals with schizoaffective disorder may respond better to ECT than do those with schizophrenia. Catatonia, which can be associated with both schizophrenia and mood disorders, is highly responsive to ECT (Krystal and Coffey 1997), even when this condition is associated with a wide variety of medical conditions (American Psychiatric Association 2001).

ECT also may be a useful treatment for Parkinson's disease when medication management fails or is not tolerated (Krystal and Coffey 1997); such patients may be at increased risk for developing cognitive side effects and delirium with ECT (Figiel et al. 1990).

Response to Electroconvulsive Therapy in Older Adults

Multiple prospective studies suggest that ECT is a highly effective acute treatment for major depression in elderly individuals (Stek et al. 2003; van der Wurff et al. 2003). Furthermore, one study indicated that ECT has a significant effect on the longitudinal course of major depression in older adults, in terms of both efficacy and morbidity and mortality rates (Philibert et al. 1995). These data provide support for a role for ECT in the practice of geriatric psychiatry.

Continuation or Maintenance Electroconvulsive Therapy

Although ECT is a highly effective treatment for several neuropsychiatric conditions, it is not a cure in the sense that it does not ensure that future episodes will not occur (American Psychiatric Association 2001). Also, evidence indicates that the relapse rate of major depressive disorder may be particularly high for older adults (Huuhka et al. 2004). As a result, it is important to institute some form of continuation or maintenance therapy. This point is underscored by the findings from a study by Sackeim and colleagues (2001), in which approximately 80% of the patients who were successfully treated with ECT for major depression relapsed within 6 months. Most commonly, continuation or maintenance pharmacotherapy is instituted after a successful course of ECT. Nevertheless, prophylactic pharmacotherapy has not been found to be universally effective, and approximately 50%–60% of depressed patients will relapse within a year of the end of the ECT course when given typical continuation or maintenance pharmacotherapy (Sackeim et al. 2001). One study suggested that rather than single-agent therapy, more aggressive pharmacotherapy—specifically, the combination of nortriptyline and lithium—is associated with a decrease in the relapse rate to about 40% 6 months after ECT (Sackeim et al. 2001).

An alternative to continuation or maintenance pharmacotherapy is continuation or maintenance ECT. Kellner and colleagues (2006) reported similar 6-month outcomes for patients who received maintenance bilateral ECT and for patients who received a combination of lithium and nortriptyline pharmacotherapy. A more recent trial by Navarro and colleagues (2008) showed a benefit for the combination of ECT and antidepressant pharmacotherapy compared with medication alone. At present, pharmacotherapy is usually instituted after a successful course of ECT unless at least one of the following conditions exists: 1) prophylactic pharmacotherapy has failed in the past, 2) the patient is intolerant of medications, 3) the patient has a medical illness that contraindicates medication management, or 4) the patient has a preference for prophylactic ECT (American Psychiatric Association 2001).

When to Recommend an Index Electroconvulsive Therapy Course

In general, the decision about whether to recommend ECT for a given patient should rest on a careful assessment of risks and benefits (American Psychiatric Association 2001). First-line treatment with ECT should be considered when an urgent need for response exists in a patient with major depression or mania. This situation typically occurs when the presenting condition threatens the patient's life because of suicidality, malnutrition, dehydration, or inability to comply with treatment of a critical medical problem. In addition, the first-line use of ECT should be considered when ECT is deemed to be safer than pharmacotherapy (Weiner et al. 2000) or when a patient has preferentially responded to ECT in prior episodes (American Psychiatric Association 2001).

The secondary use of ECT is undertaken following either medication intolerance or lack of response to pharmacotherapy. Unfortunately, no currently accepted definition exists for medication failure. Operationally, practitioners take into account the number of medications tried, treatment duration, dosage administered, symptom severity, tolerance of pharmacotherapy, expected risks of ECT, and patient preference (American Psychiatric Association 2001).

Risks of Electroconvulsive Therapy and Its Use in Patients With Neurological and Medical Disorders

Because the decision about whether to pursue a course of ECT should involve an evaluation of both the expected risks and the benefits of ECT, it is important to be able to carry out an assessment of the likelihood of potential risks for each patient.

Mortality

It has been estimated that the overall mortality rate for ECT is approximately 1 death per 80,000 treatments (American Psychiatric Association 2001). In addition, some studies have suggested that depressed inpatients who receive ECT have a lower mortality rate after discharge than do individuals who receive other types of treatment (Philibert et al. 1995). It is important to understand, however, that the likelihood of ECT-related death in high-risk populations—most commonly in older adults (see the following sections)—can be substantially higher than that mentioned earlier. Still, even in such situations, the risk of undertaking ECT may be lower than the risk of not doing it.

Cognitive Side Effects

The most important side effect with ECT is cognitive dysfunction, which appears to be a key factor limiting the use of this treatment modality (Ingram et al. 2008). The most common cognitive side effects are anterograde amnesia (difficulty retaining new information) and retrograde amnesia (difficulty recalling information learned in the past). Anterograde amnesia typically resolves within a few weeks after the treatment course, whereas retrograde amnesia tends to resolve more slowly (American Psychiatric Association 2001).

Both the degree and the duration of objective and subjective memory side effects of ECT vary substantially among individuals who receive ECT. Several factors can affect objective memory side effects of ECT (Ingram et al. 2008). Compared with unilateral placement of stimulus electrodes, bilateral placement increases the risk of amnesia, including in elderly populations (Stoppe et al. 2006). In addition, greater risk is associated with higher stimulus intensity (compared with the seizure threshold), larger numbers of ECT treatments, higher dosages of anesthetic, and more frequent treatments.

Other Risks With Electroconvulsive Therapy

It is important to identify individuals at risk for medical complications with ECT and to be aware of the modifications in ECT technique that may minimize risks. Elderly individuals referred for ECT frequently have preexisting medical illnesses (Christopher 2003; Weiner and Krystal 2001). No illnesses should be considered "absolute" contraindications to its use (American Psychiatric Association 2001). The decision about whether to pursue a course of ECT always should involve a careful weighing of the risks and benefits of carrying out ECT with those of not using it. Conditions for which evidence suggests increased risks with ECT are discussed in the following subsections.

Central Nervous System Disorders

The primary central nervous system (CNS) risks of ECT stem from the increase in intracranial and intravascular pressure that can occur with ECT seizures (Krystal and Coffey 1997). Despite these increases in pressure, the CNS complication rate is generally quite low. Some CNS disorders leave individuals more vulnerable to increases in pressure compared with those in the general ECT population. These include the presence of any space-occupying CNS lesions (Krystal and Coffey 1997). Although brain tumors were once considered an absolute contraindication to ECT, several reports described successful ECT in individuals with small, slow-growing lesions (Krystal and Coffey 1997).

Notwithstanding the transient hypertension that occurs with ECT, intracranial hemorrhages are extremely rare (Krystal and Coffey 1997). Nonetheless, individuals with recent strokes, arteriovenous malformations, and aneurysms are considered to be at increased risk. Use of prophylactic antihypertensive agents at the time of ECT should be considered for individuals with a history of hemorrhagic stroke; however, this may be counterproductive in individuals following cerebral ischemic events. Other adverse CNS conditions associated with ECT include prolonged seizures (lasting longer than 3 minutes) and status epilepticus (American Psychiatric Association 2001). Morbidity associated with prolonged seizures can be minimized by rapidly administering antiepileptic drugs to terminate such events.

Cardiovascular Disorders

Fluctuations in pulse and blood pressure that occur during ECT treatments may be associated with cardiovascular complications. Immediately after the stimulus, an increase in parasympathetic tone occurs, which can lead to a sudden but transient decrease in heart rate, often presenting as a brief period of asystole. The subsequent induced seizure, however, is associated with a sympathetic surge that markedly increases both blood pressure and heart rate. This sympathetic surge is then followed by a relative increase in parasympathetic tone as the induced seizure ends.

Despite these autonomic fluctuations, cardiovascular complications from ECT rarely occur in individuals without preexisting cardiovascular risk factors (Takada et al. 2005). The risk is increased in those with recent myocardial infarction, uncompensated congestive heart failure, severe valvular disease, unstable aneurysm, unstable angina or active cardiac ischemia, uncontrolled hypertension, high-grade atrioventricular block, symptomatic ventricular arrhythmia, and supraventricular arrhythmia with uncontrolled ventricular rate (American Psychiatric Association 2001). For patients with these conditions, a consultation with a cardiologist is recommended. An assessment of functional cardiac status (such as a stress test) should be considered in 1) men younger than 60 and women younger than 70 with definite angina, 2) men older than 60 and women older than 70 with probable angina, 3) all patients with angina and two risk factors for myocardial infarction, and 4) those with clinically significant extracardiac vascular disease (Applegate 1997).

For individuals with coronary artery disease, anticholinergic medications such as atropine can be used to decrease the occurrence and severity of bradycardia, β-adrenergic blockers can be used to decrease the cardiac workload, and nitrates or calcium channel blockers may be used to decrease the risks of ischemia (Weiner et al. 2000). Typically, medications for the treatment of coronary artery disease at the time of referral for ECT are maintained throughout the ECT course, including administration before ECT on treatment days (Applegate 1997).

Arrhythmias may increase the risks of ECT (Takada et al. 2005). In particular, individuals with atrial fibrillation may experience spontaneous cardioversion with ECT that may lead to an embolic event. As a result, echocardiography (to rule out a mural thrombus) and the use of anticoagulants should be considered.

Other Medical Disorders

Patients with diabetes are more likely than other ECT patients to have problems stemming from the need to fast from midnight until the time of the ECT treatment. Insulin doses may need to be adjusted, and pretreatment intravenous glucose administration can be considered if indicated (Weiner et al. 2000).

In individuals with hyperkalemia, prolonged paralysis and associated apnea induced by succinylcholine may be seen, and the use of paralytic agents other than succinylcholine should be considered when the abnormality cannot be corrected.

Thrombophlebitis carries with it the risk of embolism with ECT, a risk that is generally easily avoided with the use of anticoagulant medications, such as warfarin, with a goal of achieving an International Nor-

malized Ratio (prothrombin time normalized to the laboratory control value) between 1.5 and 2.5 (Petrides and Fink 1996).

Patients with asthma or chronic obstructive pulmonary disease have an increased risk of posttreatment bronchospasm, which should be mitigated by the use of bronchodilators (Weiner et al. 2000).

Complications of aspiration in patients with gastroesophageal reflux may be diminished with the use of a pretreatment histamine-2 antagonist the night before and the morning of treatment (Weiner et al. 2000). Fecal impaction may be a risk factor for intestinal rupture with ECT. Consequently, it is important to address constipation, which is particularly common in the elderly population.

Urinary retention could, in theory, lead to bladder rupture with ECT. As a result, it has been recommended that patients void before ECT, and urinary catheterization should be considered in those with significant difficulty urinating.

Musculoskeletal conditions—such as osteoporosis, unstable fractures, and loose or damaged teeth—are common in older adults. Patients with osteoporosis or with recent or unstable fractures are at risk for bone damage during the induced convulsion. This risk can be addressed by using an increased dose of succinylcholine to ensure good neuromuscular relaxation. The use of a mouth guard at the time of ECT is always necessary to avoid oral trauma.

Adverse Effects in Older Adults

Advanced age itself does not appear to increase the medical risks of ECT. As a group, however, older adults have a higher frequency of comorbid medical and neurological conditions that increase the risks of treatment, as outlined earlier. In addition, several studies have reported that older adults tend to have more cognitive impairment with ECT (see American Psychiatric Association 2001; Sackeim et al. 2007).

The greater frequency of comorbid medical and neurological disease in elderly persons also increases the risks associated with pharmacological management of their neuropsychiatric conditions. Manly et al. (2000) compared the frequency of side effects associated with ECT and with pharmacotherapy in a group of depressed patients older than 75 years and reported that ECT resulted in fewer side effects and greater efficacy. This study underscores that ECT may be both the safest and the most effective option for many older adults.

Pre–Electroconvulsive Therapy Evaluation

Basic Components of the Evaluation

Each pre-ECT evaluation should be carried out by an individual clinically privileged to administer ECT in conjunction with an anesthesia provider. This evaluation should include 1) a thorough psychiatric history and examination, including history of response to ECT and other treatments; 2) a medical history and examination, with special attention paid to cardiovascular, respiratory, neurological, and musculoskeletal systems; 3) a history of dental problems and examination for loose or missing teeth; and 4) a history of personal and family experiences with anesthesia. Laboratory tests are generally performed, although no agreed-on routine set of tests to carry out in each case is available. The most commonly administered pre-ECT tests include a complete blood count, serum chemistry (including sodium and potas-

sium), and electrocardiogram (American Psychiatric Association 2001; Tess and Smetana 2009). A chest radiograph is indicated in the setting of cardiovascular or pulmonary disease or when the patient has a history of smoking (Weiner et al. 2000).

The decision about whether to pursue testing of cerebral function and structure should be made on an individual basis, guided by the history and examination. In addition, spinal radiographs should be considered in individuals with known or suspected spinal disease.

Informed Consent

The collaborative aspect of decision making has been formalized as the legal doctrine of informed consent. No patient with the capacity to give voluntary consent should be treated with ECT without his or her written, informed consent. Although there is no clear consensus about how to determine capacity to give consent, capacity generally has been interpreted as evidence that the patient can understand information about the procedure and can act responsibly on the basis of this information (American Psychiatric Association 2001). The process of determining capacity and any specific procedures regarding informed consent may be specified by applicable state statutes. Because of the increased likelihood of cognitive dysfunction in older adults, capacity to consent is of particular concern.

Written consent should be obtained before a course of ECT, if an unusually large number of treatments become necessary, and before initiating continuation or maintenance ECT (American Psychiatric Association 2001). The consent form should include 1) a list of treatment alternatives; 2) a description of how, when, and where ECT will be carried out; 3) options regarding electrode placement; 4) the typical range of number of treatments; 5) a statement that there is no guarantee that the treatment will be successful; 6) a statement that continuation or maintenance treatment will be necessary; 7) a discussion of possible risks, including death, cardiac dysfunction, confusion, and memory impairment; 8) a statement that the consent also applies to any emergency treatment when the patient is unconscious; 9) a listing of patient requirements during the ECT course, such as taking nothing by mouth after midnight before treatment; 10) a statement that there has been an opportunity to ask questions and who to contact with further questions; and 11) a statement that consent is voluntary and can be withdrawn at any time (American Psychiatric Association 2001).

Informed consent involves more than just signing a consent form; it requires a consent discussion with the patient or surrogate (and, if possible, a significant other). The consent discussion should include any significant differences in likelihood of benefit or extent of risk from that depicted in the consent form, and mention of such discussion should be briefly documented in the patient's medical record.

Management of Medications

Medications that are needed to decrease medical risks should be continued. Other medications may be added to decrease risks based on the pre-ECT evaluation. Nonpsychotropic medications that are not protective should be withheld until after the treatment on ECT days or—if they interfere with or increase the risks of ECT—should be discontinued.

Regarding use of psychotropic medications during the ECT course, there are considerable differences of opinion and great variation in practice, although compelling evidence exists for the use of antipsychotic agents in schizophrenic individuals receiving ECT (American Psychiatric Association 2001). The literature regarding antidepressant medication as a means to augment the ECT response is unclear, although it does not appear that this combination is associated with significantly increased risk (Loo et al. 2010).

The following psychotropic medications should be avoided or maintained at the lowest possible levels: 1) lithium—it may increase the risks for delirium or prolonged seizures; 2) benzodiazepines—their anticonvulsant properties may decrease efficacy (but can be reversed with flumazenil at the time of ECT) (Krystal et al. 1998); 3) antiepileptic drugs—their anticonvulsant properties may decrease efficacy, but they may be needed in those with epilepsy or with very brittle bipolar disorder (in which case they should be withheld the night before and the morning of treatment if possible); and 4) bupropion and clozapine—they may increase the risk of prolonged seizures (the dosage should be kept at low to moderate levels).

Electroconvulsive Therapy Technique

Inpatient Versus Outpatient Administration

Although ECT traditionally has been an inpatient treatment modality, it also may be offered on an outpatient basis (American Psychiatric Association 2001). Even when inpatient treatments are initially required, consideration should be given to switching to an outpatient mode when it is clinically feasible.

Anesthetic Considerations

ECT is a procedure involving general anesthesia. Airway management, the administration of medications necessary for anesthesia, and the handling of medical emergencies are the responsibility of the anesthesia provider (American Psychiatric Association 2001). Appropriate medical backup should be present for high-risk cases.

The patient is ventilated by mask with 100% oxygen throughout the procedure. General anesthesia is usually provided by intravenous methohexital, typically 1 mg/kg (American Psychiatric Association 2001; Saito 2005). Because seizure threshold (the amount of electricity necessary to induce a seizure) appears to increase with age, difficulties in seizure induction can be experienced with older adults, particularly late in an index ECT course. In such situations, methohexital dosage can be slightly diminished by concurrent use of a short-acting sedative narcotic such as remifentanil, or the anesthetic itself can be switched to one with fewer anticonvulsant properties (e.g., etomidate or ketamine).

After loss of consciousness, the muscle relaxant succinylcholine is administered intravenously, at a typical dose of 1 mg/kg (American Psychiatric Association 2001). When the patient's muscles are relaxed (ascertainable by disappearance of relaxant-induced fasciculations and loss of deep tendon reflexes or twitch response to a peripheral nerve stimulator), the electrical stimulus can be delivered.

An anticholinergic medication, such as glycopyrrolate, may be administered before anesthesia to minimize the risk of stimulus-related asystole and postictal oral secretions. When seizure-related hypertension and tachycardia are severe or when prophylaxis is indicated on the basis of preexisting cardiovascular disease, β-blocking medications (e.g., labetalol) are often used. When necessary, postictal agitation or delirium can be managed with the use of intravenous mi-

dazolam (1 mg) or haloperidol (2–5 mg), as well as by providing reassurance and maintaining a quiet, low-light environment for the postictal recovery process.

With older adults, lower dosages of medications may be indicated because of altered metabolism or tolerance.

Physiological Monitoring

During ECT, vital signs and pulse oximetry are monitored throughout the procedure and until stabilization occurs. After spontaneous respiration resumes and vital signs and oxygen saturation are trending toward baseline, the patient is moved to a postanesthesia care unit or area, where monitoring of vital signs and oxygenation continues.

Both motor and electroencephalographic representations of seizure activity are monitored during ECT. To allow monitoring of the motor response, a blood pressure cuff is placed around the ankle and inflated to more than 200 mm Hg just before administration of the muscle relaxant, preventing ictal muscle activity distal to the cuff. Ictal electroencephalographic recordings are made after placing recording leads on the head. Such recording can be accomplished by placing one pair of recording electrodes over the left prefrontal and left mastoid areas and the other pair over the homologous areas on the right.

Stimulus Electrode Placement

The three major types of stimulus electrode placement are bitemporal, bifrontal, and unilateral nondominant (the right side for the great majority of individuals). Bitemporal ECT involves placement of both stimulus electrodes over the frontotemporal regions, with the center of the electrode approximately 1 inch above the midpoint of a line transecting the external canthus of the eye and the tragus of the ear. Bifrontal electrode placement involves locating the center of the stimulus electrodes approximately 5 cm superior to each external canthus. The preferred type of unilateral nondominant placement involves location of one electrode over the right frontotemporal area (as above) and the other over the right centroparietal area, just to the right of the vertex of the scalp, a point defined by the intersection of lines between the inion and the nasion and between the tragi of both ears.

Significant controversy exists over the choice of stimulus electrode placement (American Psychiatric Association 2001). Although unilateral ECT appears to be effective in many patients as long as stimulus intensity is sufficient (see the following subsection, "Stimulus Dosing"), some patients may preferentially respond to bitemporal ECT. However, ECT-associated amnesia is greater with bitemporal ECT. A reasonable trade-off is to use unilateral ECT initially, unless an urgent response is necessary or the patient has indicated a preference for or has shown a past preferential response to bitemporal ECT. With bifrontal electrode placement, the newest of the three techniques, data are mixed (Kellner et al. 2010).

The choice of stimulus electrode placement is particularly challenging in older individuals, for whom an urgent need for a rapid response is often present, yet in whom adverse cognitive effects are of concern. One recent study reported that high-dosage unilateral ECT was as effective in older individuals as bitemporal ECT (Stoppe et al. 2006), although the placement controversy remains unresolved.

Stimulus Dosing

All contemporary U.S. ECT devices use a bidirectional, constant-current, brief-pulse stimulus waveform. Recently, these devices also have incorporated the use of the ultra-brief-pulse stimulus, defined as a pulse duration of less than 0.5 ms, which is considered a more efficient way to induce seizures (Loo et al. 2007). The paradigm for the choice of stimulus dose intensity, however, appears to be as controversial as the choice of electrode placement. The disagreement centers on whether to dose with respect to an empirically determined seizure threshold estimate obtained at the first treatment (dose-titration technique) or to use a formula based on factors such as age, gender, and electrode placement to make this decision (formula-based technique) (American Psychiatric Association 2001).

We have found that the dose-titration technique is better in that it offers a more precise means to determine the patient's seizure threshold (which can vary manyfold) (Coffey et al. 1995).

Stimulus intensity for unilateral ECT should be between 2.5 and 8 times the seizure threshold (McCall et al. 2000). However, it is important to note that increasing stimulus intensity also increases the severity of ECT-associated amnesia, although to a lesser degree than with a switch to bilateral ECT. Stimulus intensity is less of an issue with bilateral ECT, in which a stimulus 1.5 times the seizure threshold appears to be sufficient. However, stimulus intensity is of most concern with ultrabrief-pulse ECT, regardless of electrode placement (Sackeim et al. 2008).

Determination of Seizure Adequacy

The ictal electroencephalogram manifests the typical electroencephalographic features of a grand mal seizure, with chaotic polyspike activity marking the tonic portion of the seizure and repetitive polyspike and slow-wave discharges during the clonic component. During the immediate postictal period, a relative suppression (i.e., flattening) of electroencephalographic activity typically can be seen (Weiner et al. 1991).

Compelling evidence indicates that not all seizures are equally potent from a therapeutic perspective. With unilateral ECT, barely suprathreshold seizures—despite having identical durations as seizures from more moderately suprathreshold stimuli—are only minimally therapeutic (Sackeim et al. 1993). On the basis of findings that seizures with higher stimulus intensity have attributes such as higher amplitude, greater regularity in shape, and greater postictal electroencephalographic suppression (Krystal et al. 1995) and that such features are associated with the therapeutic response to ECT, a growing interest has developed in the possibility that electroencephalographically based stimulus dosing may one day be feasible. ECT device manufacturers in the United States have incorporated "seizure quality" features into their devices, although their utility for routine clinical use remains to be established (see American Psychiatric Association 2001; Rasmussen et al. 2007).

Frequency and Number of Electroconvulsive Therapy Treatments

In the United States, ECT is typically administered three times a week, with an index course usually lasting between 6 and 12 treatments, although more or fewer treatments are sometimes necessary. The frequency of ECT may be reduced to twice a week or even once a week if amnesia or confusion becomes a major problem. In general, the treatments are stopped when a therapeutic plateau occurs— that is, when the patient has reached a maximum level of response. If no substantial im-

provement occurs by the sixth treatment, consideration should be given to making alterations in the ECT technique, such as switching stimulus electrode placement or increasing stimulus intensity. If no response occurs after 8–10 treatments, alternative treatment modalities should be considered. At present, these modalities generally would involve combination pharmacotherapy with multiple agents of different classes.

Maintenance Therapy

The conditions for which ECT is used are typically recurrent. The risk of relapse, particularly during the first 2–3 months, is extremely high, necessitating an aggressive program of maintenance treatment to minimize the likelihood of relapse. This maintenance treatment may be pharmacological or in the form of continued ECT (at a greatly lowered frequency).

Pharmacological Maintenance Therapy

With major depression, evidence suggests that a combination of antidepressant and mood stabilizer may be more effective in maintaining remission than an antidepressant drug alone (Sackeim et al. 2001). Maintenance pharmacotherapy following ECT treatment of mania or schizophrenia has not been well studied. In the absence of applicable data, an aggressive regimen of different drug classes should be considered.

Maintenance Electroconvulsive Therapy

The high relapse rate following ECT, even with pharmacological maintenance therapy, has created renewed interest in the practice of maintenance ECT. A random-ized trial of maintenance ECT versus phar-macotherapy in patients treated for major depression found that the efficacy of main-tenance ECT over a 6-month period was comparable to that obtained by combina-tion pharmacotherapy with both lithium and nortriptyline (Kellner et al. 2006).

Although no guidelines for a mainte-nance ECT regimen have been established, practitioners typically start with weekly treat-ments for 2–4 weeks, followed by another 1–2 months of biweekly treatments, followed by 3-week and then 4-week intervals; however, in practice, the frequency is often influenced by patient response (Lisanby et al. 2008).

In terms of cognitive effects, mainte-nance ECT is significantly better tolerated than index ECT treatments.

Future of Electroconvulsive Therapy

The use of ECT has persisted for 70 years, despite the development of many alternative treatment options. Future alternatives to ECT include not only new psychopharma-cological agents but also new electromag-netic therapies such as transcranial magnetic stimulation, vagal nerve stimulation, and deep brain stimulation (Wyche et al. 2007). Whether any of these new experimental techniques will partially or even fully re-place ECT remains to be established. In the meantime, a clear role remains for ECT in the treatment of a variety of disorders—most notably, major depression, for which older adults are at a particularly high risk.

Key Points

- Electroconvulsive therapy (ECT) is the most rapid and effective treatment for major depressive episodes in older adults.

- Major risks of ECT are largely a function of medical comorbidity.

- An index ECT treatment course can be ended once a therapeutic plateau has been reached.

- The risk for relapse after an acute course of ECT is high, and aggressive continuation treatment is needed.

References

American Psychiatric Association: The Practice of ECT: Recommendations for Treatment, Training, and Privileging. Washington, DC, American Psychiatric Press, 2001

Applegate RJ: Diagnosis and management of is-chemic heart disease in the patient sched-uled to undergo electroconvulsive therapy. Convuls Ther 13:128–144, 1997

Christopher EJ: Electroconvulsive therapy in the medically ill. Curr Psychiatry Rep 5:225–230, 2003

Coffey CE, Lucke J, Weiner RD, et al: Seizure threshold in electroconvulsive therapy, I: ini-tial seizure threshold. Biol Psychiatry 37:713–720, 1995

Endler NS: The origins of electroconvulsive therapy. Convuls Ther 4:5–23, 1988

Figiel GS, Coffey CE, Djang WT, et al: Brain magnetic resonance imaging findings in ECT-induced delirium. J Neuropsychiatry Clin Neurosci 2:53–58, 1990

Husain MM, Rush AJ, Fink M, et al: Speed of response and remission in major depressive disorder with acute electroconvulsive therapy (ECT): a Consortium for Research in ECT (CORE) report. J Clin Psychiatry 65:485–491, 2004

Huuhka M, Korpisammal L, Haataja R, et al: One-year outcome of elderly inpatients with major depressive disorder treated with ECT and antidepressants. J ECT 20:179–185, 2004

Ingram A, Saling MM, Schweitzer I: Cognitive side effects of brief pulse electroconvulsive therapy: a review. J ECT 24:3–9, 2008

Kellner CH, Knapp RG, Petrides G, et al: Continuation electroconvulsive therapy vs pharmacotherapy for relapse prevention in major depression: a multisite study from the Consortium for Research in Electroconvulsive Therapy (CORE). Arch Gen Psychiatry 63:1337–1344, 2006

Kellner CH, Tobias KG, Wiegand J: Electrode placement in electroconvulsive therapy (ECT): a review of the literature. J ECT 26:175–180, 2010

Krystal AD, Coffey CE: Neuropsychiatric considerations in the use of electroconvulsive therapy. J Neuropsychiatry Clin Neurosci 9:283–292, 1997

Krystal AD, Weiner RD, Coffey CE: The ictal EEG as a marker of adequate stimulus intensity with unilateral ECT. J Neuropsychiatry Clin Neurosci 7:295–303, 1995

Krystal AD, Watts BV, Weiner RD, et al: The use of flumazenil in the anxious and benzodiazepine-dependent ECT patient. J ECT 14:5–14, 1998

Lisanby SH, Sampson S, Husain MM, et al: Toward individualized post-electroconvulsive therapy care: piloting the Symptom-Titrated, Algorithm-Based Longitudinal ECT (STABLE) intervention. J ECT 241:79–82, 2008

Loo C, Sheehan P, Pigot M, et al: A report on mood and cognitive outcomes with right unilateral ultrabrief pulsewidth (0.3 ms) ECT and retrospective comparison with standard pulsewidth right unilateral ECT. J Affect Disord 103:277–281, 2007

Loo CK, Kaill A, Paton P, et al: The difficult-to-treat electroconvulsive therapy patient—strategies for augmenting outcomes. J Affect Disord 124:219–227, 2010

Manly DT, Oakley SP Jr, Bloch RM: Electroconvulsive therapy in old-old patients. Am J Geriatr Psychiatry 8:232–236, 2000

McCall WV, Reboussin DM, Weiner RD, et al: Titrated moderately suprathreshold vs fixed high-dose right unilateral electroconvulsive therapy: acute antidepressant and cognitive effects. Arch Gen Psychiatry 57:438–444, 2000

Mukherjee S, Sackeim HA, Schnur DB: Electroconvulsive therapy of acute mania episodes: a review of 50 years' experience. Am J Psychiatry 151:169–176, 1994

Navarro V, Gasto C, Torres X, et al: Continuation/maintenance treatment with nortriptyline versus combined nortriptyline and ECT in late-life psychotic depression: a two-year randomized study. Am J Geriatr Psychiatry 16:498–505, 2008

Petrides G, Fink M: Atrial fibrillation, anticoagulation, and ECT. Convuls Ther 12:91–98, 1996

Petrides G, Fink M, Husain MM, et al: ECT remission rates in psychotic versus nonpsychotic depressed patients: a report from CORE. J ECT 17:244–253, 2001

Philibert RA, Richards L, Lynch CF, et al: Effect of ECT on mortality and clinical outcome in geriatric unipolar depression. J Clin Psychiatry 56:390–394, 1995

Rasmussen KG, Varghese R, Stevens SR, et al: Electrode placement and ictal EEG indices in electroconvulsive therapy. J Neuropsychiatry Clin Neurosci 19:453–457, 2007

Rosenbach ML, Hermann RC, Dorwart RA: Use of electroconvulsive therapy in the Medicare population between 1987 and 1992. Psychiatr Serv 48:1537–1542, 1997

Sackeim HA, Prudic J, Devanand DP, et al: Effects of stimulus intensity and electrode placement on the efficacy and cognitive effects of electroconvulsive therapy. N Engl J Med 328:839–846, 1993

Sackeim HA, Haskett RF, Mulsant BH, et al: Continuation pharmacotherapy in the prevention of relapse following electroconvulsive therapy: a randomized controlled trial. JAMA 285:1299–1307, 2001

Sackeim HA, Prudic J, Fuller R, et al: The cognitive effects of electroconvulsive therapy in community settings. Neuropsychopharmacology 32:244–254, 2007

Sackeim HA, Prudic J, Nobler MS, et al: Effects of pulse width and electrode placement on the efficacy and cognitive effects of electroconvulsive therapy [published erratum appears in Brain Stimul 1:A2, 2008]. Brain Stimul 1:71–83, 2008

Saito S: Anesthesia management for electroconvulsive therapy: hemodynamic and respiratory management. J Anesth 19:142–149, 2005

Shorter E, Healy D: Shock Therapy: A History of Electroconvulsive Treatment in Mental Illness. New Brunswick, NJ, Rutgers University Press, 2007

Stek ML, Wurff van der FFB, Hoogendijk WJG, et al: Electroconvulsive therapy for the depressed elderly. Cochrane Database of Systematic Reviews 2003, Issue 2. Art. No.: CD003593. DOI: 10.1002/14651858. CD003593.

Stoppe A, Louza M, Rosa M, et al: Fixed high-dose electroconvulsive therapy in the elderly with depression: a double-blind, randomized comparison of efficacy and tolerability between unilateral and bilateral electrode placement. J ECT 22:92–99, 2006

Takada JY, Solimene MC, da Luz PL, et al: Assessment of the cardiovascular effects of electroconvulsive therapy in individuals older than 50 years. Braz J Med Biol Res 38:1349–1357, 2005

Tess AV, Smetana GW: Medical evaluation of patients undergoing electroconvulsive therapy. N Engl J Med 360:1437–1444, 2009

Tharyan P, Adams CE: Electroconvulsive therapy for schizophrenia. Cochrane Database of Systematic Reviews 2005, Issue 2. Art. No.: CD000076. DOI: 10.1002/14651858. CD000076.pub2.

UK ECT Review Group: Efficacy and safety of electroconvulsive therapy in depressive disorders: a systematic review and meta-analysis. Lancet 361:799–808, 2003

van der Wurff FB, Stek ML, Hoogendijk WJ, et al: The efficacy and safety of ECT in depressed older adults: a literature review. Int J Geriatr Psychiatry 18:894–904, 2003

Weiner RD, Krystal AD: Electroconvulsive therapy, in Treatments of Psychiatric Disorders, 3rd Edition. Edited by Gabbard GO, Rush AJ. Washington, DC, American Psychiatric Press, 2001, pp 1267–1293

Weiner RD, Coffey CE, Krystal AD: The monitoring and management of electrically induced seizures. Psychiatr Clin North Am 14:845–869, 1991

Weiner RD, Coffey CE, Krystal AD: Electroconvulsive therapy in the medical and neurologic patient, in Psychiatric Care of the Medical Patient, 2nd Edition. Edited by Stoudemire A, Fogel BS, Greenberg D. New York, Oxford University Press, 2000, pp 419–428

Wyche MC, O'Reardon J, Carpenter LL: Neurostimulation therapies for depression: acute and long-term outcomes. Depression: Mind and Body 3:106–114, 2007

Suggested Readings

Abrams R: Electroconvulsive Therapy, 4th Edition. New York, Oxford University Press, 2002

American Psychiatric Association: The Practice of ECT: Recommendations for Treatment, Training, and Privileging. Washington, DC, American Psychiatric Press, 2001

Dukakis K, Tye L: Shock: The Healing Power of Electroconvulsive Therapy. New York, Avery, 2006

Endler NS: Holiday of Darkness, Revised. Toronto, ON, Wall & Davis, 1990

Fink M: Electroshock: Restoring the Mind. New York, Oxford University Press, 1999

Mankad MV, Beyer JL, Weiner RD, Krystal AD: Clinical Manual of Electroconvulsive Therapy. Washington, DC, American Psychiatric Publishing, 2010

CHAPTER 18

INDIVIDUAL AND GROUP PSYCHOTHERAPY

THOMAS R. LYNCH, PH.D.
DAWN E. EPSTEIN, B.S.
MORIA J. SMOSKI, PH.D.

Psychotherapy has been shown to be an effective treatment for several mental disorders seen in older adults. As a treatment modality, it can be particularly useful for older adult psychiatric patients who cannot or will not tolerate medication or who are dealing with stressful conditions, interpersonal difficulties, limited levels of social support, or recurrent episodes of a disorder. However, it has been estimated that only 10% of older adults in need of psychiatric services actually receive professional care, and there has been minimal use of mental health services in this age group (Lebowitz et al. 1997; Weissman et al. 1981). African American older adults seek out professional mental health care about one-half as often as their white counterparts do, turning to informal support networks as a means of coping (Conner et al. 2010). Older adults report a longer delay in initiation of mental health treatment than do younger cohort groups (Wang et al. 2005).

Many practitioners assume that older individuals have negative attitudes toward psychotherapy, but research on attitudes toward treatment in elderly samples is not conclusive. Contrary to clinical lore, grow-

The author M.J.S. was supported by K23-MH087754.

ing descriptive research suggests that older individuals may prefer counseling over medication treatment (Connor et al. 2010; Gum et al. 2006). Older adults also have been shown to report a greater number of positive attitudes toward mental health professionals and to be less concerned than younger adults about stigma attached to seeking treatment for depression (Rokke and Scogin 1995). However, older adults prefer that mental health treatment be provided in a primary care context rather than through specialty clinics; favor therapists who understood their existential and spiritual concerns and values; and, as result of their unique sociohistorical context, often feel more comfortable receiving care from practitioners who are of the same race, ethnicity, and religion as themselves (Bartels et al. 2004; Chen et al. 2006; Gum et al. 2010; Hinrichsen 2006; Snodgrass 2009). Whenever possible, patient preferences or biases regarding treatment should be considered before referral for psychotherapy.

As discussed in more detail in the sections on specific disorders, older adults will respond to many of the therapeutic interventions used with younger populations. For example, highly effective treatments originally developed in younger adult populations, such as cognitive-behavioral therapy (CBT) for mood and anxiety disorders and dialectical behavior therapy (DBT) for personality disorders, have been successfully modified for older adult populations. Given the higher incidence of confounding factors in older adult populations (e.g., declines in sensory functions and speed of processing), age-specific adaptations of standard therapy procedures are advisable. For instance, the pace of therapy should be slower, and fonts for written material should be larger. Providing memory aids such as handouts and

session summaries also can be very helpful. Accounting for unique cohort-based differences (e.g., sociohistorical environment, norms and commonly held beliefs, role expectations, illness beliefs, and culture) and age-specific stressors (e.g., chronic illness and disability; loss of loved ones and, consequently, sources of support; and caregiving responsibilities) is also advisable. In-home mental health services may be a valuable option for those who lack reliable transportation and/or have a medical or physical disability. Alternatively, telephone and Internet-based interventions also may help older adults overcome common treatment barriers (Alexander et al. 2010). Thorough pretreatment assessment and modifications specific to the individual's strengths and deficits can help to circumvent age-related pitfalls in psychological treatment (Knight and Poon 2008; Snodgrass 2009; Yang et al. 2009).

In this chapter, we review the theoretical and empirical evidence for psychotherapy in older adults, giving consideration to both individual and group-based therapies. The material is organized by type of disorder and, for each disorder, by type of therapy. When possible, we evaluate the evidence with respect to quality of data, generalizability, and long-term effects of treatment.

Depression

Individual Cognitive-Behavioral Therapies

The "family" of cognitive-behavioral therapies is widely effective for major depressive disorder. Cognitive therapies focus on problematic thoughts that may perpetuate depression and aim to change and adapt cognitive patterns away from automatic negative thoughts. More purely behavioral interventions are derived from classic learning theory in which problematic behaviors are viewed as the result of specific antecedent stimuli and consequential events that reinforce, punish, or maintain behavioral responses (e.g., Dougher and Hackbert 1994). Recent component analysis research suggests that behavioral activation and automatic thought modification have equal effectiveness and that both components used together are no more effective in preventing relapse than when used alone (Dimidjian et al. 2006; Gortner et al. 1998; Jacobson et al. 1996). In addition, an increasing amount of data suggests that the salient mechanism of change in cognitive therapy is the development of metacognition (i.e., responding to negative thoughts as transitory events rather than as an inherent aspect of self or as necessarily true) rather than change in the dysfunctional attitude per se (Teasdale et al. 2002). However, CBT is more effective than a talk therapy control intervention in augmenting medication treatment in older adults, suggesting that warmth and attention, both defining features of the talking control intervention, are not sufficient mediators of change (Serfaty et al. 2009). Regardless of mechanistic explanations of change, cognitive-behavioral interventions have been the most frequently studied therapies and have repeatedly been found useful in treating depression in older adults (Koder et al. 1996; Scogin and McElreath 1994; Serfaty et al. 2009; Thompson and Gallagher 1984; Thompson et al. 1987).

Several variants of CBT are effective in reducing depressive symptoms in older adults. Exercise therapy, which uses many of the techniques of behavioral activation, appears to be more effective than psycho-education in reducing depressive symptoms (Singh et al. 2001) and may even be comparable to medication use (sertraline) in

older adults (Babyak et al. 2000; Blumenthal et al. 2007). Group-based exercise interventions also may help to increase older adults' level of social integration and, as a result, reduce depressogenic symptoms and increase psychological well-being (Fox et al. 2007; Salmon 2001). Another variant, problem-solving therapy (PST), is based on a model in which ineffective coping under stress is hypothesized to lead to a breakdown of problem-solving abilities and subsequent depression (Nezu 1987; Thompson and Gallagher 1984). Patients are taught a structured multistage format for solving problems in an attempt to increase coping and buffer factors that maintain and aggravate depression (Hegel et al. 2002). PST has been found to be effective in treating depression in populations with (Areán et al. 2010) or without (Areán et al. 1993) executive function deficits and can be successfully implemented in a primary care setting (Areán et al. 2010; Hegel et al. 2002; Mynors-Wallis 2001; Unützer et al. 2001; Williams et al. 2000).

Group-Based Cognitive-Behavioral Psychotherapies

Although originally designed to be implemented as an individual therapy, CBT has been successfully modified for a group format. Group-based CBT has been found to be more effective than a wait-list control condition and slightly more effective than a psychodynamic group therapy (Jarvik et al. 1982; Steuer 1984). It also can be used as an effective augmentation of pharmacotherapy in outpatient (Beutler et al. 1987; but see Wilkinson et al. 2009) and inpatient (Brand and Clingempeel 1992) settings. DBT, another treatment approach that combines cognitive and behavioral strategies, teaches specific skills to increase mindfulness, interpersonal effectiveness, emotion regulation, and distress tolerance. Originally designed to treat chronically suicidal younger adult women, DBT has been modified for use in several difficult-to-treat conditions, including chronic depression in older individuals (Lynch et al. 2003). In a recent study in older adults with comorbid depression and personality disorders, DBT plus medication showed a faster reduction in depressive symptoms when compared with medication alone (Lynch et al. 2007).

In summary, group-based cognitive-behavioral interventions appear promising for use with depressed older adults. Group therapy also may offer advantages for many elderly individuals; it is generally less expensive than individual treatment, and the social network provided by group therapy may provide significant therapeutic benefits to elders experiencing a loss of interpersonal relationships through the death of friends and spouses.

Interpersonal Psychotherapy

Interpersonal psychotherapy (IPT) is a problem-focused, manualized treatment that focuses on four components that are hypothesized to lead to or maintain depression: 1) grief (e.g., death of a spouse), 2) interpersonal disputes (e.g., conflict with adult children), 3) role transitions (e.g., retirement), and 4) interpersonal deficits (e.g., lack of assertiveness skills). Whatever its etiology, depression is seen to persist in a social context. Techniques used in treatment include role-playing, communication analysis, clarification of the patient's wants and needs, and links between affect and environmental events (Hinrichsen 1997, 2008). Separate treatment manuals for interpersonal therapy in late life and interpersonal

maintenance therapy for older individuals have been developed that include adaptations specific for use in elderly patients, such as flexibility in length of sessions, long-standing role disputes, and the need to help the patient with practical problems (Frank et al. 1993).

Controlled trials in populations of depressed adults have documented the efficacy of IPT for the treatment of acute depression (Bruce et al. 2004; Frank and Spanier 1995; Hinrichsen 1997), and IPT in the acute treatment of major depressive disorder was as effective as nortriptyline (Sloane et al. 1985). Of additional importance are findings that elderly patients receiving IPT were less likely to drop out of treatment than were those taking nortriptyline because of the medication's side effects, with combined IPT and medication management emerging as the most effective treatment strategy for maintaining treatment gains (Reynolds et al. 1999).

Other Psychotherapeutic Techniques

Various other psychotherapeutic techniques used for the treatment of late-life depression boast less empirical support but warrant mentioning: bibliotherapy, life review and reminiscence psychotherapy, and psychodynamic psychotherapy. Bibliotherapy, or book therapy, emphasizes a skills acquisition approach via selected readings from books and has been shown to be efficacious in the treatment of mild to moderate depression (Floyd et al. 2004; Jamison and Scogin 1995; Naylor et al. 2010; Scogin et al. 1989, 1990). Individuals with depression read books such as *Feeling Good* (Burns 1980) to enhance behavioral skills that combat depression or to modify dysfunctional thoughts. A study by Naylor and colleagues (2010) compared a physician-delivered behavioral prescription to read *Feeling Good* and a usual care control for depression in a primary care setting. Dysfunctional attitudes and depressive symptoms were similarly reduced in both treatment groups, and perceived life satisfaction and enjoyment increased. Bibliotherapy might be a viable alternative for those who cannot afford the cost of medication, are partial or nonresponders, are reluctant to engage in tertiary psychiatric or psychological care, or experience adverse side effects.

Life review and reminiscence psychotherapy are both based on the patient reexperiencing personal memories and significant life experiences. These interventions have been empirically supported as effective therapies in the treatment of late-life depression, with reminiscence therapy showing reductions in depressive symptoms comparable to those with CBT in a meta-analysis performed by Pinquart and colleagues (2007). Reminiscence therapy is often administered in a group setting with the goal of improving one's self-esteem and sense of social cohesiveness. For a comprehensive review of reminiscence therapy and mental health, see Westerhof et al. (2010).

Psychodynamic psychotherapy is based on psychoanalytic theory, which views current interpersonal and emotional experience as having been influenced by early childhood experience (Bibring 1952). Revised conceptualizations have emphasized how relationships are internalized and transformed into a sense of self (e.g., Kohut and Wolf 1978; Mahler 1952). During therapy, patients are encouraged to develop insight into past experiences and how these experiences influence their current relationships. Although short-term psychodynamic ther-

apy has been less studied for older adults than other treatments have (e.g., CBT, IPT), there have been several indications that short-term psychodynamic therapy, particularly as conducted by Gallagher-Thompson and Steffen (1994), Gallagher-Thompson et al. (1990), Thompson et al. (1987), and colleagues, is an effective means to treat depression in samples of older adults. These interesting results call for additional controlled trials comparing different treatment modalities, continued component analysis research, and continued research that examines which type of treatment works best with which type of patient.

Anxiety Disorders

Individual Cognitive-Behavioral Therapies

Anxiety disorders are among the most prominent mental disorders of late life, with generalized anxiety disorder (GAD) being the most commonly diagnosed anxiety disorder (Blazer et al. 1991). For a comprehensive review of anxiety disorders in older adults, see Wolitzky-Taylor et al. (2010). Anxiety disorders in late life have been associated with significant distress, increased morbidity and health-related activity limitations, memory deficits, and significant reductions in health-related quality of life. Although pharmacotherapy for late-life anxiety is quite effective, unwanted side effects can limit its utility (Stanley et al. 2009; Wetherall et al. 2011). Research on evidence-based treatments for late-life anxiety is still in its infancy; however, CBT appears to be the best-equipped form of psychotherapy to manage the diagnostic and treatment issues that exist in older populations with GAD (Ayers et al. 2007; Stanley and Novy 2000; Stanley et al. 1996,

2004; Wetherell et al. 2003). CBT has been found to be effective for a range of anxiety symptoms (Barrowclough et al. 2001), with effectiveness comparable to that of medication management (Gorenstein et al. 2005); an additional benefit is that CBT can be used to augment medications (Wetherall et al. 2011). Findings from a meta-analysis (Covin et al. 2008) support the conclusion that CBT for GAD is highly effective in reducing the cardinal symptom of GAD: pathological worry.

In one example of a randomized trial of GAD treatment, Stanley and colleagues (2003a) compared the efficacy of CBT with that of a minimal contact condition. The researchers' treatment protocol included education training, relaxation training, cognitive restructuring, and exposure to anxiety-provoking stimuli. CBT participants reported a significant within-group improvement in the severity of GAD symptoms postintervention and at a 12-month follow-up. These findings suggest that CBT not only may provide effective immediate therapy but also may promote long-term gains in the management of GAD. Several other randomized trials also have supported the use of CBT for the treatment of GAD (Mohlman et al. 2003; Stanley et al. 1996, 2003b; Wetherell et al. 2003), including in primary care settings (Stanley et al. 2009). Adapting CBT to use in primary care facilities will provide treatment where older adults are most likely to look for it and will facilitate collaboration between CBT therapists and prescription providers. This integration also may be a cost-effective treatment option, as has been the case in primary care psychotherapy for depression.

Although CBT has strong promise for treating GAD in older adults, further empirical research must be conducted to verify its efficacy in this population and to determine mediators and moderators of treatment response. For example, it appears that CBT is not effective in older adults who have consistently low executive function abilities but is effective in individuals whose executive functioning improves along with their psychological symptoms (Mohlman and Gorman 2004). In addition, and in contrast to younger adult populations, older individuals with more severe anxiety at baseline as well as psychiatric comorbidities showed the greatest benefit from treatment (Wetherell et al. 2005). A greater understanding of the mechanisms and predictors of treatment response will help further refine CBT as an effective treatment for late-life anxiety disorders.

Relaxation Training

The most frequently used and the most well-substantiated treatments for anxiety in older adults are based on behavioral therapies, including relaxation training. Work by DeBerry (1982a, 1982b; DeBerry et al. 1989) showed that progressive muscle relaxation and meditation relaxation techniques reduced anxiety symptoms more effectively than treatment control conditions in older adults. Scogin et al. (1992) assessed the use of progressive muscle relaxation and imaginal relaxation. General symptom improvements were maintained at a 1-month follow-up, and gains in treatment responders were maintained in a 1-year follow-up assessment (Rickard et al. 1984). Relaxation training has some advantages for treating mild anxiety in older adults. The strategies can be taught in brief individual or group sessions. Theoretically, the strategies can be delivered during a regular visit to a primary care physician. As with many behavioral strategies, relaxation training has the advantage of masquerading as skills training for patients who might avoid traditional psychotherapy. Also, patients with cognitive deficits, who may have difficulty with more cognitively based strategies, may benefit from purely behavioral strategies.

Substance Use Disorders

Cognitive-Behavioral Therapies

Limited research is available on the prevalence of substance use disorders in older people, and much less is available on their treatment. With the exception of alcohol use and prescription drug abuse, most substance use in late life is thought to represent an extension of substance use from earlier periods of life into late life (Oslin et al. 2000). Although medical comorbidity becomes an increasing factor in older adults, most substance use in late life is presumed to differ from younger populations' use, because of cohort differences more than developmental differences. Treatment research on substance use in the older population, specifically illicit drug use, is lagging but is greatly needed. The baby-boom cohort is approaching old age and is larger than previous cohorts. Moreover, rates of heavy alcohol use and illicit drug use are higher among this cohort than among earlier cohorts (Gfroerer et al. 2003; Lofwall et al. 2008; Wu and Blazer 2011). It has been projected that 5.7 million older adults will need treatment for a substance abuse problem in 2020—a substantial increase from approximately 2.8 million in 2002–2006 (Han et al. 2009; Wu and Blazer 2011).

Research on effective therapy for alcohol-related disorders in older adults is sparse. In the review literature, standard treatment for older adults is to mainstream them into therapeutic groups for adults of any age, such as Alcoholics Anonymous. This treatment choice has not been empirically validated for older adults, and in fact some researchers suggest that older adults will show better treatment gains in peer support groups and age-specific treatment protocols (Dupree et al. 1984; Schonfeld et al. 2000). Wu and Blazer (2011) recommend that substance abuse treatment protocols be age-specific, supportive and nonconfrontational, directive, and geared toward the development of interpersonal skills for increased social support.

Although some previous comprehensive cognitive-behavioral interventions have shown promise, they are also plagued with high dropout rates (Schonfeld et al. 2000). Schonfeld and colleagues (2010) assessed the effectiveness of the Florida Brief Intervention and Treatment for Elders (BRITE) project—a low-cost approach for older individuals at risk for illicit and nonillicit substance abuse and misuse. Prescription medication misuse and alcohol abuse were most prevalent in the sample. The treatment protocol consisted of a brief home-based intervention of one to five sessions that included motivational interviewing, education about relevant substances and consequences of substance use and misuse, reasons to quit drinking, and medication management. After graduation from the brief intervention, participants completed a 16-session cognitive-behavioral treatment. The BRITE approach resulted in a significant reduction in depression and suicide risk, as well as alcohol and prescription medication misuse (Schonfeld et al. 2010).

As in other Axis I disorders, such as depression and GAD, brief interventions in primary care have received increasing attention for the treatment of alcohol use in older adults. Because primary care physicians are most likely to identify overuse of alcohol in their patients, this is a natural area in which to develop treatment protocols. Brief counseling by the treating physician has been found to be significantly more effective in reducing alcohol misuse in older adults than has providing a general health booklet (Fleming et al. 1999).

The empirical studies described earlier provide the groundwork for further research in this area. Age-specific CBT techniques show promise for the treatment of alcohol abuse in older adults. One avenue of research might examine group interventions to take advantage of peer support, whereas a second avenue of research might investigate primary care interventions to take advantage of older adults' relationships with their physicians. However, despite a growing awareness that addictive disorders are common among older populations, it remains unclear whether treatments that have shown success in younger age groups (with the exception of brief alcohol interventions) can be applied with equal success among older adults (Oslin 2005). It is clear that more research is needed in this area.

Personality Disorders

Cognitive-Behavioral Therapies

Personality disorders are enduring patterns of inner experience (e.g., cognition, affect, impulse control) and behavior (e.g., interpersonal difficulties) that have an onset in adolescence or early adulthood, are stable over time, deviate considerably from normal cultural expectations, and cause distress

or impairment in functioning. Meta-analyses have concluded that the prevalence rate of personality disorder is between 10% and 20% in the older adult community (Abrams 1996; Abrams and Horowitz 1999), which is essentially analogous to the 13% prevalence rate among younger age groups (Torgersen et al. 2001). Overall, the emotionally constricted/risk-averse disorders in Clusters A (paranoid and schizoid personality disorders) and C (obsessive-compulsive, avoidant, and dependent personality disorders) are the most commonly diagnosed in late life (Abrams 1996; Abrams and Horowitz 1999; Kenan et al. 2000; Morse and Lynch 2004), and there are also high rates of the not otherwise specified category compared with other individual personality disorder diagnoses (Abrams 1996; Abrams and Horowitz 1999; Kenan et al. 2000). In addition, personality disorder rates are even higher (approximately 30%) among depressed older adult samples (Abrams 1996; Thompson et al. 1988).

Personality psychopathology generally has been associated with poorer response to treatment—with either antidepressants or psychotherapy—among older adults (Abrams et al. 1994; Lynch et al. 2007; Thompson et al. 1988; Zweig 2008; but see Gum et al. 2007; for a review, also see Gradman et al. 1999). Depressed older adult patients with comorbid personality disorder are four times more likely to experience maintenance or reemergence of depressive symptoms compared with those without personality disorder diagnoses (Morse and Lynch 2004). Despite this, minimal controlled studies of the treatment of personality disorders in late life have been done.

The only published randomized clinical trial specifically targeting personality disorders in older adults was conducted by Lynch et al. (2007). The study focused on providing standard DBT in both group and individual sessions following Linehan's (1993) manual, with depressed older adults who had at least one comorbid personality disorder and who failed an 8-week selective serotonin reuptake inhibitor trial. Compared with a medication-only condition, participants who received DBT plus medication management reached the level of remission more quickly than did the medication management alone plus clinical management group and showed improvements in interpersonal sensitivity and aggression (Lynch et al. 2007). Adaptations of standard DBT focusing on the most common personality disorders in older adults (e.g., paranoid personality disorder, obsessive-compulsive personality disorder) are in development, with treatment targets that include reducing rigidity, cognitive inflexibility, emotional constriction, and risk aversion (Lynch and Cheavens 2008).

Despite the promising nature of these findings, most of the empirical evidence suggests that the presence of a personality disorder in an older adult seriously compromises treatment. In addition, rates of personality disorders among older adults may be only slightly lower than in younger age groups, and subsyndromal personality disorders may be more prevalent in older populations relative to younger ones (Abrams and Bromberg 2006). It appears that psychotherapy interventions likely will be enhanced when they target the unique behavioral, cognitive, and interpersonal dynamics associated with personality disorders in older adults.

Dementia

The development of psychosocial interventions for dementia is a complicated area of research. Unlike some of the other disorders discussed in this chapter, dementia is unlikely to remit as a result of psychotherapy. Researchers in this area have struggled to find distinct goals and outcomes on which to focus. Because the dementia as a whole is not expected to abate, researchers have chosen specific variables to focus on in older adults with dementia, such as global quality of life, affective states, disruptive behavioral symptoms, functional impairment, and prevention of self-harm.

Because of the cognitive deterioration experienced by dementia patients, most empirical research on interventions for dementia is based on behavioral strategies and may target caregivers as well as, or in lieu of, the patients themselves. Studies of psychosocial interventions can be categorized by the treatment outcome goals and by the intervention targets. Typical targets include cognitive functioning, affect, and problematic behaviors, with interventions often attempting to address multiple targets. Reviews of empirically supported interventions by Teri et al. (2005b) and Livingston et al. (2005) provide overviews of current treatment approaches. Treatments that specifically target the physical or sensory environment (such as managing ambient lighting levels or obscuring windows and doors to reduce cues for wandering) also may be effective in managing problem behaviors but are beyond the scope of this chapter.

Cognitive Stimulation Therapy

Cognitive symptoms such as disorientation and confusion can cause distress and injury in patients and increased stress in caregivers. One proposed psychotherapeutic technique to cope with the cognitive symptoms of dementia is cognitive stimulation therapy. Derived from reality-orientation therapy, which aims to continuously reorient patients' attention to the current situation and surroundings by repeating who they are and where they are, cognitive stimulation therapy focuses on improving information-processing abilities. Treatment can take place in formal groups or through training of professional or lay caregivers to administer intervention activities during the course of day-to-day activities. Several randomized controlled studies have found improved performance in patients receiving cognitive stimulation therapy, whether as a stand-alone intervention (Hayslip et al. 2009; Quayhagen et al. 1995; Spector et al. 2001, 2003) or as an augmentation of cholinesterase inhibitor medication (Onder et al. 2005). Cognitive abilities were generally preserved and/or improved in the treatment groups relative to the control subjects (Onder et al. 2005; Spector et al. 2003). Relative improvements in mood (Spector et al. 2001) and behavior (Quayhagen et al. 1995) were observed, but not all studies showed improvements in these areas (e.g., Onder et al. 2005; Quayhagen et al. 2000; Spector et al. 2003). Overall, cognitive stimulation therapy appears to be a promising approach to preserving cognitive function in older adults with dementia, but further study is necessary to determine its influence on mood and/or problem behaviors.

Behavioral Therapies

Individuals with dementia are often at risk for anxiety, depression, or other negative affective states. Several behavioral therapies involving a combination of caregiver training in problem solving and communication and structured behavioral activation for patients have been found to be effective in reducing depressive symptoms (Beck et al. 2004; McCallion et al. 1999; Proctor et al. 1999; Teri et al. 1997, 2003). Behavioral therapy also has a strong history of controlling patients' problem behaviors, such as aggression, withdrawal, or resistance. These therapies generally train those who care for individuals with dementia—whether in the community or in inpatient facilities—to manage patient behavior via principles of operant conditioning. The behavioral interventions found to be effective in reducing depressive symptoms also have been found to be helpful in reducing problem behaviors (Bourgeois et al. 2002; Proctor et al. 1999; Teri et al. 1997, 2003, 2005a). For example, stimulus preference assessment can be used to identify effective reinforcers for use in individualized behavioral management protocols, which have been found to reduce agitation in residents of long-term care facilities (Feliciano et al. 2009).

Progressively Lowered Stress Threshold–Based Caregiver Training

Another set of treatments with growing empirical support is based on the progressively lowered stress threshold (PLST) theory (Hall and Buckwalter 1987). From this perspective, the disease processes underlying dementia progressively lower the patient's ability to cope with stressors such as fatigue, change in routine, or physical illness. Treatment consists of educating and training caregivers in managing the patient's environment to minimize such stressors. PLST-based training is effective in reducing patient problem behaviors (Gerdner et al. 2002; Huang et al. 2003) and caregiver distress over patient behavior problems (Gerdner et al. 2002). Although further research is necessary to match the empirical validation of behavioral therapies for problem behaviors in dementia, the PLST approach shows great promise.

Several well-supported, broad-based psychosocial interventions are available to manage cognitive, affective, and behavioral challenges in elders with dementia. Although none of these interventions offers a cure, they are important tools for symptom management that have the potential to benefit both patients and their caregivers.

Conclusion

It is evident that psychotherapy offers significant promise for the treatment of psychopathology in elderly persons and at times may be the treatment of choice in terms of both efficacy and patient prefer-
ence. We encourage practitioners to select treatments that have been tested with randomized clinical trials rather than basing their choices on theoretical preference or ease of application. The use of treatments without this type of empirical support can slow or reduce recovery.

Future research should continue to examine the beneficial effects of strategies combining medication and psychotherapy. In addition, research examining the mechanisms of change and issues associated with treatment response by disorder and type of therapy remains to be more fully developed. Finally, continued research is needed to focus on populations with treatment-resistant illnesses such as personality disorders, substance dependence, and comorbid disorders.

Key Points

- Psychotherapy is a good option for treating mental disorders in older adults who have trouble tolerating medications, who prefer psychotherapy over medication treatment, or who have conditions for which psychotherapy is the most effective treatment.

- Modifications of traditional therapies may be necessary to compensate for age-related problems with vision, hearing, mobility, and cognition.

- Effective treatments for depression include several different individual and group cognitive-behavioral therapies, interpersonal psychotherapy, and short-term psychodynamic therapy.

- The most common anxiety disorders among older adults are generalized anxiety disorder and anxiety disorder not otherwise specified. Behavioral treatments such as relaxation training and cognitive-behavioral therapy are the most effective treatments for these disorders.

- Personality pathology is associated with poorer treatment response than other comorbid conditions such as depression and anxiety. Few treatments targeting personality disorder in older adults have been tested. One promising and empirically validated treatment is a modification of dialectical behavior therapy for older adults.

- Dementia is unlikely to abate as a result of psychotherapy, but treatments targeting patients and their caregivers are effective in improving global quality of life, affective states, disruptive behavioral symptoms, and functional impairment.

References

Abrams RC: Personality disorders in the elderly. Int J Geriatr Psychiatry 11:759–763, 1996

Abrams RC, Bromberg CE: Personality disorders in the elderly: a flagging field of inquiry. Int J Geriatr Psychiatry 21:1013–1017, 2006

Abrams RC, Horowitz SV: Personality disorders after age 50: a meta-analytic review of the literature, in Personality Disorders in Older Adults: Emerging Issues in Diagnosis and Treatment. Edited by Rosowsky E, Abrams RC. Mahwah, NJ, Erlbaum, 1999, pp 55–68

Abrams RC, Rosendahl E, Card C, et al: Personality disorder correlates of late and early onset depression. J Am Geriatr Soc 42:727–731, 1994

Alexander CL, Arnkoff DB, Glass CR: Bringing psychotherapy to primary care: innovations and challenges. Clinical Psychology: Science and Practice 17:191–214, 2010

Areán PA, Perri MG, Nezu AM, et al: Comparative effectiveness of social problem-solving therapy and reminiscence therapy as treatments for depression in older adults. J Consult Clin Psychol 61:1003–1010, 1993

Areán PA, Raue P, Mackin RS, et al: Problem solving therapy and supportive therapy in older adults with major depression and executive dysfunction. Am J Psychiatry 167:1391–1398, 2010

Ayers CR, Sorrell JT, Thorp SR, et al: Evidence-based psychological treatments for late-life anxiety. Psychol Aging 22:8–17, 2007

Babyak M, Blumenthal JA, Herman S, et al: Exercise treatment for major depression: maintenance of therapeutic benefit at 10 months. Psychosom Med 62:633–638, 2000

Barrowclough C, King P, Colville J, et al: A randomized trial of the effectiveness of cognitive-behavioral therapy and supportive counseling for anxiety symptoms in older adults. J Consult Clin Psychol 69:756–762, 2001

Bartels SJ, Coakley EH, Zubritsky C, et al: Improving access to geriatric mental health services: a randomized trial comparing treatment engagement with integrated versus enhanced referral care for depression, anxiety, and at-risk alcohol use. Am J Psychiatry 161:1455–1462, 2004

Beck AT, Freeman A, Davis DD: Cognitive Therapy of Personality Disorders, 2nd Edition. New York, Guilford, 2004

Beutler LE, Scogin F, Kirkish P, et al: Group cognitive therapy and alprazolam in the treatment of depression in older adults. J Consult Clin Psychol 55:550–556, 1987

Bibring E: [The problem of depression.] Psyche 6:81–101, 1952

Blazer D, George LK, Hughes D: The epidemiology of anxiety disorders: an age comparison, in Anxiety in the Elderly: Treatment and Research. Edited by Salzman C, Lebowitz BD. New York, Springer, 1991, pp 17–30

Blumenthal JA, Babyak MA, Doraiswamy PM, et al: Exercise and pharmacotherapy in the treatment of major depressive disorder. Psychosom Med 69:587–596, 2007

Bourgeois MS, Schulz R, Burgio LD, et al: Skills training for spouses of patients with Alzheimer's disease: outcomes of an intervention study. Journal of Clinical Geropsychology 8:53–73, 2002

Brand E, Clingempeel WG: Group behavioral therapy with depressed geriatric inpatients: an assessment of incremental efficacy. Behav Ther 23:475–482, 1992

Bruce ML, Ten Have TR, Reynolds CF, et al: Reducing suicidal ideation and depressive symptoms in depressed older primary care patients. JAMA 291:1081–1091, 2004

Burns D: Feeling Good. New York, New American Library, 1980

Chen H, Coakley EH, Cheal K, et al: Satisfaction with mental health services in older primary care patients. Am J Geriatr Psychiatry 14:371–379, 2006

Conner KO, Lee B, Mayers V, et al: Attitudes and beliefs about mental health among African American older adults suffering from depression. J Aging Stud 24:266–277, 2010

Covin R, Ouimet AJ, Seeds PM, et al: A meta-analysis of CBT for pathological worry among clients with GAD. J Anxiety Disord 22:108–116, 2008

DeBerry S: The effects of meditation-relaxation on anxiety and depression in a geriatric population. Psychotherapy: Theory, Research and Practice 19:512–521, 1982a

DeBerry S: An evaluation of progressive muscle relaxation on stress related symptoms in a geriatric population. Int J Aging Hum Dev 14:255–269, 1982b

DeBerry S, Davis S, Reinhard KE: A comparison of meditation-relaxation and cognitive/behavioral techniques for reducing anxiety and depression in a geriatric population. J Geriatr Psychiatry 22:231–247, 1989

Dimidjian S, Hollon SD, Dobson KS, et al: Randomized trial of behavioral activation, cognitive therapy, and antidepressant medication in the acute treatment of adults with major depression. J Consult Clin Psychol 74:658–670, 2006

Dougher MJ, Hackbert L: A behavior-analytic account of depression and a case report using acceptance-based procedures. Behav Anal 17:321–334, 1994

Dupree LW, Broskowski H, Schonfeld LI: The Gerontology Alcohol Project: a behavioral treatment program for elderly alcohol abusers. Gerontologist 24:510–516, 1984

Feliciano L, Steers ME, Elite-Marcandonatou A, et al: Applications of preference assessment procedures in depression and agitation management in elders with dementia. Clin Gerontol 32:239–259, 2009

Fleming MFM, Manwell LB, Barry KLP, et al: Brief physician advice for alcohol problems in older adults: a randomized community-based trial. J Fam Pract 48:378–384, 1999

Floyd M, Scogin F, McKendree-Smith NL, et al: Cognitive therapy for depression: a comparison of individual psychotherapy and bibliotherapy for depressed older adults. Behav Modif 28:297–318, 2004

Fox KR, Stathi A, McKenna J, et al: Physical activity and mental well-being in older people participating in the Better Ageing Project. Eur J Appl Physiol 100:591–602, 2007

Frank E, Spanier C: Interpersonal psychotherapy for depression: overview, clinical efficacy, and future directions. Clinical Psychology Science and Practice 2:349–369, 1995

Frank E, Frank N, Cornes C, et al: Interpersonal psychotherapy in the treatment of late-life depression, in New Applications of Interpersonal Psychotherapy. Edited by Klerman GL, Weissman MM. Washington, DC, American Psychiatric Press, 1993, pp 167–198

Gallagher-Thompson D, Steffen AM: Comparative effects of cognitive-behavioral and brief psychodynamic psychotherapies for depressed family caregivers. J Consult Clin Psychol 62:543–549, 1994

Gallagher-Thompson D, Hanley-Peterson P, Thompson LW: Maintenance of gains versus relapse following brief psychotherapy for depression. J Consult Clin Psychol 58:371–374, 1990

Gerdner LA, Buckwalter KC, Reed D: Impact of a psychoeducational intervention on caregiver response to behavioral problems. Nurs Res 51:363–374, 2002

Gfroerer J, Penne M, Pemberton M, et al: Substance abuse treatment need among older adults in 2020: the impact of the aging baby-boom cohort. Drug Alcohol Depend 69:127–135, 2003

Gorenstein EE, Kleber MS, Mohlman J, et al: Cognitive-behavioral therapy for management of anxiety and medication taper in older adults. Am J Geriatr Psychiatry 13:901–909, 2005

Gortner ET, Gollan JK, Dobson KS, et al: Cognitive-behavioral treatment for depression: relapse prevention. J Consult Clin Psychol 66:377–384, 1998

Gradman TJ, Thompson LW, Gallagher-Thompson D: Personality disorders and treatment outcome, in Personality Disorders in Older Adults: Emerging Issues in Diagnosis and Treatment. Edited by Rosowsky E, Abrams RC. Mahwah, NJ, Erlbaum, 1999, pp 69–94

Gum AM, Areán PA, Hunkeler E, et al: Depression treatment preferences in older primary care patients. Gerontologist 46:14–22, 2006

Gum AM, Arean PA, Bostrom A: Low-income depressed older adults with psychiatric co-morbidity: secondary analyses of response to psychotherapy and case management. Int J Geriatr Psychiatry 22:124–130, 2007

Gum AM, Ayalon L, Greenberg JM, et al: Preferences for professional assistance for distress in a diverse sample of older adults. Clin Gerontol 33:136–151, 2010

Hall GR, Buckwalter KC: Progressively lowered stress threshold: a conceptual model for care of adults with Alzheimer's disease. Arch Psychiatr Nurs 1:399–406, 1987

Han B, Gfroerer JC, Colliver JD, et al: Substance use disorder among older adults in the United States in 2020. Addiction 104:88–96, 2009

Hayslip B, Paggi K, Poole M, et al: The impact of mental aerobics training on memory impaired older adults. Clin Gerontol 32:389–394, 2009

Hegel MTP, Barrett JE, Cornell JE, et al: Predictors of response to problem solving treatment of depression in primary care. Behav Ther 33:511–527, 2002

Hinrichsen GA: Interpersonal psychotherapy for depressed older adults. J Geriatr Psychiatry 30:239–257, 1997

Hinrichsen GA: Why multicultural issues matter for practitioners working with older adults. Professional Psychology: Research and Practice 37:29–35, 2006

Hinrichsen GA: Interpersonal psychotherapy as a treatment for depression in late life. Professional Psychology: Research and Practice 39:306–312, 2008

Huang HL, Shyu YIL, Chen MC, et al: A pilot study on a home-based caregiver training program for improving caregiver self-efficacy and decreasing the behavioral problems of elders with dementia in Taiwan. Int J Geriatr Psychiatry 18:337–345, 2003

Jacobson NS, Dobson KS, Truax PA, et al: A component analysis of cognitive-behavioral treatment for depression. J Consult Clin Psychol 64:295–304, 1996

Jamison C, Scogin F: The outcome of cognitive bibliotherapy with depressed adults. J Consult Clin Psychol 63:644–650, 1995

Jarvik LF, Mintz J, Steuer JL, et al: Treating geriatric depression: a 26-week interim analysis. J Am Geriatr Soc 30:713–717, 1982

Kenan MM, Kendjelic EM, Molinari VA, et al: Age-related differences in the frequency of personality disorders among inpatient veterans. Int J Geriatr Psychiatry 15:831–837, 2000

Knight BG, Poon CYM: Contextual adult life span theory for adapting psychotherapy with older adults. Journal of Rational-Emotive and Cognitive-Behaviour Therapy 26:232–249, 2008

Koder DA, Brodaty H, Anstey KJ: Cognitive therapy for depression in the elderly. Int J Geriatr Psychiatry 11:97–107, 1996

Kohut H, Wolf ES: The disorders of the self and their treatment: an outline. Int J Psychoanal 59:413–425, 1978

Lebowitz BD, Pearson JL, Schneider LS, et al: Diagnosis and treatment of depression in late life: consensus statement update. JAMA 278:1186–1190, 1997

Linehan MM: Cognitive-Behavioral Treatment of Borderline Personality Disorder. New York, Guilford, 1993

Livingston G, Johnston K, Katona C, et al: Systematic review of psychological approaches to the management of neuropsychiatric symptoms of dementia. Am J Psychiatry 162:1996–2021, 2005

Lofwall MR, Schuster A, Strain EC: Changing profile of abused substances by older persons entering treatment. J Nerv Ment Dis 196:898–905, 2008

Lynch TR, Cheavens JS: Dialectical behavior therapy for co-morbid personality disorders. J Clin Psychol 64:154–167, 2008

Lynch TR, Morse JQ, Mendelson T, et al: Dialectical behavior therapy for depressed older adults: a randomized pilot study. Am J Geriatr Psychiatry 11:33–45, 2003

Lynch TR, Cheavens JS, Cukrowicz KC, et al: Treatment of older adults with co-morbid personality disorder and depression: a dialectical behavior therapy approach. Int J Geriatr Psychiatry 22:131–143, 2007

Mahler MS: On child psychosis and schizophrenia: autistic and symbiotic infantile psychoses. Psychoanal Study Child 7:286–305, 1952

McCallion P, Toseland RW, Freeman K: An evaluation of a family visit education program. J Am Geriatr Soc 47:203–214, 1999

Mohlman J, Gorman JM: The role of executive functioning in CBT: a pilot study with anxious older adults. Behav Res Ther 43:447–465, 2004

Mohlman J, Gorenstein EE, Kleber M, et al: Standard and enhanced cognitive-behavior therapy for late-life generalized anxiety disorder: two pilot investigations. Am J Geriatr Psychiatry 11:24–32, 2003

Morse JQ, Lynch TR: A preliminary investigation of self-reported personality disorders in late life: prevalence, predictors of depressive severity, and clinical correlates. Aging Ment Health 8:307–315, 2004

Mynors-Wallis LM: Pharmacotherapy is more effective than psychotherapy for elderly people with minor depression or dysthymia. Evidence-Based Healthcare 5:61, 2001

Naylor EV, Antonuccio DO, Litt M, et al: Bibliotherapy as a treatment for depression in primary care. J Clin Psychol Med Settings 17:258–271, 2010

Nezu AM: A problem-solving formulation of depression: a literature review and proposal of a pluralistic model. Clin Psychol Rev 7:121–144, 1987

Onder G, Zanetti O, Giocobini E, et al: Reality orientation therapy combined with cholinesterase inhibitors in Alzheimer's disease: randomised controlled trial. Br J Psychiatry 187:450–455, 2005

Oslin DW: Evidence-based treatment of geriatric substance abuse. Psychiatr Clin North Am 28:897–911, 2005

Oslin DW, Katz IR, Edell WS, et al: Effects of alcohol consumption on the treatment of depression among elderly patients. Am J Geriatr Psychiatry 8:215–220, 2000

Pinquart M, Duberstein PR, Lyness JM: Effects of psychotherapy and other behavioral interventions on clinically depressed older adults: a meta-analysis. Aging Ment Health 11:645–657, 2007

Proctor R, Burns A, Powell HS, et al: Behavioural management in nursing and residential homes: a randomised controlled trial. Lancet 354:26–29, 1999

Quayhagen MP, Quayhagen M, Corbeil RR, et al: A dyadic remediation program for care recipients with dementia. Nurs Res 44:153–159, 1995

Quayhagen MP, Quayhagen M, Corbeil RR, et al: Coping with dementia: evaluation of four nonpharmacologic interventions. Int Psychogeriatr 12:249–265, 2000

Reynolds CF 3rd, Frank E, Perel JM, et al: Nortriptyline and interpersonal psychotherapy as maintenance therapies for recurrent major depression: a randomized controlled trial in patients older than 59 years. JAMA 281:39–45, 1999

Rickard HC, Scogin F, Keith S: A one-year follow-up of relaxation training for elders with subjective anxiety. Gerontologist 34:121–122, 1984

Rokke PD, Scogin F: Depression treatment preferences in younger and older adults. Journal of Clinical Geropsychology 1:243–257, 1995

Salmon P: Effects of physical exercise on anxiety, depression, and sensitivity to stress: a unifying theory. Clin Psychol Rev 21:33–61, 2001

Schonfeld L, Dupree LW, Dickson-Fuhrmann E, et al: Cognitive-behavioral treatment of older veterans with substance abuse problems. J Geriatr Psychiatry Neurol 13:124–129, 2000

Schonfeld L, King-Kallimanis BL, Duchene DM, et al: Screening and brief intervention for substance misuse among older adults: The Florida BRITE Project. Am J Public Health 100:108–114, 2010

Scogin F, McElreath L: Efficacy of psychosocial treatments for geriatric depression: a quantitative review. J Consult Clin Psychol 62:69–73, 1994

Scogin F, Jamison C, Gochneaur K: Comparative efficacy of cognitive and behavioral bibliotherapy for mildly and moderately depressed older adults. J Consult Clin Psychol 57:403–407, 1989

Scogin F, Jamison C, Davis N: Two-year follow-up of bibliotherapy for depression in older adults. J Consult Clin Psychol 58:665–667, 1990

Scogin F, Rickard HC, Keith S, et al: Progressive and imaginal relaxation training for elderly persons with subjective anxiety. Psychol Aging 7:419–424, 1992

Serfaty MA, Hayworth D, Blanchard M, et al: Clinical effectiveness of individual cognitive behavioral therapy for depressed older people in primary care: a randomized controlled trial. Arch Gen Psychiatry 66:1332–1340, 2009

Singh NA, Clements KM, Fiatarone Singh MA: The efficacy of exercise as a long-term antidepressant in elderly subjects: a randomized, controlled trial. J Gerontol A Biol Sci Med Sci 56:M497–M504, 2001

Sloane RB, Staples FR, Schneider LSM: Interpersonal therapy versus nortriptyline for depression in the elderly: case reports and discussion, in Clinical and Pharmacological Studies of Psychiatric Disorders. Edited by Burrows G, Norman TR, Dennerstein L. London, John Libbey, 1985, pp 344–346

Snodgrass J: Toward holistic care: integrating spirituality and cognitive behavioral therapy for older adults. Journal of Religion, Spirituality and Aging 21:219–236, 2009

Spector A, Orrell M, Davies S, et al: Can reality orientation be rehabilitated? Development and piloting of an evidence-based programme of cognition-based therapies for people with dementia. Neuropsychol Rehabil 11:377–379, 2001

Spector A, Thorgrimsen L, Woods B, et al: Efficacy of an evidence-based cognitive stimulation therapy programme for people with dementia: randomised controlled trial. Br J Psychiatry 183:248–254, 2003

Stanley MA, Novy DM: Cognitive-behavior therapy for generalized anxiety in late life: an evaluative overview. J Anxiety Disord 14:191–207, 2000

Stanley MA, Beck JG, Glassco JD: Treatment of generalized anxiety in older adults: a preliminary comparison of cognitive-behavioral and supportive approaches. Behav Ther 27:565–581, 1996

Stanley MA, Beck JG, Novy DM, et al: Cognitive behavioral treatment of late-life generalized anxiety disorder. J Consult Clin Psychol 71:309–319, 2003a

Stanley MA, Hopko DR, Diefenbach GJ, et al: Cognitive-behavioral therapy for older adults with late-life anxiety disorder in primary care: preliminary findings. Am J Geriatr Psychiatry 11:92–96, 2003b

Stanley MA, Diefenbach GJ, Hopko DR: Cognitive behavioral treatment for older adults with generalized anxiety disorder: a therapist manual for primary care settings. Behav Modif 28:73–117, 2004

Stanley MA, Wilson NL, Novy DM, et al: Cognitive behavior therapy for generalized anxiety disorder among older adults in primary care: a randomized clinical trial. JAMA 301:1480–1487, 2009

Steuer JL: Cognitive-behavioral and psychodynamic group psychotherapy in treatment of geriatric depression. J Consult Clin Psychol 52:180–189, 1984

Teasdale JD, Moore RG, Hayhurst H, et al: Metacognitive awareness and prevention of relapse in depression: empirical evidence. J Consult Clin Psychol 70:275–287, 2002

Teri L, Logsdon RG, Uomoto J, et al: Behavioral treatment of depression in dementia patients: a controlled clinical trial. J Gerontol B Psychol Sci Soc Sci 52:P159–P166, 1997

Teri L, Gibbons LE, McCurry SM, et al: Exercise plus behavioral management in patients with Alzheimer disease: a randomized controlled trial. JAMA 290:2015–2022, 2003

Teri L, McCurry SM, Logsdon RG, et al: Training community consultants to help family members improve dementia care: a randomized controlled trial. Gerontologist 45:802–811, 2005a

Teri L, McKenzie G, LaFazia D: Psychosocial treatment of depression in older adults with dementia. Clinical Psychology: Science and Practice 12:303–316, 2005b

Thompson LW, Gallagher D: Efficacy of psychotherapy in the treatment of late-life depression. Advances in Behaviour Research and Therapy 6:127–139, 1984

Thompson LW, Gallagher D, Breckenridge JS: Comparative effectiveness of psychotherapies for depressed elders. J Consult Clin Psychol 55:385–390, 1987

Thompson LW, Gallagher D, Czirr R: Personality disorder and outcome in the treatment of late-life depression. J Geriatr Psychiatry 21:133–146, 1988

Torgersen S, Kringlen E, Cramer V: The prevalence of personality disorders in a community sample. Arch Gen Psychiatry 58:590–596, 2001

Unützer JM, Katon WM, Williams JWJ, et al: Improving primary care for depression in late life: the design of a multicenter randomized trial. Med Care 39:785–799, 2001

Wang PS, Berglund P, Olfson M, et al: Failure and delay in initial treatment contact after first onset of mental disorders in the national comorbidity survey replication. Arch Gen Psychiatry 62:629–640, 2005

Weissman MM, Myers JK, Thompson WD: Depression and its treatment in a U.S. urban community—1975–1976. Arch Gen Psychiatry 38:417–421, 1981

Westerhof GJ, Bohlmeijer E, Webster JD: Reminiscence and mental health: a review of recent progress in theory, research and interventions. Aging and Society 30:697–721, 2010

Wetherell JL, Gatz M, Craske MG: Treatment of generalized anxiety disorder in older adults. J Consult Clin Psychol 71:31–40, 2003

Wetherell JL, Hopko DR, Diefenbach GJ, et al: Cognitive-behavioral therapy for late-life generalized anxiety disorder: who gets better? Behav Ther 36:147–156, 2005

Wetherell JL, Stoddard JA, White KS, et al: Augmenting antidepressant medication with modular CBT for geriatric generalized anxiety disorder: a pilot study. Int J Geriatr Psychiatry 26:869–875, 2011

Wilkinson P, Alder N, Juszczak E, et al: A pilot randomised controlled trial of a brief cognitive behavioural group intervention to reduce recurrence rates in late life depression. Int J Geriatr Psychiatry 24:68–75, 2009

Williams JW Jr, Barrett J, Oxman T, et al: Treatment of dysthymia and minor depression in primary care: a randomized controlled trial in older adults. JAMA 284:1519–1526, 2000

Wolitzky-Taylor KB, Castriotta N, Lenze EJ, et al: Anxiety disorders in older adults: a comprehensive review. Depress Anxiety 27:190–211, 2010

Wu LT, Blazer DG: Illicit and nonmedical drug use among older adults: a review. J Aging Health 23:481–504, 2011

Yang JA, Garis J, Jackson C, et al: Providing psychotherapy to older adults in home: benefits, challenges, and decision-making guidelines. Clin Gerontol 32:333–346, 2009

Zweig RA: Personality disorder in older adults: assessment challenges and strategies. Professional Psychology: Research and Practice 39:298–305, 2008

Suggested Readings

Barrowclough C, King P, Colville J, et al: A randomized trial of the effectiveness of cognitive-behavioral therapy and supportive counseling for anxiety symptoms in older adults. J Consult Clin Psychol 69:756–762, 2001

Bartels SJ, Coakley EH, Zubritsky C, et al: Improving access to geriatric mental health services: a randomized trial comparing treatment engagement with integrated versus enhanced referral care for depression, anxiety, and at-risk alcohol use. Am J Psychiatry 161:1455–1462, 2004

Bruce ML, Ten Have TR, Reynolds CF, et al: Reducing suicidal ideation and depressive symptoms in depressed older primary care patients. JAMA 291:1081–1091, 2004

Lebowitz BD, Pearson JL, Schneider LS, et al: Diagnosis and treatment of depression in late life: consensus statement update. JAMA 278:1186–1190, 1997

Livingston G, Johnston K, Katona C, et al: Systematic review of psychological approaches to the management of neuropsychiatric symptoms of dementia. Am J Psychiatry 162:1996–2021, 2005

Lynch TR, Cheavens JS, Cukrowicz KC, et al: Treatment of older adults with co-morbid personality disorder and depression: a dialectical behavior therapy approach. Int J Geriatr Psychiatry 22:131–143, 2007

Mohlman J, Gorman JM: The role of executive functioning in CBT: a pilot study with anxious older adults. Behav Res Ther 43:447–465, 2004

Oslin DW: Evidence-based treatment of geriatric substance abuse. Psychiatr Clin North Am 28:897–911, 2005

Thompson LW, Coon DW, Gallagher-Thompson D, et al: Comparison of desipramine and cognitive/behavioral therapy in the treatment of elderly outpatients with mild-to-moderate depression. Am J Geriatr Psychiatry 9:225–240, 2001

Unützer JM, Katon W, Callahan CM, et al: Collaborative care management of late-life depression in the primary care setting: a randomized controlled trial. JAMA 228:2836–2845, 2002

CHAPTER 19

WORKING WITH FAMILIES OF OLDER ADULTS

LISA P. GWYTHER, M.S.W.
DIANE E. MEGLIN, M.S.W., L.C.S.W., D.C.S.W.

No single model exists for working with families of older adults. Clinicians need to provide both patients and families with individualized family assessment and treatment, taking into account issues of diversity and heterogeneity. Despite the need for family-specific treatment, patterns of family issues consistently emerge that are based on trajectories of psychiatric illness. Perhaps the most specific guidance in the literature comes from meta-analyses of clinical research on families of older adults with progressive degenerative dementias (Gallagher-Thompson and Coon 2007; Pinquart and Sorenson 2006).

Over the course of an older adult's degenerative dementia, families will confront depression, delusions, agitation, behavioral changes, and other psychiatric symptoms in their cognitively impaired relative (Lyketsos et al. 2000; Tractenberg et al. 2002). The burden on the family can be great, information can be insufficient, and doubt can be overwhelming. Families caring for older members with dementia need reminders from psychiatrists to focus on maintaining family quality of life as well as quality of care within the constraints imposed by psychiatric, functional, and behavior changes (Hughes et al. 1999).

Lisa P. Gwyther gratefully acknowledges support for preparing this manuscript from grant P30-AG028377 from the National Institute on Aging to the Joseph and Kathleen Bryan Alzheimer's Disease Research Center at Duke University Medical Center.

Family Care for Older Adults With Dementia

Certain trends have emerged from studies of family care in dementia. A shift is occurring away from the direct provision of care by families toward more long-distance care or family care coordination. Dementia care frequently precipitates the family's first experience with seeking help from agencies and other family members. Increasing evidence shows that the lack of an available and affordable long-term care system is pushing the limits of family capacity and solidarity.[1]

Family care is universally preferred, based in strong family values that cross cultural and ethnic lines. Yet exclusive reliance on family care has well-documented personal and social costs. Family caregivers may become overwhelmed, exhausted, depressed, or anxious. Many family caregivers report loss of pleasure, motivation, friends, activities, privacy, intimacy, or identity. Gradual and sometimes sudden loss of the person "as he once was" can precipitate significant grief in family members.

Despite this apparent investment of families in care for older adults, some families never comprehend the minimal safety risks associated with dementia care. Elder mistreatment—whether abuse or passive or active neglect—may be associated with ex-ceeding these family limits (Fulmer et al. 2005). Family members may feel powerless and overwhelmed when they cannot predictably control the symptoms and course of dementia. The role of the psychiatrist with the family becomes one of assessment of tolerance limits, education, treatment of psychiatric consequences of caregiver burden, and management of family expectations of the disease course and of themselves.

Increasing dependency, loss, and grief are realities of family care in Alzheimer's disease, but not all family outcomes are negative or burdensome. Although depression is the most frequently reported psychiatric symptom among caregivers of Alzheimer's disease patients, some families express pride in their care as a legacy of their commitment to family values.

Goals in Working With Families of Older Adults

Clinical goals with families of older adults will vary with presenting problems and family resources. Common goals, however, are to normalize variability, address safety issues, mobilize secondary family support, facilitate appropriate decision making at care transitions, and help family members to accept help or let go of direct care as necessary. In essence, the family is forced to

---

[1] In November 2007, Evercare, a health care coordination program, in collaboration with the National Alliance for Caregiving (NAC), released their findings from a comprehensive survey on the personal financial costs of family caregiving. Although not limited to families caring for a person with dementia, the data revealed that for as many as 17 million people in the United States, costs (including food, household goods, clothing, travel, transportation, medical copayments, and medications) averaged more than 10% of caregivers' own household incomes. The financial burden of family care is clearly a significant factor, and its implications need to be addressed by practitioners as well as policy makers (see www.evercarehealthplans.com/pdf/CareGiversStudy.pdf).

adapt to a new state of "normal" in their family life, often with resistance from the member with dementia. Well-timed psychiatric help in interpreting the family's and the elder's reluctance to accept new realities can promote appropriate decision making and help smooth care transitions.

Other goals in working with family caregivers include treatment of their own mood, substance abuse, or anxiety disorders. Additionally, goals include providing individual and family treatment around issues of grief, loss, or conflict in family relationships that limit the effectiveness of care. In general, family work should enhance the effectiveness of family care and coping, the self-efficacy of caregivers (Fortinsky et al. 2002a), and the family's satisfaction with their preferred levels of involvement.

Psychiatrists should be especially alert to escalating anxiety, self-neglect, suicidal ideation, depression, or anger in caregivers, as well as signs of abuse or neglect of the patient. These indications should prompt immediate recommendations for treatment, respite, or relinquishment of primary care responsibility. Exigent negative caregiver outcomes on which to focus therapy include decrements in mental health, social participation, personal or family time, and loss of privacy.

Interdisciplinary Partnerships

Focused work with families of older adults holds great potential for positive outcomes, particularly in the context of an interdisciplinary partnership or team (Fortinsky et al. 2002b). Research suggests that social workers' individual and family counseling with spouse caregivers can mobilize and sustain community and secondary family support, reduce and prevent further primary caregiver depression, preserve caregiver self-reported health, change negative appraisals of behavioral symptoms, and even delay nursing home placement by more than a year compared with a control group (Mittelman et al. 1996, 2004, 2007).

Psychiatrists may work collaboratively with social workers or nurses. These mental health professionals can provide timely or sustained assistance during the particularly vulnerable times of care transitions (Gwyther 2005). Over time, the social worker or nurse may provide care management and monitor family capacity while educating the family about symptoms and helping with care transitions (Callahan et al. 2006).

Some families initially will resist referrals to a social worker but may become more amenable if the social worker is described as an expert consumer guide or family consultant. The family consultant can help families learn how to be their own case managers. The consultant may serve as a teacher, coach, advocate, counselor, cheerleader, or support person who can provide energy and a fresh perspective to promote family resilience.

Referrals to well-developed and validated psychoeducational group treatment programs have had equally positive results (Hepburn et al. 2007; Ostwald et al. 1999). Participation in peer counseling or support groups can have positive outcomes for active caregiver participants (Pillemer and Suitor 1996).

Another way to monitor goals in the psychiatric treatment of families of older adults is to base treatment on known precipitants of the breakdown of family care. Major precipitants of placement include both patient and caregiver factors (Yaffe et al. 2002). One of the patient factors that strongly predicts nursing home placement is disruptive psychiatric and behavioral symptoms. Changes in behavior and personality are also major causes of caregiver burden and depression. To the extent that psychiatric consultation is available to the older adult for treatment of psychiatric symptoms, and to the extent the family can be taught nonpharmacological approaches (see Goforth and Gwyther, Chapter 15, "Agitation and Suspiciousness," in this volume), the health of the family and caregivers and effective home care for the older adult can be preserved.

The Family as Information Seeker

Many family caregivers do not seek a diagnosis until psychiatric symptoms (e.g., suspiciousness) emerge or personality changes (e.g., uncharacteristic irritability) disrupt family life. Unfortunately, the patient is most likely to resist an evaluation once these symptoms have emerged. Psychiatrists typically are reluctant to speak with family members without the consent of the patient. An evaluation can be facilitated if the psychiatrist agrees to see the patient about a less threatening symptom such as headaches, loss of interest, or low energy.

Diagnostic Office Visits

Although the patient is entitled to time alone with the psychiatrist initially, later time alone with family informants is invaluable to the psychiatrist as he or she assesses the effects of functional loss and other family stressors. Most family caregivers prefer to talk privately

with the psychiatrist to avoid confronting the older adult about his or her symptoms and declining capacity. It may be helpful to have two family members accompany the patient for an evaluation. One family member can distract or sit with the older adult while another speaks privately with the psychiatrist.

Initial Communication With Older Adults and Their Families

Initially, communication with patients and their family members will likely be in response to the common emotional reactions to learning that the patient has a diagnosis of degenerative dementia. Elders and family members may express doubt about the diagnosis. Rather than confront their doubt or denial, it may be helpful for the psychiatrist to suggest that they behave as if the diagnosis of Alzheimer's disease has been confirmed while awaiting confirmation based on symptoms or progression of the disease. Asking directly about common early changes, such as difficulty handling money or increased irritability, may highlight expectable changes. Explaining the symptoms of apathy and loss of executive function can help families understand why their efforts to persuade the elder to try harder at tasks are likely to prove frustrating and futile.

Initial family sessions often elicit fear from family caregivers about their interdependent future or risks of heritability. Frustration is another common theme that emerges in early family treatment. Family caregivers frequently express frustration with the elder's obsessive need for repetition and reassurance. Clinicians can help families cope by offering information to clear up misconceptions about the presumed intentionality of the elder's resistance. Additionally, the elder's confabulations are typical and predictable attempts to fill in gaps for a failing memory. Encouraging the family to get angry at the disease rather than at professionals, the services, or one another can be extremely helpful. Families should be reminded that conflict among their members will only limit needed help (Coon et al. 2003). It is important for the family to understand that the elder's realistic dependency does not imply weakness of character or lack of will.

Fatigue and exhaustion are also common issues. Encouraging rest, exercise, and energy economies can be helpful for family members. Another common theme in family work is the guilt that family members feel about losing patience. They appreciate reminders from clinicians that everyone experiences regret based on unique but certain limits.

After the psychiatric evaluation, key themes, tailored to the family's capacity to understand or use them, should be highlighted and repeated in writing for distant or absent family members. Older couples in first marriages are generally more comfortable facing threatening health information together. Spouses of older adults with Alzheimer's disease often are put off by attempts to separate them from their impaired spouse. Providing the same information to both spouses at the same time helps older couples preserve their couple identity and accept the psychiatric recommendations as a mutual and shared adaptive challenge.

Assessing the Family of an Older Adult

A targeted assessment of the family of an older adult may result in referrals to Alzheimer's Association services, private or public geriatric care management, family or peer counseling, home help, day programs, assisted living, or nursing home care. Cultural values, expectations, and health beliefs will influence how and when families decide to pursue referrals, as well as their receptivity to family treatment by psychiatrists.

One of the most useful ways to elicit a picture of family functioning is to ask the family to describe a typical day. Clues about how much time the patient is left alone and about potential safety risks come from such open-ended questions. The psychiatrist should probe further if the caregiver hints about increased use of alcohol or psychoactive medications in response to stress.

The psychiatrist should encourage or support positive activities such as regular exercise, social stimulation, and secondary family support. A husband caring for his wife may be frustrated by her loss of interest in cooking. A suggestion to try regular restaurant meals at a familiar diner may conserve his energy and better meet the couple's nutritional and social needs.

It is wise to assess the home and neighborhood environment. People with dementia are easy targets for exploitation by telephone and mail fraud and people who come to the door. High-crime neighborhoods pose additional risks. An older adult who spends his or her time at the corner store buying alcohol and cigarettes may be especially vulnerable.

The psychiatrist should ask specifically about the primary caregiver's health. The psychiatrist should be alert to offhand comments such as "I'm fine as long as he can drive me to chemotherapy." The caregiver should be asked about his or her sleep and how it is affected by the older adult's sleep pattern. Many family caregivers will report being frustrated, overwhelmed, edgy, or exhausted but will deny having depression, anxiety, or psychiatric symptoms. Although psychiatrists are well advised to respond promptly to poorly controlled rage or suicidal or violent threats, skillful probing may be required to elicit frank symptoms (Rabins et al. 2006).

A brief review of family relationships may further elicit new or resurfacing family conflict that can complicate care. The psychiatrist must be alert to reports by family caregivers of exacerbated somatic symptoms or chronic illnesses of their own that they may not attribute to caregiver burden.

Another key to effective family assessment is to ask about other family commitments and responsibilities. Cultural expectations must be carefully assessed along with each family member's subjective perceptions of financial resources. When paid or formal services are needed, family decision making is often related to subjective perceptions of future financial adequacy rather than the objective cost or affordability of services. Some family members may be saving for a rainy day, whereas others may value preserving their inheritance above meeting the elder's current care needs.

It is wise to assess family strengths, skills, and goals. For example, some families may cope well with providing care for incontinence, or end-of-life care, but may be unable to tolerate the disruptive behaviors or sleep patterns of moderate dementia. Families who have coped with chronic mental illness or substance abuse in other family members may have well-developed coping strategies or support systems (such as Alcoholics Anonymous) that help them adapt to care for an impaired elder.

Finally, assessment should include some review of the family's experience with previous and current help from family members or paid services. Some key assessment areas include the adequacy, quality, cost, dependability, and perceptions about the type and quality of help.

Selecting Interventions for Families of Older Adults

Families of persons with dementia need a continuing source of reliable information. Referrals to the Alzheimer's Association (800-272-3900; www.alz.org) and the Alzheimer's Disease Education and Referral Center of the National Institute on Aging (800-438-4380; www.nia. nih.gov/ alzheimers) meet this need.

Multidimensional interventions have been shown to enhance positive caregiver outcomes (Belle et al. 2006; Gitlin et al. 2010). The most effective multidimensional interventions for family caregivers emphasize psychological and/or skill-building strategies for problem solving and behavior change over purely educational approaches. Effective multidimensional approaches are flexible and tailored to individual risk factors, are timed to key transition points or stressors in care trajectories (McCurry et al. 2005a), and are offered in sufficient dosages or amounts of assistance over time to ensure sustained or long-term outcomes. Combining individual and family counseling, family education, support group participation, and sustained availability of a care manager is associated with decreased caregiver burden and depression; decreases in the elderly patient's disruptive symptoms; and increased caregiver satisfaction, subjective well-being, and self-efficacy (Sorensen et al. 2002). Although interventions with dementia caregivers appear effective in meta-analyses, effects are small and domain-specific rather than global (McCurry et al. 2005b). For example, a reasonable multimodal approach to treating an elderly person's disruptive agitation could include treatment of depression in the elder or in the family caregiver with pharmacological and nonpharmacological strategies; participation by the family caregiver in psychoeducational, skills training, or caregiver support groups; and participation by the elder and the family caregiver in structured exercise programs (Teri et al. 2003).

Referrals to support groups should be balanced and participation not oversold. Research on participation in support groups documents specific benefits from experiential similarity, consumer information, coping and survivor models, expressive or advocacy outlets, and (for some participants) the creation of substitute family or social outlets. Indeed, early studies of support group participation showed that participants knew more about Alzheimer's disease and services (although participants did not necessarily use that information) and that participants felt less isolated and misunderstood than nonparticipants. However, the benefits of support group participation have realistic limits.

Online information can be quite useful for seeking resources at care transition points as well. Online guides to choosing a nursing home are available at medicare.gov, and state ombudsman offices also offer online information about local facilities. Online discussion boards and caregiver- or Alzheimer's disease–focused discussion groups can be helpful as well.

Educational Strategies With Families of Older Adults

Many families are too overwhelmed at a first psychiatric consultation to absorb information or instructions. Teachable moments with families come at crisis points with specific psychiatric symptoms, such as when accusations of family theft or spousal infidelity occur or when the older adult asks his or her spouse to find his "real" wife or husband.

A medicine metaphor is appropriate. The timing and "dosing" of information may enhance effective use of that information in adapting care over time. Some families have read or heard inaccurate or partially correct information about symptoms that can be easily corrected, such as myths about all older men with dementia becoming sexual predators. Just like medication management in geriatrics, the maxim "start low and go slow" applies equally well to family education about dementia. Overwhelming families with too many treatment suggestions or referrals is just as likely to lead to poor compliance as is changing multiple medication regimens all at once. Finally, information should be presented in hopeful terms, such as "Treating your depression should have positive effects on your husband's mood as well" or "Many families surprise themselves with their resilience."

The presentation of information in a timed and dosed manner also offers opportunities for repetition of key themes. The key messages for family caregivers listed in Table 19–1 can be presented at intervals and in "doses" that are based on the frequency of contact with the family, the family's need to know, and the family's capacity to understand. Assessing caregiver vulnerability can be facilitated by asking family members to self-assess their pressure points or signs of increasing caregiver overload (Kaufer et al. 1998).

Responding to Families Over the Course of Progressive Impairment

Clinical red flags may signal imminent danger resulting from the caregiver's precarious health. Unsubtle hints may be a caregiver's

TABLE 19–1. Key messages for family caregivers

1. Be willing to listen to the older adult, but understand that you cannot fix or do everything he or she may want or need. Know that it will not necessarily get easier, but things will change, and the experience will change you forever.

2. You are living with a situation you did not create, and your choices are limited by circumstances beyond your control. Seek options that are good enough for now.

3. You can only do what seems best at the time. Identify what you can and will tolerate, then set limits and call in reinforcements. Doubts are inevitable.

4. Find someone with whom you can be brutally honest, express those doubts and negative feelings, and move on.

5. Solving problems is much easier than living with the solutions. It is tempting for distant relatives to second-guess or criticize. Hope for the best, but plan for the worst.

6. It is not always possible to compare how one person handles things with how another relative would handle them if the positions were reversed.

7. The older adult is not unhappy or upset because of what you have done. He or she is living with unwanted dependency. Sick people often take out their frustration on close family members.

8. Considering what is best for your family involves compromise among competing needs, loyalties, and commitments. Everyone may get some of what he or she needs. Think twice before giving up that job, club, or church group. Make realistic commitments, and avoid making promises that include the words always, never, or forever.

9. Find ways to let your older relative give to or help you. He or she needs to feel purposeful, appreciated, and loved.

10. Take time to celebrate small victories when things go well.

comments such as "sometimes I feel like just letting him wander away." Pursuing these threads with standard clinical protocols is certainly warranted.

Other issues surface when working with families of moderately impaired older adults. Isolation of the caregiver and elder is common as friends drop off in response to disruptive behavioral symptoms or the need for constant supervision of the older adult. Families need to be reminded that being vulnerable does not make older people grateful or lovable and that cabin fever among cohabitating elders and family caregivers is a real threat to mental health and safety. Families are especially sensitive to elders who confuse

or mistake family identities or suggest that family members are impostors. Making suggestions that family caregivers say something like "I'll try to do it like your mother would" may help them understand and respond to accusations of this type.

Family members need to be warned not to give up cherished activities—social engagement has positive mental health effects at any age, and maintenance of a strong religious faith or community has been shown to have positive effects on elders and family caregivers. Expressive outlets such as sports, the arts, or advocacy can help families cope with frustration and anger. Prayer, meditation, exercise, massage, and yoga, in combination with active treatment of depression or anxiety, are all worthy treatment recommendations. An elder's participation at an adult day center can be presented to the family as a source of social stimulation for the elder and a stress-reduction strategy for the family caregiver (Gitlin et al. 2006; Zarit et al. 1998).

Helping Families Assess Capacity of Older Adults

Many families turn to psychiatrists to assess the judgment and decision-making capacity of older adults, whether it is related to handling money, making health decisions, living alone, or driving.

Money-handling and health care decisions should be addressed soon after diagnosis to ensure time for patients to select a surrogate. Often families seek psychiatric consultation when family conflict surfaces over the patient's selection of a surrogate or the surrogate's handling of the older adult's funds. Questions about whether the patient had sufficient capacity at the time he or she wrote a will or assigned power of attorney can become adversarial and unrelated to family treatment.

Effective work with families regarding financial capacity is done early with a preventive focus. It is wise for one family member to make sure bills are paid. This can be done with different levels of involvement of the patient, from making decisions about which bills to pay to signing checks (Widera et al. 2011)

Assessment of and Limitations on Driving

Families can be encouraged to assess driving capacity based on observations of current driving (e.g., incorrect signaling, confusion about exits, getting lost, stopping in traffic for no apparent reason), with reminders that dementia affects judgment, reaction time, and problem solving. Psychiatric assessment of the elderly patient along with current observations from the family will provide direction regarding when driving should be limited. Unfortunately, by the time a decline in driving abilities is evident, many patients cannot adequately report or judge their safety on the road. Anonymous reports to the Department of Motor Vehicles may lead to required testing or removal of the patient's license, but the absence of a license rarely stops a determined older adult with dementia.

Psychiatrists may suggest a range of successful ways to limit driving, such as the following:

- A prescription reminder to stop driving can be tempered with a qualifier such as "until the end of your treatment." The patient's forgetfulness can be put to work for the psychiatrist. However, patients have been known to keep driving, making comments such as "That doctor doesn't know anything."
- Shaving the patient's keys, substituting another key, removing a distributor cap, or otherwise disabling a car can sometimes reduce the need to confront the patient with lost skills. However, patients have been known to fix the car, replace the keys, or even buy a new car while the old one was "in the shop."
- The car could be sold, moved to an undisclosed location, or put up on blocks. One family of a taxi driver put the taxi on blocks in the backyard to help the patient remember that it was broken.
- The family can also work on solutions that limit the need for driving—delivery

services, senior vans, or offers of regular rides to church or for visits. Some families find that a charge account with a taxi service works best. Other families appeal to the person's altruism and suggest giving the car to a grandchild for school or work, and that grandchild agrees to provide escorted rides in exchange.

Addressing Questions of Capacity to Live Alone

Families may go to extremes to keep an older adult with dementia in a familiar environment, allowing values of autonomy and choice to temporarily trump safety. In addition to performing a psychiatric assessment of the patient's cognition, judgment, functional impairment, and decision-making capacity, the psychiatrist can suggest that the family consider the following questions:

- Can the person with dementia use the telephone to call for help from a family member or to call 911? Will he or she respond inappropriately to telemarketers? Have mysterious packages or bills for unusual items begun appearing? Does he or she make repetitive calls every few minutes to the police or the same family member at work or at home?
- Can the family member with dementia get to the store or to his or her regular activities? Does he or she overbuy or underbuy certain items?
- Can the individual handle money and pay bills, or if not, is he or she willing to let others do this for him or her?
- Can he or she take medicine appropriately, on time, and in correct doses? Does he or she self-medicate or risk overdoses of unnecessary medications?
- Is he or she bathing, changing clothes, and dressing appropriately for the weather?

- Is he or she leaving the house after dark or traveling in dangerous areas alone? Does he or she let strangers in or buy from or contribute to questionable causes based on visits to his or her home?
- Is he having problems positioning his body to use a toilet, or is he urinating in wastebaskets or plants?
- Is he or she falling or getting lost by wandering outside a safe area?
- Are there significant changes in his or her appetite, weight, sleep, appearance, or eating habits?
- Is discreet surveillance by neighbors, friends, or family readily available?

The question of discreet surveillance is paramount. Persons with moderate dementia may live alone successfully if they have regular contact with, surveillance by, or checking from neighbors or family members. Environmental demand varies considerably and must be assessed along with patient variables.

Families and Institutionalization of the Older Adult

Family stress does not stop at the door of the nursing home—ample evidence shows that families experience the greatest burden, disruption, and conflict in the time immediately before and after nursing home placement. Family members may seek psychiatric services to deal with guilt, grief, and often anger toward the nursing facility, reimbursement system, and one another. Many families are disappointed by the lack of medical or psychiatric treatment available to residents of nursing homes. Families should be encouraged to work with the facility and the nursing home ombudsman while dealing with their affective, anxiety, and grief symptoms.

Conclusion

Work with families of older adults is about adaptation to change and loss. Much of psychiatric treatment of families helps them modify expectations for new dependency while learning to forgive themselves and others for inevitable doubts and mistakes. Interdisciplinary partnerships and teamwork with the Alzheimer's Association or with nurses or social workers offer the most effective and efficient models for psychiatric services to families of older adults. There is often as much need for "timed and dosed"

patient and family education as there is need for treatment of specific psychiatric symptoms or syndromes of the elder or family members. Families will expect psychiatrists to provide active treatment and monitoring of psychiatric symptoms, reassurance, interpretation of information, and referrals. In addition, it is always helpful to acknowledge losses and contributions to care by individual family members, to encourage caregiver self-care, to offer authoritative absolution for inevitable mistakes, and to offer decisional support, especially with transitions in care or with end-of-life care.

Key Points

- Psychiatric treatment for families helps them modify expectations about the newly dependent family member and learn to forgive themselves and others for inevitable doubts and mistakes.

- Interdisciplinary partnerships and teamwork with the Alzheimer's Association or with social workers or nurses offer the most effective and efficient models for psychiatric services to families of older adults.

- Psychiatrists should provide active treatment and monitoring of family caregivers' psychiatric symptoms, outline reasonable expectations, and offer families information about outcomes of treatment.

- It is helpful to acknowledge family caregivers' losses and their contributions to care. It is also important to encourage their own self-care and to offer them expert decisional support during transitions in care.

References

Belle SH, Burgio L, Burns R, et al: Enhancing the quality of life of dementia caregivers from different ethnic or racial groups: a randomized, controlled trial. Ann Intern Med 145:727–738, 2006

Callahan CM, Boustani MA, Unverzagt FW, et al: Effectiveness of collaborative care for older adults with Alzheimer disease in primary care: a randomized controlled trial. JAMA 295:2148–2157, 2006

Coon DW, Thompson L, Steffen A, et al: Anger and depression management: psychoeducational skill training intervention for women caregivers of a relative with dementia. Gerontologist 43:678–689, 2003

Fortinsky RH, Kercher K, Burant CJ: Measurement and correlates of family caregiver self-efficacy for managing dementia. Aging Ment Health 6:153–160, 2002a

Fortinsky RH, Unson CG, Garcia RI: Helping family caregivers by linking primary care physicians with community-based dementia care services. Dementia 1:227–240, 2002b

Fulmer T, Paveza G, Van de Weerd C, et al: Dyadic vulnerability and risk profiling for elder neglect. Gerontologist 45:525–534, 2005

Gallagher-Thompson D, Coon DW: Evidence-based psychological treatments for distress in family caregivers of older adults. Psychol Aging 22:37–51, 2007

Gitlin LN, Reever K, Dennis MP, et al: Enhancing quality of life of families who use adult day services: short-and long-term effects of the Adult Day Services Plus Program. Gerontologist 46:630–639, 2006

Gitlin LN, Winter L, Dennis MP, et al: A biobehavioral home-based intervention and the well-being of patients with dementia and their caregivers: the COPE randomized trial. JAMA 304:983–991, 2010

Gwyther LP: Family care and Alzheimer's disease: what do we know? What can we do? N C Med J 66:39–44, 2005

Hepburn K, Lewis M, Tornatore J, et al: The Savvy Caregiver program: the demonstrated effectiveness of a transportable dementia caregiver psychoeducation program. J Gerontol Nurs 33:30–36, 2007

Hughes SL, Giobie-Harder A, Weaver FM, et al: Relationships between caregiver burden and health-related quality of life. Gerontologist 39:534–545, 1999

Kaufer DI, Cummings JL, Christine D, et al: Assessing the impact of neuropsychiatric symptoms in Alzheimer's disease: the Neuropsychiatric Inventory Caregiver Distress Scale. J Am Geriatr Soc 46:210–215, 1998

Lyketsos CG, Steinberg M, Tschanz JT, et al: Mental and behavioral disturbances in dementia: findings from the Cache County Study on Memory in Aging. Am J Psychiatry 157:708–714, 2000

McCurry SM, Gibbons LE, Logsdon RG, et al: Nighttime insomnia treatment and education for Alzheimer's disease: a randomized controlled trial. J Am Geriatr Soc 53:793–802, 2005a

McCurry SM, Logsdon R, Gibbons LE: Training community consultants to help family members improve dementia care: a randomized controlled trial. Gerontologist 45:802–811, 2005b

Mittelman MS, Ferris SH, Shulman E, et al: A family intervention to delay nursing home placement of patients with Alzheimer disease: a randomized controlled trial. JAMA 276:1725–1731, 1996

Mittelman MS, Roth DL, Haley WE, et al: Effects of a caregiver intervention on negative caregiver appraisals of behavior problems in patients with Alzheimer's disease: results of a randomized trial. J Gerontol B Psychol Sci Soc Sci 59:P27–P34, 2004

Mittelman MS, Roth DL, Clay OJ, et al: Preserving health of Alzheimer caregivers: impact of a spouse caregiver intervention. Am J Geriatr Psychiatry 15:780–789, 2007

Ostwald SK, Hepburn KW, Caron W, et al: Reducing caregiver burden: a randomized psychoeducational intervention for caregivers of persons with dementia. Gerontologist 39:299–309, 1999

Pillemer K, Suitor JJ: "It takes one to help one": effects of similar others on the well-being of caregivers. J Gerontol B Psychol Sci Soc Sci 51:S250–S257, 1996

Pinquart M, Sorensen S: Helping caregivers of persons with dementia: which interventions work and how large are the effects? Int Psychogeriatr 18:577–595, 2006

Rabins PV, Lyketsos C, Steele C: Practical Dementia Care. Oxford, UK, Oxford University Press, 2006

Sorensen S, Pinquart M, Duberstein P, et al: How effective are interventions with caregivers? An updated meta-analysis. Gerontologist 42:356–372, 2002

Teri L, Gibbons LE, McCurry SM, et al: Exercise plus behavioral management in patients with Alzheimer's disease: a randomized controlled trial. JAMA 290:2015–2022, 2003

Tractenberg RE, Weiner MF, Thal LJ: Estimating the prevalence of agitation in community-dwelling persons with Alzheimer's disease. J Neuropsychiatry Clin Neurosci 14:11–18, 2002

Widera E, Steenpass V, Marson D, et al: Finances in the older patient with cognitive impairment: "He didn't want me to take over." JAMA 305:698–706, 2011

Yaffe K, Fox P, Newcomer R, et al: Patient and caregiver characteristics and nursing home placement in patients with dementia. JAMA 287:2090–2097, 2002

Zarit SH, Stephens MA, Townsend A, et al: Stress reduction for family caregivers: effects of adult day care use. J Gerontol B Psychol Sci Soc Sci 53:S267–S277, 1998

Suggested Readings

Belle SH, Burgio L, Burns R, et al: Enhancing the quality of life of dementia caregivers from different ethnic or racial groups: a randomized, controlled trial. Ann Intern Med 145:727–738, 2006

Gallagher-Thompson D, Coon DW: Evidence-based psychological treatments for distress in family caregivers of older adults. Psychol Aging 22:37–51, 2007

Mittelman MS, Roth DL, Clay OJ, et al: Preserving health of Alzheimer caregivers: impact of a spouse caregiver intervention. Am J Geriatr Psychiatry 15:780–789, 2007

Pinquart M, Sorensen S: Helping caregivers of persons with dementia: which interventions work and how large are the effects? Int Psychogeriatr 18:577–595, 2006

Rabins PV, Lyketsos C, Steele C: Practical Dementia Care. Oxford, UK, Oxford University Press, 2006

CHAPTER 20

CLINICAL PSYCHIATRY IN THE NURSING HOME

JOEL E. STREIM, M.D.

Nursing homes provide long-term care for elderly patients with chronic illness and disability as well as rehabilitation and convalescent care for individuals recovering from acute illness. As documented in previous reviews (Streim and Katz 2009), clinical studies have consistently provided evidence that the diagnosis, management, and treatment of mental disorders are important components of nursing home care. The delivery of mental health services in nursing homes continues to be shaped by several factors, including growing scientific knowledge, availability of new treatments, evolving federal regulations, public dissemination of survey data, and changes in the medical marketplace. In this chapter, I review current information on the psychiatric problems that are common in the nursing home, discuss current trends affecting clinical care,

and present a conceptual model for the organization of mental health services in the nursing home setting.

Prevalence of Psychiatric Disorders

Epidemiological studies conducted between 1986 and 1993 uniformly reported high prevalence rates for psychiatric disorders among nursing home residents. Rovner et al. (1990a) reported the prevalence of psychiatric disorders among individuals newly admitted to a proprietary chain of nursing homes to be 80.2%. Parmelee et al. (1989) found psychiatric disorders diagnosed according to DSM-III-R (American Psychiatric Association 1987) criteria in 91% of the residents of a large urban geriatric center. On the basis of psychiatric interviews of subjects in randomly selected samples, other investigators found prevalence rates of DSM-III (American Psychiatric Association 1980) or DSM-III-R disorders to be as high as 94% (Chandler and Chandler 1988; Rovner et al. 1986; Tariot et al. 1993). Although some studies reported lower rates, those investigations used less rigorous methods for sampling or diagnosis (Burns et al. 1988; Custer et al. 1984; German et al. 1986; National Center for Health Statistics 1987; Teeter et al. 1976). In one study, case ascertainment by review of selected medical records revealed a 68% prevalence of psychiatric diagnoses (Linkins et al. 2006), suggesting that chart documentation of mental disorders by nursing home clinicians may underestimate the actual rates of mental disorders. A more recent review of epidemiological studies and the 2004 National Nursing Home Survey calculated that the median prevalence of dementia among nursing home residents was 58%, the median prevalence of behavioral and psychological symptoms of dementia was 78%, the median prevalence of major depression was 10%, and the prevalence of depressive symptoms was 29% (Seitz et al. 2010). These prevalence data, whether based on clinical interviews or chart review, suggest that nursing homes are de facto neuropsychiatric institutions, although they were not originally intended for this purpose. The challenge of providing long-term care services in nursing homes is therefore complicated by the extensive psychiatric comorbidity found in this setting (Reichman and Conn 2010).

Cognitive Disorders and Behavioral Disturbances

In all studies, the most common psychiatric disorder was dementia, with prevalence rates of 50%–75% (Chandler and Chandler

1988; Katz et al. 1989; Parmelee et al. 1989; Rovner et al. 1986, 1990a; Tariot et al. 1993; Teeter et al. 1976). Alzheimer's disease (DSM-III-R primary degenerative dementia) accounted for about 50%–60% of cases of dementia, and vascular dementia accounted for about 25%–30% (Barnes and Raskind 1980; Rovner et al. 1986, 1990a). Other causes of dementia were reported with lower prevalence and greater variability between sites. The prevalence rates of frontotemporal and Lewy body dementia have not been ascertained in nursing home populations.

Delirium is common in nursing homes and occurs primarily in patients made more vulnerable by a dementing illness. Available studies indicated that approximately 6%–7% of residents were delirious at the time of evaluation (Barnes and Raskind 1980; Rovner et al. 1986, 1990a). However, this figure probably underestimates the number of patients who have cognitive impairment associated with reversible toxic or metabolic factors. In one study, investigators found that nearly 25% of impaired residents had potentially reversible conditions (Sabin et al. 1982); another study found that 6%–12% of residential care patients with dementia actually improved in cognitive performance over the course of 1 year (Katz et al. 1991). A large study of residents with severe cognitive impairment found improvement at 6-month follow-up in 14% of the sample, associated with the following baseline findings: higher function, antidepressant medication use, and falls (Buttar et al. 2003). In the nursing home, as in other settings, a common reversible cause of cognitive impairment may be cognitive toxicity from drugs used to treat medical or psychiatric disorders. For residents admitted to the nursing home for post–acute care rehabilitation, unresolved delirium is associated with poor functional recovery (Kiely et al. 2007).

The clinical features of dementing disorders include treatable behavioral and psychological symptoms of dementia—such as hallucinations, delusions, depression, anxiety, and agitation—that can contribute to disability. Combined 1-year prevalence of psychosis, agitation, and depression has been estimated between 76% and 82% (Ballard et al. 2001), and 2-year prevalence of neuropsychiatric symptoms was found to be 96.6% in residents with dementia (Wetzels et al. 2010). In nursing home populations, psychotic symptoms have been reported in approximately 25%–50% of residents with a primary dementing illness (Berrios and Brook 1985; Chandler and Chandler 1988; Rovner et al. 1986, 1990a; Teeter et al. 1976). Clinically significant depression is seen in approximately 25% of patients with dementia; one-third of such patients have symptoms of secondary major depression (Parmelee et al. 1989; Rovner et al. 1986, 1990a). Dementia complicated by mixed agitation and depression accounts for more than one-third of complicated dementia cases in nursing home populations and is associated with multiple psychiatric and medical needs, psychotropic drug use, and hospital admissions (Bartels et al. 2003).

Data from the Medical Expenditures Panel Survey (MEPS) indicate that 30% of nursing home residents have behavior problems, including 11.8% with verbal abuse, 9.1% with physical abuse, 14.5% with socially inappropriate behavior, 12.5% with resistance to care, and 9.4% with wandering (Krauss and Altman 1998). A more recent prospective cohort study of nursing home residents with dementia found a point prevalence of agitation or aggression ranging

from 20.5% to 29.1%, with a 2-year cumulative prevalence of 53.8%; a point prevalence of irritability ranging from 21.4% to 28.2%, with a 2-year cumulative prevalence of 58.1%; and a point prevalence of aberrant motor behavior fluctuating between 18.8% and 26.5%, with a cumulative prevalence of 50.4% (Wetzels et al. 2010). Most psychiatric consultations in long-term care settings are for the evaluation and treatment of behavioral disturbances such as pacing and wandering, verbal abusiveness, disruptive shouting, physical aggression, destructive acts, and resistance to necessary care (Fenton et al. 2004; Loebel et al. 1991). Behavioral disturbances most frequently occur in individuals with dementia, often in those with psychotic symptoms—an association that remains even after controlling for level of cognitive impairment (Rovner et al. 1990b). Agitation and hyperactivity also can be caused by agitated depression (Heeren et al. 2003) as well as delirium, sensory deprivation or overload, occult physical illness, pain, constipation, urinary retention, and adverse drug effects (including akathisia caused by neuroleptics) (Cohen-Mansfield and Billig 1986). Depressive symptoms are associated with disruptive vocalizations in nursing home residents, even after controlling for gender, age, and cognitive status (Dwyer and Byrne 2000). In a subsequent study that compared verbal and physical nonaggressive agitation, verbal agitation was found to be correlated with female gender, depressed affect, poor performance of activities of daily living (ADLs), and impaired social functioning (Cohen-Mansfield and Libin 2005).

In addition to agitation, symptoms such as apathy, inactivity, and withdrawal occur among nursing home residents with and without a diagnosis of depression. Apathy has been found to increase over time, with a

2-year cumulative incidence of 42.1% (Wetzels et al. 2010). Although these symptoms are less disturbing to staff and less frequently lead to psychiatric consultation (Fenton et al. 2004), they can be disabling and may be associated with decreases in socialization and self-care.

Depression

Among community-dwelling elderly persons in the United States and Europe, depression increases the risk of nursing home admission (Ahmed et al. 2007; Harris and Cooper 2006; Onder et al. 2007), and this association remains after controlling for age, physical illness, and functional status (Harris 2007). Among those who reside in nursing homes, depressive disorders represent the second most common psychiatric diagnosis. Most studies in U.S. nursing homes show depression prevalence rates of 15%–50%, depending on the population studied and the instruments used, whether major depression or depressive symptoms are being reported, and whether primary depression and depression occurring secondary to dementia are considered together or separately (Baker and Miller 1991; Chandler and Chandler 1988; Hyer and Blazer 1982; Katz et al. 1989; Kaup et al. 2007; Lesher 1986; Levin et al. 2007; Parmelee et al. 1989; Rovner et al. 1986, 1990a, 1991; Tariot et al. 1993; Teeter et al. 1976). Approximately 6%–10% of all nursing home residents, and 20%–25% of those who are cognitively intact, meet DSM-III or DSM-III-R criteria for major depression; the latter figure is an order of magnitude greater than rates among community-dwelling elderly persons (Blazer and Williams 1980; Kramer et al. 1985).

Parmelee et al. (1992a) reported that the 1-year incidence of major depression was 9.4% and that patients with preexisting minor depression were at increased risk; the incidence of minor depression among those who were euthymic at baseline was 7.4%. These data show that minor or subsyndromal depression in nursing home residents appears to be a risk factor for major depression and might represent an opportunity for preventive treatment in this population.

Depression among nursing home residents tends to be persistent. Although there may be moderate decreases in self-rated depression during the initial 2 weeks to 6 months following nursing home admission (Engle and Graney 1993; Smalbrugge et al. 2006), Ames and colleagues (1988) found that only 17% of the patients with diagnosable depressive disorders had recovered after an average 3.6 years of follow-up. Smalbrugge and colleagues (2006) found persistence of symptoms in two-thirds of nursing home residents at 6-month follow-up, although rates were significantly higher in those patients with more severe symptoms at baseline.

Evidence for morbidity associated with depression comes from studies that showed an increase in pain complaints among residents with depression (Parmelee et al. 1991) and an association between depression and biochemical markers of subnutrition (Katz et al. 1993). Depression in nursing home residents, both those with and those without dementia, is associated with disability (Kaup et al. 2007). Among individuals admitted to nursing homes for post–acute care rehabilitation, those with depression have poorer functional outcomes (Webber et al. 2005). In addition to its association with morbidity and disability, depression has been found to be associated with an increase in mortality rate, with effect sizes ranging from 1.6 to 3 (Ashby et al. 1991; Katz et al.

1989; Parmelee et al. 1992b; Rovner et al. 1991; Sutcliffe et al. 2007). In addition to the high level of complexity that characterizes major depression among nursing home residents, the evidence of heterogeneity in these patients may reflect the existence of clinically relevant subtypes of depression. The treatment study by Katz et al. (1990) reported that measures of self-care deficits and serum levels of albumin were highly intercorrelated and that both predicted a lack of response to treatment with nortriptyline. Therefore, although this study determined that major depression is a specific, treatable disorder—even in long-term care patients with medical comorbidity—there is also evidence in this setting for a treatment-relevant subtype of depression characterized by high levels of disability and low levels of serum albumin. This latter condition may be related to failure to thrive in infants, as discussed by Braun et al. (1988) and by Katz et al. (1993). As described later in this chapter, evidence also indicates that depression may be different in nursing home residents with dementia, compared with those who are depressed and cognitively intact. Depressed residents with dementia have been found to have poorer response to treatment with noradrenergic and serotonergic antidepressant drugs (Magai et al. 2000; Oslin et al. 2000; Streim et al. 2000).

Progress in Treatment of Psychiatric Disorders in the Nursing Home

An appreciation of the unique characteristics of nursing home populations—particularly the extremes of old age and the high prevalence rates of cognitive impairment, psychiatric and medical comorbidity, and

disability, all in the context of residential long-term care institutions—has led to increased recognition that results of efficacy studies conducted in general adult outpatient populations may not be readily generalizable to nursing home residents. This recognition points to the need for treatment studies conducted specifically with nursing home patients. Although the number of randomized controlled studies is limited, the body of literature on treatment outcomes in the nursing home is growing.

Nonpharmacological Management of Behavioral Disturbances

Since 1990, numerous studies have been published describing nonpharmacological interventions for behavioral disturbances associated with dementia in the nursing home setting. Few of these were randomized controlled trials. The reader is referred to comprehensive reviews of these studies by Cohen-Mansfield (2001), Snowden and colleagues (2003), and Livingston and colleagues (2005). Several nonpharmacological interventions have been shown to be effective, although only behavior management therapies, specific types of caregiver and residential care staff education, and possibly cognitive stimulation appear to have lasting effectiveness (Livingston et al. 2005). One promising approach combined enhanced activities, guidelines for the use of psychotropic medication, and educational rounds for nursing home staff (Rovner et al. 1996). In a randomized clinical trial, this approach was shown to reduce the prevalence of problem behaviors and the use of antipsychotic drugs and physical restraints. Activities matched to skills and interests of residents with dementia also have been shown to reduce agitation and negative affect (Kolanowski et al. 2005). Individualized consultation for staff nurses about the management of patients with dementia also was shown to diminish the use of physical restraints (Evans et al. 1997). Reductions in agitation were observed in a study of a daytime physical activity intervention combined with a nighttime program to decrease noise and sleep-disruptive nursing care practices (Alessi 1999). Bright light therapy has been demonstrated to increase observed nocturnal sleep time but not to improve agitated behavior in nursing home residents with dementia (Lyketsos et al. 1999). Although some studies have claimed that aromatherapy with lavender oil is effective in reducing agitated behaviors, results have not been consistently replicated when controlling for nonolfactory aspects of treatment in residents with severe dementia (Snow et al. 2004). Other programs seek to reduce behavioral difficulties through individualized modifications in the physical environment (van Weert et al. 2005).

Psychotherapy

The evidence for the efficacy of psychotherapy in other settings suggests that it may be of value for treating mental disorders of aging in nursing home residents whose cognitive abilities allow them to participate. Bharucha and colleagues (2006) identified and reviewed 18 controlled "talk" psychotherapy studies conducted in nursing home populations and found that most showed at least short-term benefits on measures of mood, hopelessness, perceived control, self-esteem, or other psychological variables. However, the investigators noted that interpretation of the findings of many of these studies was limited by small sample sizes, variable study entry criteria, short duration

of trials, heterogeneous outcome assessment methods, and lack of detail on intervention methods. Controlled research studies of psychotherapeutic interventions has included studies of task-oriented versus insight-oriented therapy (Moran and Gatz 1987); reality orientation (Baines et al. 1987); reminiscence groups (Baines et al. 1987; Chao et al. 2006; Goldwasser et al. 1987; McMurdo and Rennie 1993; Orten et al. 1989; Politis et al. 2004; Rattenbury and Stones 1989; Youssef 1990); exercise, activity, and progressive relaxation group therapies (Bensink et al. 1992; McMurdo and Rennie 1993); supportive group psychotherapy (Goldwasser et al. 1987; Williams-Barnard and Lindell 1992); validation therapy (Tondi et al. 2007; Toseland et al. 1997); cognitive or cognitive-behavioral group therapies (Abraham et al. 1992; Zerhusen et al. 1991); focused visual imagery therapy (Abraham et al. 1997); and a psychosocial activity intervention (Beck et al. 2002). With the exception of the investigations by Abraham and colleagues, patients in most of these studies were not selected on the basis of specific psychiatric symptoms or syndromes but rather on the basis of age, cognitive status, or mobility.

Some of these studies reported improvements on measures of communication, behavior, cognitive performance, mood, social withdrawal, physical function, somatic preoccupation, self-esteem, perceived locus of control, quality of life, and life satisfaction. Overall, there is a paucity of research on the outcomes of well-described psychotherapies among nursing home residents who have well-characterized psychiatric disorders. Nevertheless, the available evidence from nursing home research, considered together with outcomes of psychotherapy for older adults in other clinical settings, suggests that psychotherapy should be regarded as an important component of mental health treatment for the more cognitively intact nursing home residents with depression.

Pharmacotherapy

Pharmacological treatments are commonly used in nursing homes for dementia and its associated psychological and behavioral symptoms and for depression. For a more comprehensive review of the evidence for pharmacological treatment of neuropsychiatric symptoms of dementia, the reader is referred to the article by Sink and colleagues (2005) and a meta-analysis that included several nursing home studies and examined mortality risk (Schneider et al. 2005).

Some earlier studies provided evidence for the efficacy of antipsychotic drugs in managing agitation and related symptoms in nursing home residents with dementia, but the effect sizes were often modest, and high placebo response rates were common (Barnes et al. 1982; Schneider et al. 1990; Sunderland and Silver 1988). Subsequently, several multicenter, randomized, double-blind, placebo-controlled clinical trials demonstrated that some of the atypical antipsychotic agents had efficacy for the treatment of psychotic symptoms and agitated behavior in nursing home residents with dementia. These clinical trials included published studies of risperidone (Brodaty et al. 2003; Katz et al. 1999), olanzapine (Meehan et al. 2002; Street et al. 2000), quetiapine (Zhong et al. 2007), and aripiprazole (Mintzer et al. 2007). Secondary analyses of data from the nursing home trials of risperidone showed that it had antipsychotic effects and also had independent effects on aggression or agitation. Other studies of atypical antipsychotic drugs in nursing home residents with dementia failed to demonstrate statistically significant benefits on the a priori designated primary outcome measures related to psychosis or behavioral disturbances (De Deyn et al. 1999, 2005; Mintzer et al. 2006; Streim et al. 2008), although some of these studies found possible benefits on secondary behavioral measures. The widespread interest in studying atypical antipsychotics for treatment in elderly nursing home residents was partly attributable to the expectation that these agents would be better tolerated than conventional antipsychotics in this population. For example, early follow-up studies had suggested that risperidone might cause less tardive dyskinesia compared with typical antipsychotic medications (Jeste et al. 2000).

These controlled clinical trials have examined only the acute effects of treatment, typically for 6–12 weeks of treatment, and little is known about the effectiveness of treatment for longer periods. However, evidence suggests that the need for and benefit from antipsychotic drug treatment changes over the course of months in nursing home patients with dementia. Several double-blind, placebo-controlled studies of antipsychotic drug discontinuation reported that most patients who had been receiving longer-term treatment could be withdrawn from these agents without reemergence of psychosis or agitated behaviors (Bridges-Parlet et al. 1997; Cohen-Mansfield et al. 1999; Ruths et al. 2004). Therefore, it is important to reevaluate periodically the need for continuing antipsychotic drug treatment.

Since 2003, analyses of safety data from randomized controlled studies of atypical antipsychotic drugs in elderly patients with dementia, including the aforementioned nursing home studies, have found significantly increased risks of cerebrovascular adverse events and mortality in this population. Although elevated risks were not found in every study, pooled analyses showed that the rate of cerebrovascular adverse events (including stroke and transient ischemic attacks) is greater than with placebo. These findings led to regulatory warnings in the United States, Canada, and the United Kingdom regarding the safety of these drugs in elderly patients with dementia.

The U.S. Food and Drug Administration (FDA) also warned that elderly patients with dementia-related psychosis who are given atypical antipsychotics have a risk of death between 1.6 and 1.7 times greater than those who are given placebo (4.5% vs. 2.6%), with a reminder that atypical antipsychotics are not FDA-approved for the treatment of dementia-related psychosis. Consistent with this FDA warning, a meta-analysis by Schneider et al. (2005), which examined results of 15 randomized controlled trials, many of which were conducted in nursing home patients, found that the risk of mortality was 3.5% in elderly patients taking atypical antipsychotics compared with 2.3% in patients taking placebo. Wang et al. (2005) found a significantly higher adjusted risk of death in elderly patients taking conventional antipsychotics compared with those taking atypical antipsychotic medications, regardless of whether the patients had dementia or resided in a nursing home. The investigators suggested that conventional antipsychotic medications should not be used to replace atypical agents discontinued in response to FDA warnings.

In light of the concerns about risks of antipsychotic medications in elderly nursing home residents with dementia, experts in the field have suggested that nonpharmacological approaches should be considered first when treating noncognitive behavioral symptoms. However, for those nursing home patients whose behavioral symptoms do not respond to nonpharmacological interventions, the decision to use an atypical antipsychotic should be based on a careful assessment of individual risk-benefit profile.

Five randomized clinical trials evaluated the efficacy of mood-stabilizing anticonvulsant drugs for the treatment of agitation and aggression in nursing home residents. The first of these was a study of carbamazepine that showed it to be effective for agitation and aggression but not for psychotic symptoms such as delusions and hallucinations (Tariot et al. 1998). In this study, nursing reports indicated that less staff time was required for patient care in the group taking carbamazepine. Another trial of carbamazepine found high rates of improvements in patients receiving carbamazepine or placebo, with no significant between-group differences (Olin et al. 2001). Several placebo-controlled studies evaluated divalproex with few encouraging results, including one trial that was discontinued before completion because of adverse effects in the drug treatment group. Overall, these studies failed to provide evidence for efficacy in reducing agitated behavior (Porsteinsson et al. 2001; Tariot et al. 2001b, 2005). It is of note that the tolerability of divalproex was limited by somnolence, weakness, and diminished oral intake in this population of elderly nursing home subjects with dementia.

Acetylcholinesterase inhibitors have been shown to delay the decline in cognitive function in patients with mild to severe Alzheimer's disease, although few studies have been conducted specifically in nursing home samples. One randomized clinical trial of donepezil in nursing home residents showed effects on cognitive performance that were comparable to those observed in less impaired outpatients (Tariot et al. 2001a). A subsequent study reported that donepezil improves cognition and preserves function in Alzheimer's disease patients with severe dementia residing in nursing homes (Winblad et al. 2006). These studies also examined the effects of donepezil on behavioral disturbances, as a secondary outcome measure, and did not find significant benefits. Tariot et al. (2004) reported significant improvement on Neuropsychiatric Inventory scores with the *N*-methyl-D-aspartate receptor antagonist memantine, but this agent has not been studied prospectively in the nursing home setting. Survival analyses in an observational study have suggested that the addition of memantine to a cholinesterase inhibitor can delay the time to nursing home placement (Lopez et al. 2009).

Only four randomized clinical trials have evaluated the effects of antidepressants in nursing home residents. The first study, which was placebo controlled, showed a positive response to nortriptyline for treatment of major depression in a long-term care population with high levels of medical comorbidity (Katz et al. 1990). In the second study, patients were randomly assigned to receive regular or low-dosage nortriptyline, and significant plasma level–response relations were documented in cognitively intact patients (Streim et al. 2000). These findings again confirmed the validity of the diagnosis of depression in nursing home residents in the context of significant medical comorbidity and disability. However, in patients with dementia, the plasma level–response relation was significantly different, suggesting that the depression occurring in dementia might be a treatment-relevant subtype of depression or a distinct disorder. A controlled antidepressant trial in nursing

home residents with late-stage Alzheimer's disease showed no significant benefits of sertraline over placebo (Magai et al. 2000). Available open-label studies of the efficacy of selective serotonin reuptake inhibitors (SSRIs) in nursing home residents with depression have had mixed results, some consistent with the findings of Magai et al. (2000), suggesting that SSRIs may be less effective for depression in patients with dementia than in those who are cognitively intact (Oslin et al. 2000; Rosen et al. 2000; Trappler and Cohen 1996, 1998).

Although the SSRIs might be expected to be well tolerated by frail elderly nursing home patients because of their side-effect profile, evidence indicates that these drugs can cause serious adverse events in this population. Thapa et al. (1998) found that the use of SSRIs was associated with a nearly twofold increase in the risk of falls in nursing home residents, comparable with the risk found with tricyclic antidepressant drugs. Investigators in the United Kingdom reported that antidepressant use was associated with better physical functioning but also with greater frequency of falls in residential care patients (Arthur et al. 2002). A randomized, double-blind comparison trial found that venlafaxine was less well tolerated compared with sertraline in frail nursing home patients without conferring more treatment benefits, as might be expected from an agent with mixed serotonergic and noradrenergic effects (Oslin et al. 2003).

History of Deficient Mental Health Care as an Impetus for Nursing Home Reform

Although psychiatric disorders are extraordinarily common among nursing home residents, and efficacious treatments exist, psychiatric services are often not adequate. Historically, nursing home design, staffing, programs, services, and funding have not evolved to meet the needs of patients with mental disorders (Reichman and Conn 2010; Streim and Katz 1994). This mismatch of psychiatric needs and available treatment led not only to neglect but also to inappropriate treatment; psychiatric problems were often mismanaged by using physical or chemical restraints.

Physical Restraints

A 1977 survey of American nursing home residents showed that 25% of 1.3 million people were being restrained by geriatric chairs, cuffs, belts, or similar devices, primarily in an attempt to control behavioral symptoms (National Center for Health Statistics 1979). Other early surveys found rates of restraint as high as 85%. Patient factors predicting the use of restraints, in addition to agitation and behavior problems, include age, cognitive impairment, risk of injuries to self (e.g., from falls) or others (e.g., from combative behavior), physical frailty, the presence of monitoring or treatment devices, and the need to promote body alignment. Institutional and systemic factors associated with restraint use include pressure to avoid litigation, staff attitudes, insufficient staffing, and the availability of restraint devices. Potential adverse effects include an increased risk of falls and other injuries (Capezuti et al. 1996) as well as functional decline, skin breakdown, physiological effects of immobilization stress, disorganized behavior, and demoralization. Although mechanical restraints frequently have been used in attempts to control agitation, they do not in fact decrease behavioral disturbances (Werner et al. 1989), and cross-national studies indicated that nursing home residents can be managed without such measures (Cape 1983; Evans and Strumpf 1989; Innes and Turman 1983).

Misuse of Psychotropic Drugs

Concerns about inadequate and inappropriate care also have focused on the overuse of psychotropic drugs in nursing home residents, especially the misuse of these drugs as "chemical restraints" to control patient behaviors. Studies in the 1970s and 1980s reported that approximately 50% of residents had orders for psychotropic medications, with 20%–40% being given antipsychotic drugs, 10%–40% given anxiolytics or hypnotics, and 5%–10% given antidepressants (Avorn et al. 1989; Beers et al. 1988; Buck 1988; Burns et al. 1988; Cohen-Mansfield 1986; Custer et al. 1984; DeLeo et al. 1989; Ray et al. 1980; Teeter et al. 1976; Zimmer et al. 1984). Psychotropic drugs were frequently prescribed without adequate regard for the residents' psychiatric diagnosis or medical status. In one study, Zimmer et al. (1984) reported that only 15% of the residents being given psychotropic drugs had received a psychiatric consultation. Other studies reported that 21% of patients without a psychiatric diagnosis were receiving psychotropic medication (Burns et al. 1988), that physicians'—as opposed to patients'—characteristics predicted drug dosages (Ray et al. 1980), and that psychotropic drugs often were prescribed in the absence of any documentation of the patient's mental status in the clinical record (Avorn et al. 1989).

The greatest concerns about inappropriate overprescribing of medications have related to the misuse of antipsychotic drugs as chemical restraints to control residents' behaviors. In light of concerns about balancing safety and efficacy of antipsychotic drugs in managing psychosis and agitation in nursing home residents with dementia, patients with nonpsychotic behavior problems may be more appropriately managed with other medications, behavioral treatments, interpersonal approaches, or environmental interventions. Moreover, it is important to note that although all the evidence for the efficacy of antipsychotic medications comes from short-term studies, these medications are frequently prescribed for long-term treatment. In this context, concerns about overuse of antipsychotic drugs were supported by findings from drug discontinuation studies (cited earlier). One classic double-blind study of neuroleptic withdrawal found that only 16% of the patients who had been receiving medications on a chronic basis experienced significant deterioration when the drugs were withdrawn (Barton and Hurst 1966). A subsequent small-scale withdrawal study in patients who had been receiving neuroleptics for several months showed that 22% experienced increased agitation on withdrawal, indicating a need for continued treatment, but that 22% were unchanged and 55% actually showed improvement (Risse et al. 1987).

Inadequate Treatment of Depression

Although the focus of public concern and regulatory scrutiny in the 1970s and 1980s was on overprescription of antipsychotic medications in patients with dementia, undertreatment of other psychiatric conditions in the nursing home also has been a serious problem. The Institute of Medicine Committee on Nursing Home Regulation (1986) report "Improving the Quality of

Care in Nursing Homes," which did much to stimulate nursing home reform in the United States, highlighted problems both in the overuse of antipsychotic drugs and in the underuse of antidepressants for treatment of affective disorders. Similarly, in reviewing epidemiological studies on the use of psychotropics in nursing homes, Murphy (1989) noted that antidepressants were the one class of drugs that appeared to be underused and that, as a result, major depression in this setting often remained untreated.

Federal Regulations and Psychiatric Care in the Nursing Home

The misuse of physical and chemical restraints was a rallying point for advocacy groups that urged the federal government to institute a process of nursing home reform. In addition, the U.S. General Accounting Office was concerned that states were admitting individuals with chronic and severe psychiatric problems to Medicaid-certified nursing homes not because the patients needed this type of care but because admission would shift a substantial portion of the costs of patients' care from the state to the federal government. Apparently in response to both sets of concerns, Congress enacted the Nursing Home Reform Act as part of the Omnibus Budget Reconciliation Act of 1987 (OBRA '87; P.L. 100-203). This legislation provided for government regulation of the operation of nursing facilities and of the care that they provide (Elon and Pawlson 1992). As part of this legislation, the Health Care Financing Administration (HCFA)— reorganized and renamed in 2001 as the Centers for Medicare and Medicaid Services

(CMS)—was empowered to issue regulations (Health Care Financing Administration 1991) that operationalize the laws and to develop guidelines (Centers for Medicare and Medicaid Services 2011) that assist federal and state surveyors in interpreting the regulations. Mental health screening, assessment, care planning, and treatment are addressed under sections of the regulations that pertain to nursing home resident assessment, resident rights and facility practices, and quality of care (Health Care Financing Administration 1991, 1992a, 1992b).

Regulations requiring comprehensive assessment for all residents (Health Care Financing Administration 1991) have led to development of a uniform Resident Assessment Instrument, which includes the Minimum Data Set (MDS) (Morris et al. 1990), an updated version of which was implemented in 2010 (Centers for Medicare and Medicaid Services 2010). This instrument must be administered on a regular basis by members of an interdisciplinary health care team (Health Care Financing Administration 1992c). Areas of assessment relevant to mental illness and behavior include mood, cognition, communication, functional status, medications, and other treatments. Responses on the MDS may indicate changes in a patient's clinical status that warrant further evaluation and possible need for changes in the treatment plan.

Regulations related to resident rights and facility practices restrict the use of physical restraints and antipsychotic medications when they are "administered for purposes of discipline or convenience and not required to treat the resident's medical symptoms" (Health Care Financing Administration 1991, p. 48,875). Regulations related to quality of care further require that residents not receive "unnecessary drugs" and specify that antipsychotic medications may not be given "unless these are necessary to treat a specific condition as diagnosed and documented in the clinical record" (p. 48,910). An *unnecessary drug* is defined as any drug that is used 1) in excessive dose (including duplicate therapy), 2) for excessive duration, 3) without adequate monitoring, 4) without adequate indications for its use, 5) in the presence of adverse consequences that indicate that it should be reduced or discontinued, or 6) for any combination of the first five reasons (Health Care Financing Administration 1991). The guidelines based on these regulations additionally limit the use of antipsychotic medications, antianxiety agents, sedative-hypnotic agents, and related medications (Centers for Medicare and Medicaid Services 2011). For each of these medication classes, the guidelines specify a list of acceptable indications, upper limits for daily dosages, requirements for monitoring treatment and adverse effects, and time frames for attempting dosage reductions and discontinuation. These guidelines are periodically updated to reflect new clinical knowledge and the availability of new drugs approved by the FDA (Centers for Medicare and Medicaid Services 2011).

To minimize concerns about federal interference with medical practice, the current guidelines include qualifying statements that recognize cases in which strict adherence to medication prescribing limits or gradual dosage reduction or discontinuation is "clinically contraindicated." Thus, the physician's options for treating nursing home residents need not be unduly restricted by the regulations if the clinical rationale—explaining that the benefits of treatment (in terms of symptom relief, improved health status, or improved functioning) outweigh the risks—is clearly documented in the medical record. Although the facility, not the physician, is accountable for compliance with the regulations, the physician's clinical reasoning and judgment play a critical role in the process of ensuring quality care.

Although much of the emphasis of the federal regulations is on eliminating inappropriate treatment, requirements are also included for the provision of necessary and appropriate care for nursing home residents with mental health problems. Under the provisions designed to ensure quality of care, federal regulations define a need for geriatric psychiatry services in nursing homes, requiring that "the facility must ensure that a resident who displays mental or psychosocial adjustment difficulties receives appropriate services to correct the assessed problem" (Health Care Financing Administration 1991, p. 48,896). More recently, acting within the scope of its responsibility as a payer, CMS developed a system for assessing the quality of care provided in nursing homes in the United States. To enable surveyors to compare individual facilities within the same state, CMS introduced quality indicators derived from MDS data (Nursing Home Quality Indicators Development Group 1999). There are 24 quality indicators in 11 different domains, including behavior and emotional problems, cognitive patterns, and psychotropic drug use.

Whenever a review in any of these areas results in a citation of deficiency, a plan of correction must be developed and submitted for approval. This system is a first step in monitoring quality of care, although the face validity of some of the quality indicators has been questioned, and the results of quality surveys may be difficult to interpret. Nevertheless, the results from every nursing home surveyed are available for public in-

spection, and consumers of nursing home services (and their families) can access the quality indicators reports online.

Changing Patterns of Psychiatric Care

Since the implementation of the Nursing Home Reform Act in 1990, there have been significant changes in nursing home care, including mental health care. Some of these changes may be attributed to the process of conducting surveys and enforcing federal regulations; however, several other factors appear to have contributed, including the dissemination of information about regulatory requirements, availability and marketing of new medications, advances in scientific knowledge from nursing home research, and cumulative effects of professional education regarding good clinical practice. Public reporting of quality indicators and increasing consumer awareness are also likely to be playing a role.

Shifts in Antipsychotic Medication Use

Studies of the effect of federal regulations in the early years after implementation showed a substantial decline in the use of antipsychotic drugs (Shorr et al. 1994) and physical restraints (Hawes et al. 1997) and increases in antidepressant use (Lantz et al. 1996). Between 1991 and 1997, a 52.2% decrease (from 33.7% to 16.1%) in the use of antipsychotic medications was reported (Hughes et al. 2000). Soon after the regulations were introduced, several investigators developed educational programs for physicians, nurses, and aides to teach practice principles consistent with federal guidelines. Studies evaluating these educational interventions reported reductions of 23%–72% in the use of anti-psychotic medication (Avorn et al. 1992; Meador et al. 1997; Ray et al. 1993; Rovner et al. 1992; Schnelle et al. 1992). Studies of the appropriateness of antipsychotic medication use, examining documentation of OBRA '87–approved diagnostic indications and appropriate target symptoms, as well as dosing within the recommended limits in the HCFA guidelines, suggested relatively high rates of compliance with OBRA '87 regulations (Llorente et al. 1998; Siegler et al. 1997).

Although the changes found by the studies generally were interpreted as an indication of improvement in care, the studies did not examine health care outcomes or effects on residents' quality of life (Snowden and Roy-Byrne 1998) and did not address concerns that reductions in medication use might have an adverse effect on patients who required antipsychotic treatment. In contrast to the declining rates of antipsychotic use in the early 1990s, Online Survey Certification and Reporting (OSCAR) data showed a reversal in this trend from 1995 to 1999, with the national rate for antipsychotic drug use in nursing homes increasing from 16% to 19.4% during that period (American Society of Consultant Pharmacists 2000). Despite this increase, a survey conducted by the Office of the Inspector General of the Department of Health and Human Services, based on data from the year 2000, found that psychotropic drugs were appropriately prescribed in 85% of 485 cases reviewed (Office of Inspector General 2001). However, the findings of the Office of the Inspector General are contra-dicted by a large retrospective analysis of Medicare databases merged to MDS assessments from the same time period (Briesacher et al. 2005). In this analysis, 27.6% of all Medicare beneficiaries in nursing homes re-ceived antipsychotic medications between 2000 and 2001; of the treated patients, only 41.8% received antipsychotic therapy within federal prescribing guidelines. A cross-sectional analysis of the 2004 National Nursing Home Survey similarly identified that 26% of the nursing home residents used antipsychotic medication; 40% of these cases were without appropriate indications for antipsychotic use (Stevenson et al. 2010).

The increased rates of antipsychotic medication use, coupled with the safety concerns related to the risk of cerebrovascular adverse events and mortality, have prompted a closer look at alternatives to antipsychotic drug treatment of behavioral disturbances in nursing home residents with dementia. A study by Fossey et al. (2006), conducted in the wake of the safety findings described earlier in this chapter, examined 12-month outcomes of an intervention that provided training and support to nursing home staff in psychosocial approaches for managing agitated behavior associated with dementia. The rate of antipsychotic medication use was 19.1% lower in the intervention homes, with no significant differences in the level of agitated or disruptive behavior between intervention and control facilities. Thus, it appears that a significant proportion of residents may be managed with less risk without a concomitant increase in behavior problems. Nevertheless, changes in the prevalence of antipsychotic medication use specifically in response to safety concerns have not yet been documented in nursing home populations.

Increase in Antidepressant Drug Use

Despite the decline in use of antipsychotic drugs in the early 1990s, it has been estimated that the overall use of psychotherapeutic medications in U.S. nursing homes actually increased, from 21.7% in 1991 to 46.1% in 1997 (Hughes et al. 2000). This increase was partly attributable to a rise in the use of antidepressants from 12.6% to 24.9% (a 97.6% increase) during that period. Rates of antidepressant use similarly increased in the United Kingdom, from 11% in 1990 to 18.9% in 1997 (Arthur et al. 2002). Since the mid-1990s, there have been continued substantial increases in the prevalence of antidepressant medication use. A study of 12 Pennsylvania nursing homes conducted a decade ago found that 47.6% of the residents were taking antidepressant agents (Datto et al. 2002), a level consistent with national rates of use over the past decade. OSCAR data from more than 12,000 U.S. nursing homes showed an increase in antidepressant prescribing from 21.9% in 1996 to 47.5% in 2006 (Hanlon et al. 2010). Prior to 1990, fewer than 15% of the residents with a known diagnosis of depression were receiving antidepressant medication (Heston et al. 1992).

Considered together, these data represent an extraordinary change in the pattern of drug use in a population that has traditionally received inadequate pharmacotherapy for depression. The dramatic increase in antidepressant prescriptions is probably due in part to the wide availability of newer antidepressants that were thought to be well tolerated by elderly nursing home residents with medical and psychiatric comorbidity. Aggressive marketing to primary care physicians also may play a role. With current antidepressant drug use rates that appear comparable to or greater than the estimated prevalence of depression in nursing homes, it is possible that a significant proportion of antidepressant prescriptions are intended for indications other than depression, such

as insomnia, pain, anxiety, or agitation. Research is needed to determine whether the reported changes in prescribing have had a positive effect on the mental health of nursing home residents with depression.

Decline in Physical Restraint Use

Although questions remain about the interpretation of trends in the use of psychotropic drugs (Lantz et al. 1996), the effect of the federal regulations on restraints appears to be positive, with several studies showing significant reductions in the use of physical restraints (Castle et al. 1997). One study found restraint use rates of 37.4% in 1990 (before OBRA '87 implementation in October 1990) and 28.1% in 1993 (after introduction of the standardized Resident Assessment Instrument required by OBRA '87) (Hawes et al. 1997). Siegler et al. (1997) found that restraint use could be significantly reduced without a resultant increase in antipsychotic or benzodiazepine use. No published evidence of an increase in fall-related injuries is associated with lower rates of physical restraint use.

Special Care Units

Encouraged by consumer demand to better meet the needs of nursing home residents with dementia, 10% of U.S. nursing homes had established special care units (SCUs) by 1991. A decade later, it was estimated that 22% of nursing homes had designated SCUs for patients with dementia. In the 2004 National Nursing Home Survey, 23.8% of the facilities reported having special programs for the management of behavior problems, although not all of these were provided exclusively on a dedicated SCU (National Center for Health Statistics 2004).

Research on the effectiveness of SCUs is difficult to interpret and generalize because of the heterogeneity of these facilities (Office of Technology Assessment 1992; Ohta and Ohta 1988). Some studies indicate that the facilities, services, and programs offered by SCUs may not be significantly better than those available on conventional nursing home units. A case-control study of 625 patients in 31 SCUs and 32 traditional units found that residence in an SCU was associated with reduced use of physical restraints but not with less use of "pharmacological restraints" (Sloane et al. 1991). A subsequent study that included data on more than 1,100 residents in 48 SCUs reported that the use of physical restraints was not different, and the likelihood of psychotropic medication use was actually greater, for patients on SCUs than for their counterparts on traditional units (Phillips et al. 2000). Although evidence suggests that mobility may be maintained for longer periods among residents of SCUs (Saxton et al. 1998), others have found that the rate of decline in ADL function is not significantly slower for SCU residents (Phillips et al. 1997). Studies showing benefits of SCUs for behavioral disturbances are limited, although one randomized clinical trial reported a reduced frequency of catastrophic reactions (Swanson et al. 1993)—sudden agitated behavior in response to overwhelming external stimuli—as a positive outcome for residence on a dementia SCU. Some studies have identified psychological benefits not only for patients (Lawton et al. 1998) but also for caregivers (Kutner et al. 1999; Wells and Jorm 1987), with evidence of increased family involvement (Hansen et al. 1988; Sloane et al. 1998).

Despite the efforts of these investigators, knowledge about the essential elements of treatment in SCUs is still insufficient, and evidence for the effectiveness of these units has not been adequately established.

Subacute Care in Nursing Homes

Over the past 30 years, many patients have been discharged to nursing homes that serve as step-down facilities, providing subacute medical treatment, convalescent care, and rehabilitation services. It has been estimated that subacute-care patients constitute about one-third of nursing home admissions in the United States.

In general, short-stay residents—patients who, after relatively brief stays in nursing homes, are discharged to the community or die—differ from long-term care patients in that they are younger; more likely to be admitted directly from an acute-care hospital; less likely to have irreversible cognitive impairment, incontinence, or ambulatory dysfunction; and more likely to have a primary diagnosis of hip fracture, stroke, or cancer. The objectives of mental health care for short-stay patients are related not so much to managing behavior problems associated with dementia as to helping patients cope with disease and disability, to searching for delirium and reversible causes of cognitive impairment, and to treating disorders such as depression and anxiety that can be impediments to rehabilitation and recovery. In short, the objectives of mental health care for these patients are similar to goals of traditional consultation-liaison psychiatry in the general hospital. As the opportunities for psychiatric intervention follow these patients from the acute-care hospital into the nursing homes, the services required may need to be more frequent or intensive than those usually available to long-term care residents. For subacute-care patients in nursing homes, an investment in psychiatric care can lead to improved participation in rehabilitation efforts, with more efficient recovery and return to independent functioning and more rapid discharge to the community. It is hoped that the benefits of mental health care, in terms of both cost offsets and improved quality of life, will provide a strong incentive for insurers, public and private, to establish reimbursement policies that facilitate such treatment.

Adequacy of Care

The high prevalence of psychiatric problems and the federal mandate to ensure quality of care define a need for geriatric mental health services in nursing homes (Smith et al. 1990). Although the OBRA '87 regulations are having the intended effect (Snowden and Roy-Byrne 1998) and have resulted in measurable improvements in patient care, concurrent improvements in access to mental health care, receipt of appropriate care, or health care outcomes have not been seen. Medicare claims data in 1992, 2 years after implementation of the Nursing Home Reform Act of 1987, indicated that only 26% of all nursing home residents and 36% of residents with a mental illness received psychiatric services (Smyer et al. 1994), and evidence shows continued low levels of mental health treatment in nursing homes (Reichman and Conn 2010; Shea et al. 2000).

Limited access to care appears to be at least part of the problem. In a survey of nursing homes across six states, conducted by Reichman et al. (1998), 47.6% of 899 respondents indicated that the frequency of on-site psychiatric consultation was inadequate. The 2004 National Nursing Home Survey similarly reported that only 40.4% of

nursing homes had mental health services available at the facility, and only 48.5% had formal contracts for psychology or psychiatry services (National Center for Health Statistics 2004). Directors of nursing judged 38% of nursing home residents as needing a psychiatric evaluation, but more than one-fourth of rural facilities and more than one-fifth of small facilities reported that no psychiatric consultant was available to them. Thus, evidence indicates that the federal requirement that patients receive services to "attain or maintain the highest practicable physical, mental, and psychosocial well-being" has not remedied the problem of access to mental health services in U.S. nursing homes (Colenda et al. 1999).

Even among patients whose mental disorders are recognized and for whom treatment is initiated, evidence shows that treatment is often inadequate. A report by Brown et al. (2002) indicated that of nursing home residents known to be depressed and receiving antidepressants, 32% were taking dosages lower than the manufacturers' recommended minimum effective dosage for treating depression. In a survey of 12 nursing homes, Datto et al. (2002) found that 47% of patients were taking antidepressants, but nearly half of these patients were still depressed. Although a small proportion of these residents may have been in the early stages of treatment, before a treatment response could reasonably be expected, it appears likely that many residents did not receive proper follow-up care with required dosage adjustments or changes in therapy for those who were not responsive to initial treatment. This finding points to a need for nursing home providers to improve adherence to practice guidelines for the follow-up care of depression.

A federal quality indicator introduced in 1999 focused on persistence of depression

(Nursing Home Quality Indicators Development Group 1999). Prescription of an antidepressant suggests that depression has been recognized and diagnosed and that the first step has been taken to manage it. However, persistence of depression in a patient who is receiving an antidepressant drug suggests that the treatment may not be adequate. Thus, if the proportion of depressed patients receiving antidepressants is high, it may indicate that the facility is doing a good job of recognizing depression and initiating treatment, but it also may suggest that it is not doing an adequate job of monitoring patients' response to treatment and modifying treatments as needed to produce optimal outcomes. Clearly, care processes need to be improved, and the federal quality indicators for depression care in the nursing home must be further refined. For a more comprehensive treatment of this subject, the reader is referred to consensus recommendations for improving the quality of mental health care in nursing homes (American Geriatrics Society and American Association for Geriatric Psychiatry 2003).

Mental Health Care in Nursing Homes: A Model for Service Delivery

The high prevalence of psychiatric disorders in nursing homes argues for the importance of establishing systems that incorporate mental health into the basic services provided (Borson et al. 1987). In addition, several factors argue for the importance of the professional components of care: 1) the complex nature of the psychiatric disorders in nursing home residents, 2) the need to evaluate medical as well as social and environmental factors as causes of mental health problems, 3) the potential benefits of specific treatments, and 4) the need for careful monitoring to assess treatment responses and prevent serious adverse effects of medications. Thus, clinical needs demand that mental health services in nursing homes have two distinct but interacting systems: one that is intrinsic to the facility and is contextual and another that is professional and is concerned primarily with the delivery of specific treatments.

It has been suggested that mental health training should be provided to facility staff to develop basic skills in assessment and clinical management that can help staff handle problems that occur when specific professional services are lacking. However, it is important to recognize that the intrinsic and the professional systems cannot readily replace each other and that adequate care requires both. Although a real need exists for staff training, a realistic goal is to develop staff skills that complement rather than replace the activities of mental health professionals. This two-system model has obvious implications with respect to the financing of mental health services in nursing homes: it establishes the need to fund mental health care both as a necessary part of the per diem costs of nursing home care and as a reimbursable professional service.

Although the intrinsic and the professional systems for mental health services are distinct, they must interact: geriatric psychiatrists and psychologists and geropsychiatric nurse practitioners can play important intrinsic roles as administrative and staff consultants, in-service educators, moderators of case conferences, participants in interdisciplinary team meetings, and contributors in other activities familiar to the consultation-liaison psychiatrist. Facility staff must be effective in recognizing problems, facilitating referral, supporting treatment, and monitoring outcome to enable the professional system to function optimally.

Intrinsic System

The intrinsic system of mental health care in nursing homes can be conceptualized as including a wide range of components: design of the environment; implementation of psychosocial programs; formulation of institutional policies and procedures for assessment, care delivery, monitoring, and quality improvement; and optimization of the ways in which staff and residents interact. The importance of the intrinsic system is recognized in nursing home regulations that require training of nursing aides; in the nursing staff assessments required for completion of the MDS; and in OBRA '87 requirements that nursing homes provide assessment, treatment planning, and services to attain or maintain the highest practicable level of mental and physical well-being for each resident. Because psychiatric disorders are common in nursing homes, nurses and aides should be knowledgeable about the nature of the cognitive and functional deficits associated with dementia and the manifestations of delirium and depression. Staff members should understand how to modify their approach to working with residents when cognitive impairment or communication deficits interfere with care. Staff also should know how to apply basic principles of behavioral psychology to identify the causes of agitation and related behavioral symptoms in patients with dementia as well as how to plan environmental and behavioral interventions.

Professional System

The intrinsic system for mental health services as just described is necessary but not sufficient to meet the needs of nursing home residents. In addition, the services of mental health professionals are important in evaluating the interactions between medical and mental health problems, in establishing psychiatric diagnoses, and in planning and administering specific treatments for mental disorders. This component of the professional system must encompass medically oriented psychiatric care, including psychopharmacological treatment. A position statement by the major provider groups in this field (American Association for Geriatric Psychiatry et al. 1992) acknowledged the history of misuse of psychotropic drugs in nursing homes, but the statement emphasized that psychopharmacological treatment of diagnosed mental disorders is an important part of the medical and mental health care of nursing home residents. The complexity of psychopharmacological treatment in frail nursing home residents with medical comorbidity requires that the skills of psychiatrists knowledgeable in geriatrics be an integral part of the professional system.

The professional system should include care with a psychosocial and a biomedical focus. For example, psychiatrists, psychologists, and psychiatric nurse practitioners and advanced practice nurses with specific expertise in behavioral treatment may be successful in evaluating the antecedents and causes of agitation and related symptoms among patients with dementia and in developing environmental and behavioral interventions, even when efforts by the facility's nursing staff have proven ineffective. Integration of the professional and intrinsic components of mental health care in the nursing home is required because of the inherent interdependence of these systems. To conduct valid assessments and make diagnoses, mental health professionals must rely on nursing home staff to report their shift-by-shift observations of residents' behavior and other clinical signs. Mental health professionals also must depend on nursing home staff to implement and monitor the treatments they prescribe. Conversely, to succeed in providing appropriate mental health care to nursing home residents, staff members in the intrinsic system must have access to ongoing consultation from, and must receive direct support from, mental health professionals who are knowledgeable in geriatrics.

Key Points

- According to the 2004 National Nursing Home Survey, 4% of Americans age 65 years or older—1.5 million people—resided in 16,100 long-term care facilities.

- Epidemiological studies have consistently shown that 80%–94% of nursing home residents have diagnosable psychiatric disorders. These prevalence data suggest that nursing homes are de facto neuropsychiatric institutions, although they were not originally intended for this purpose.

- Since the implementation of federal nursing home regulations in 1991, the rate of antipsychotic medication use has declined, and the use of antidepressants has increased. However, approximately half of nursing home residents who are receiving antidepressant medications continue to have symptoms of depression.

- Since 2003, analyses of safety data from randomized controlled studies of atypical antipsychotic drugs in elderly patients with dementia, including nursing home studies, have found significantly increased risks of cerebrovascular adverse events and mortality in this population.

- Although mechanical restraints frequently have been used in attempts to control agitation, they do not decrease behavioral disturbances, and cross-national studies have indicated that it is possible to manage nursing home residents without such measures.

- The social environment within which care is provided can have a significant effect on nursing home residents; environmental design should be viewed as a component of mental health care.

References

Abraham IL, Neundorfer MM, Currie LJ: Effects of group interventions on cognition and depression in nursing home residents. Nurs Res 41:196–202, 1992

Abraham IL, Onega LL, Reel SJ, et al: Effects of cognitive group interventions on depressed frail nursing home residents, in Depression in Long Term and Residential Care: Advances in Research and Treatment. Edited by Rubinstein RL, Lawton MP. New York, Springer, 1997, pp 154–168

Ahmed A, Lefante CM, Alam N: Depression and nursing home admission among hospitalized older adults with coronary artery disease: a propensity score analysis. Am J Geriatr Cardiol 16:76–83, 2007

Alessi CA: A randomized trial of a combined physical activity and environmental intervention in nursing home residents: do sleep and agitation improve? J Am Geriatr Soc 47:784–791, 1999

American Association for Geriatric Psychiatry, American Geriatrics Society, American Psychiatric Association: Psychotherapeutic medications in the nursing home. J Am Geriatr Soc 40:946–949, 1992

American Geriatrics Society, American Association for Geriatric Psychiatry: The American Geriatrics Society and American Association for Geriatric Psychiatry recommendations for policies in support of quality mental health care in U.S. nursing homes. J Am Geriatr Soc 51:1299–1304, 2003

American Psychiatric Association: Diagnostic and Statistical Manual of Mental Disorders, 3rd Edition. Washington, DC, American Psychiatric Association, 1980

American Psychiatric Association: Diagnostic and Statistical Manual of Mental Disorders, 3rd Edition, Revised. Washington, DC, American Psychiatric Association, 1987

American Society of Consultant Pharmacists: Fact Sheet. Alexandria, VA, American Society of Consultant Pharmacists, September 2000

Ames D, Ashby D, Mann AH, et al: Psychiatric illness in elderly residents of part III homes in one London borough: prognosis and review. Age Ageing 17:249–256, 1988

Arthur A, Matthews R, Jagger C, et al: Factors associated with antidepressant treatment in residential care: changes between 1990 and 1997. Int J Geriatr Psychiatry 17:54–60, 2002

Ashby D, Ames D, West CR, et al: Psychiatric morbidity as prediction of mortality for residents of local authority homes for the elderly. Int J Geriatr Psychiatry 6:567–575, 1991

Avorn J, Dreyer P, Connelly K, et al: Use of psychoactive medication and the quality of care in rest homes: findings and policy implications of a statewide study. N Engl J Med 320:227–232, 1989

Avorn J, Soumerai SD, Everitt DE, et al: A randomized trial of a program to reduce the use of psychoactive drugs in nursing homes. N Engl J Med 327:168–173, 1992

Baines S, Saxby P, Ehlert K: Reality orientation and reminiscence therapy. Br J Psychiatry 151:222–231, 1987

Baker FM, Miller CL: Screening a skilled nursing home population for depression. J Geriatr Psychiatry Neurol 4:218–221, 1991

Ballard CG, Margallo-Lana M, Fossey J, et al: A 1-year follow-up study of behavioral and psychological symptoms in dementia among people in care environments. J Clin Psychiatry 62:631–636, 2001

Barnes R, Raskind MA: DSM-III criteria and the clinical diagnosis of dementia: a nursing home study. J Gerontol 36:20–27, 1980

Barnes R, Veith R, Okimoto J, et al: Efficacy of antipsychotic medications in behaviorally disturbed dementia patients. Am J Psychiatry 139:1170–1174, 1982

Bartels SJ, Horn SD, Smout RJ, et al: Agitation and depression in frail nursing home elderly patients with dementia: treatment characteristics and service use. Am J Geriatr Psychiatry 11:231–238, 2003

Barton R, Hurst L: Unnecessary use of tranquilizers in elderly patients. Br J Psychiatry 112:989–990, 1966

Beck CK, Vogelpohl TS, Rasin JH, et al: Effects of behavioral interventions on disruptive behavior and affect in demented nursing home residents. Nurs Res 51:219–228, 2002

Beers M, Avon J, Soumerai SB, et al: Psychoactive medication use in intermediate-care facility residents. JAMA 260:3016–3020, 1988

Bensink GW, Godbey KL, Marshall MJ, et al: Institutionalized elderly: relaxation, locus of control, self-esteem. J Gerontol Nurs 18:30–36, 1992

Berrios GE, Brook P: Delusions and psychopathology of the elderly with dementia. Acta Psychiatr Scand 75:296–301, 1985

Bharucha AJ, Dew MA, Miller MD, et al: Psychotherapy in long-term care: a review. J Am Med Dir Assoc 7:568–580, 2006

Blazer DG, Williams CD: Epidemiology of dysphoria and depression in an elderly population. Am J Psychiatry 137:439–444, 1980

Borson S, Liptzin B, Nininger J, et al: Psychiatry and the nursing home. Am J Psychiatry 144:1412–1418, 1987

Braun JV, Wykle MH, Cowling WR: Failure to thrive in older persons: a concept derived. Gerontologist 28:809–812, 1988

Bridges-Parlet S, Knopman D, Steffes S: Withdrawal of neuroleptic medications from institutionalized dementia patients: results of a double-blind, baseline-treatment-controlled pilot study. J Geriatr Psychiatry Neurol 10:119–126, 1997

Briesacher BA, Limcangco R, Simoni-Wastila L, et al: The quality of antipsychotic drug prescribing in nursing homes. Arch Intern Med 165:1280–1285, 2005

Brodaty H, Ames D, Snowdon J, et al: A randomized placebo-controlled trial of risperidone for the treatment of aggression, agitation, and psychosis of dementia. J Clin Psychiatry 64:134–143, 2003

Brown MN, Lapane KL, Luisi AF: The management of depression in older nursing home residents. J Am Geriatr Soc 50:69–76, 2002

Buck JA: Psychotropic drug practice in nursing homes. J Am Geriatr Soc 36:409–418, 1988

Burns BJ, Larson DB, Goldstrom ID, et al: Mental disorder among nursing home patients: preliminary findings from the National Nursing Home Survey Pretest. Int J Geriatr Psychiatry 3:27–35, 1988

Buttar AB, Mhyre J, Fries BE, et al: Six-month cognitive improvement in nursing home residents with severe cognitive impairment. J Geriatr Psychiatry Neurol 16:100–108, 2003

Cape RD: Freedom from restraint. Gerontologist 23:217, 1983

Capezuti E, Evans L, Strumpf N, et al: Physical restraint use and falls in nursing home residents. J Am Geriatr Soc 44:627–633, 1996

Castle NG, Fogel B, Mor V: Risk factors for physical restraint use in nursing homes: pre- and post-implementation of the Nursing Home Reform Act. Gerontologist 37:737–747, 1997

Centers for Medicare and Medicaid Services: Nursing home quality initiatives: MDS 3.0 Technical Information. Baltimore, MD, Centers for Medicare and Medicaid, 2010. Available at: https://www.cms.gov/NursingHomeQualityInits/30_NHQIMDS30TechnicalInformation.asp#TopOfPage. Accessed November 7, 2011.

Centers for Medicare and Medicaid Services: State Operations Manual, Appendix PP—Guidance to Surveyors for Long Term Care Facilities; Rev 70, 01-07-11. Baltimore, MD, Centers for Medicare and Medicaid, 2011. Available at: https://www.cms.gov/manuals/Downloads/som107ap_pp_guidelines_ltcf.pdf. Accessed Accessed November 7, 2011.

Chandler JD, Chandler JE: The prevalence of neuropsychiatric disorders in a nursing home population. J Geriatr Psychiatry Neurol 1:71–76, 1988

Chao SY, Liu HY, Wu CY, et al: The effects of group reminiscence therapy on depression, self esteem, and life satisfaction of elderly nursing home residents. J Nurs Res 14:36–45, 2006

Cohen-Mansfield J: Agitated behaviors in the elderly: preliminary results in the cognitively deteriorated. J Am Geriatr Soc 34:722–727, 1986

Cohen-Mansfield J: Nonpharmacologic interventions for inappropriate behaviors in dementia: a review, summary, and critique. Am J Geriatr Psychiatry 9:361–381, 2001

Cohen-Mansfield J, Billig N: Agitated behaviors in the elderly: a conceptual review. J Am Geriatr Soc 34:711–721, 1986

Cohen-Mansfield J, Libin A: Verbal and physical non-aggressive agitated behaviors in elderly persons with dementia: robustness of syndromes. J Psychiatr Res 39:325–332, 2005

Cohen-Mansfield J, Lipson S, Werner P, et al: Withdrawal of haloperidol, thioridazine, and lorazepam in the nursing home: a controlled, double-blind study. Arch Intern Med 159:1733–1740, 1999

Colenda CC, Streim JE, Greene JA, et al: The impact of the Omnibus Budget Reconciliation Act of 1987 (OBRA '87) on psychiatric services in nursing homes. Am J Geriatr Psychiatry 7:12–17, 1999

Custer RL, Davis JE, Gee SC: Psychiatric drug usage in VA nursing home care units. Psychiatr Ann 14:285–292, 1984

Datto C, Oslin D, Streim J, et al: Pharmacological treatment of depression in nursing home residents: a mental health services perspective. J Geriatr Psychiatry Neurol 15:141–146, 2002

De Deyn PP, Rabheru K, Rasmussen A, et al: A randomized trial of risperidone, placebo, and haloperidol for behavioral symptoms of dementia. Neurology 53:946–955, 1999

De Deyn PP, Katz IR, Brodaty H, et al: Management of agitation, aggression, and psychosis associated with dementia: a pooled analysis including three randomized, placebo-controlled double-blind trials in nursing home residents treated with risperidone. Clin Neurol Neurosurg 107:497–508, 2005

DeLeo D, Stella AG, Spagnoli A: Prescription of psychotropic drugs in geriatric institutions. Int J Geriatr Psychiatry 4:11–16, 1989

Dwyer M, Byrne GJ: Disruptive vocalization and depression in older nursing home residents. Int Psychogeriatr 12:463–471, 2000

Elon R, Pawlson LG: The impact of OBRA on medical practice within nursing facilities. J Am Geriatr Soc 40:958–963, 1992

Engle VF, Graney MJ: Stability and improvement of health after nursing home admission. J Gerontol 48:S17–S23, 1993

Evans LK, Strumpf NE: Tying down the elderly: a review of the literature on physical restraint. J Am Geriatr Soc 37:65–74, 1989

Evans LK, Strumpf NE, Allen-Taylor SL, et al: A clinical trial to reduce restraints in nursing homes. J Am Geriatr Soc 45:675–681, 1997

Fenton J, Raskin A, Gruber-Baldini AL, et al: Some predictors of psychiatric consultation in nursing home residents. Am J Geriatr Psychiatry 12:297–304, 2004

Fossey J, Ballard C, Juszczak E, et al: Effect of enhanced psychosocial care on antipsychotic use in nursing home residents with severe dementia: cluster randomised trial. BMJ 332:756–761, 2006

German PS, Shapiro S, Kramer M: Nursing home study of eastern Baltimore epidemiologic catchment area, in Mental Illness in Nursing Homes: Agenda for Research. Edited by Harper MS, Lebowitz BD. Rockville, MD, National Institute of Mental Health, 1986, pp 21–40

Goldwasser AN, Auerbach SM, Harkins SW: Cognitive, affective, and behavioral effects of reminiscence group therapy of demented elderly. Int J Aging Hum Dev 25:209–222, 1987

Hanlon JT, Handler SM, Castle NG: Antidepressant prescribing in US nursing homes between 1996 and 2006 and its relationship to staffing patterns and use of other psychotropic medications. J Am Med Dir Assoc 11:320–324, 2010

Hansen SS, Patterson MA, Wilson RW: Family involvement on a dementia unit: the Resident Enrichment and Activity Program. Gerontologist 28:508–510, 1988

Harris Y: Depression as a risk factor for nursing home admission among older individuals. J Am Med Dir Assoc 8:14–20, 2007

Harris Y, Cooper JK: Depressive symptoms in older people predict nursing home admission. J Am Geriatr Soc 54:593–597, 2006

Hawes C, Mor V, Phillips CD, et al: The OBRA-87 nursing home regulations and implementation of the Resident Assessment Instrument: effects on process quality. J Am Geriatr Soc 45:977–985, 1997

Health Care Financing Administration: Medicare and Medicaid: Requirements for Long Term Care Facilities, Final Regulations. Fed Regist 56:48865–48921, 1991

Health Care Financing Administration: Medicare and Medicaid Programs: Preadmission Screening and Annual Resident Review. Fed Regist 57:56450–56504, 1992a

Health Care Financing Administration: Medicare and Medicaid: Resident Assessment in Long Term Care Facilities. Fed Regist 57:61614–61733, 1992b

Health Care Financing Administration: State Operations Manual: Provider Certification (Transmittal No 250). Washington, DC, Health Care Financing Administration, 1992c

Heeren O, Borin L, Raskin A, et al: Association of depression with agitation in elderly nursing home residents. J Geriatr Psychiatry Neurol 16:4–7, 2003

Heston LL, Garrard J, Makris L, et al: Inadequate treatment of depressed nursing home elderly. J Am Geriatr Soc 40:1117–1122, 1992

Hughes CM, Lapane KL, Mor V: Influence of facility characteristics on use of antipsychotic medications in nursing homes. Med Care 38:1164–1173, 2000

Hyer L, Blazer DG: Depressive symptoms: impact and problems in long term care facilities. International Journal of Behavioral Gerontology 1:33–44, 1982

Innes EM, Turman WG: Evolution of patient falls. Q Rev Biol 9:30–35, 1983

Institute of Medicine Committee on Nursing Home Regulation: Improving the Quality of Care in Nursing Homes. Washington, DC, National Academy Press, 1986

Jeste DV, Okamoto A, Napolitano J, et al: Low incidence of persistent tardive dyskinesia in elderly patients with dementia treated with risperidone. Am J Psychiatry 157:1150–1155, 2000

Katz IR, Lesher E, Kleban M, et al: Clinical features of depression in the nursing home. Int Psychogeriatr 1:5–15, 1989

Katz IR, Simpson GM, Curlik SM, et al: Pharmacological treatment of major depression for elderly patients in residential care settings. J Clin Psychiatry 51 (suppl):41–48, 1990

Katz IR, Parmelee P, Brubaker K: Toxic and metabolic encephalopathies in long-term care patients. Int Psychogeriatr 3:337–347, 1991

Katz IR, Beaston-Wimmer P, Parmelee PA, et al: Failure to thrive in the elderly: exploration of the concept and delineation of psychiatric components. J Geriatr Psychiatry Neurol 6:161–169, 1993

Katz IR, Jeste DV, Mintzer JE, et al: Comparison of risperidone and placebo for psychosis and behavioral disturbances associated with dementia: a randomized, double-blind trial. J Clin Psychiatry 60:107–115, 1999

Kaup BA, Loreck D, Gruber-Baldini AL, et al: Depression and its relationship to function and medical status, by dementia status, in nursing home admissions. Am J Geriatr Psychiatry 15:438–442, 2007

Kiely DK, Jones RN, Bergmann MA, et al: Association between delirium resolution and functional recovery among newly admitted postacute facility patients. J Gerontol A Biol Sci Med Sci 62:107–108, 2007

Kolanowski AM, Litaker M, Buettner L: Efficacy of theory-based activities for behavioral symptoms of dementia. Nurs Res 54:219–228, 2005

Kramer M, German PS, Anthony JC, et al: Patterns of mental disorders among the elderly residents of eastern Baltimore. J Am Geriatr Soc 33:236–245, 1985

Krauss NA, Altman BM: Characteristics of Nursing Home Residents, 1996. MEPS Research Findings No 5 (AHCPR Publ No 99-0006). Rockville, MD, Agency for Health Care Policy and Research, 1998

Kutner N, Mistretta E, Barnhart H, et al: Family members' perceptions of quality of life change in dementia SCU residents. J Appl Gerontol 18:423–439, 1999

Lantz MS, Giambanco V, Buchalter EN: A ten-year review of the effect of OBRA-87 on psychotropic prescribing practices in an academic nursing home. Psychiatr Serv 47:951–955, 1996

Lawton MP, Van Haitsma K, Klapper J, et al: A stimulation-retreat special care unit for elders with dementing illness. Int Psychogeriatr 10:379–395, 1998

Lesher E: Validation of the Geriatric Depression Scale among nursing home residents. Clinics in Gerontology 4:21–28, 1986

Levin CA, Wei W, Akincigil A, et al: Prevalence and treatment of diagnosed depression among elderly nursing home residents in Ohio. J Am Med Dir Assoc 8:585–594, 2007

Linkins KW, Lucca AM, Housman M, et al: Use of PASRR programs to assess serious mental illness and service access in nursing homes. Psychiatr Serv 57:325–332, 2006

Livingston G, Johnston K, Katona C, et al: Systematic review of psychological approaches to the management of neuropsychiatric symptoms of dementia. Am J Psychiatry 162:1996–2021, 2005

Llorente MD, Olsen EJ, Leyva O, et al: Use of antipsychotic drugs in nursing homes: current compliance with OBRA regulations. J Am Geriatr Soc 46:198–201, 1998

Loebel JP, Borson S, Hyde T, et al: Relationships between requests for psychiatric consultations and psychiatric diagnoses in long-term care facilities. Am J Psychiatry 148:898–903, 1991

Lopez OL, Becker JT, Wahed AS, et al. Long-term effects of the concomitant use of memantine with cholinesterase inhibition in Alzheimer disease. J Neurol Neurosurg Psychiatry 80:600–607, 2009

Lyketsos CG, Lindell Veiel L, Baker A, et al: A randomized, controlled trial of bright light therapy for agitated behaviors in dementia patients residing in long-term care. Int J Geriatr Psychiatry 14:520–525, 1999

Magai C, Kennedy G, Cohen CI, et al: A controlled clinical trial of sertraline in the treatment of depression in nursing home patients with late-stage Alzheimer's disease. Am J Geriatr Psychiatry 8:66–74, 2000

McMurdo MET, Rennie L: A controlled trial of exercise by residents of old people's homes. Age Ageing 22:11–15, 1993

Meador KG, Taylor JA, Thapa PB, et al: Predictors of antipsychotic withdrawal or dose reduction in a randomized controlled trial of provider education. J Am Geriatr Soc 45:207–210, 1997

Meehan KM, Wang H, David SR, et al: Comparison of rapidly acting intramuscular olanzapine, lorazepam, and placebo: a double-blind, randomized study in acutely agitated patients with dementia. Neuropsychopharmacology 26:494–504, 2002

Mintzer J, Greenspan A, Caers I, et al: Risperidone in the treatment of psychosis of Alzheimer disease: results from a prospective clinical trial. Am J Geriatr Psychiatry 14:280–291, 2006

Mintzer JE, Tune LE, Breder CD, et al: Aripiprazole for the treatment of psychoses in institutionalized patients with Alzheimer dementia: a multicenter, randomized, double-blind, placebo-controlled assessment of three fixed doses. Am J Geriatr Psychiatry 15:918–931, 2007

Moran JA, Gatz M: Group therapies for nursing home adults: an evaluation of two treatment approaches. Gerontologist 27:588–591, 1987

Morris JN, Hawes C, Fries BE, et al: Designing the national Resident Assessment Instrument for nursing homes. Gerontologist 30:293–307, 1990

Murphy E: The use of psychotropic drugs in long-term care (editorial). Int J Geriatr Psychiatry 4:1–2, 1989

National Center for Health Statistics: The National Nursing Home Survey (DHEW Publ No PHS-79-1794). Hyattsville, MD, National Center for Health Statistics, 1979

National Center for Health Statistics: Use of Nursing Homes by the Elderly: Preliminary Data From the 1985 National Nursing Home Survey (DHHS Publ No PHS-87-1250). Hyattsville, MD, National Center for Health Statistics, 1987

National Center for Health Statistics: The National Nursing Home Survey. Hyattsville, MD, National Center for Health Statistics, 2004. Available at: http://cdc.gov/nchs/nnhs.htm. Accessed December 26, 2007.

Nursing Home Quality Indicators Development Group: Facility Guide for the Nursing Home Quality Indicators. National Data System. September 28, 1999. Available at: http://www.cms.hhs.gov/MinimumData Sets20/Downloads/CHSRA% 20QI%20Fact% 20Sheet.pdf. Accessed August 6, 2008.

Office of Inspector General: Psychotropic Drug Use in Nursing Homes (Publ No OEI-02-00-00490). Washington, DC, U.S. Department of Health and Human Services, 2001. Available at: http://oig.hhs.gov/oei/reports/oei-02-00-00490. pdf. Accessed July 17, 2003.

Office of Technology Assessment: Special Care Units for People With Alzheimer's and Other Dementias: Consumer Education, Research, Regulatory, and Reimbursement Issues (OTA-H-543). Washington, DC, U.S. Government Printing Office, August 1992

Ohta RJ, Ohta BM: Special units for Alzheimer's disease patients: a critical look. Gerontologist 28:803–808, 1988

Olin JT, Fox LS, Pawluczyk S, et al: A pilot randomized trial of carbamazepine for behavioral symptoms in treatment-resistant outpatients with Alzheimer disease. Am J Geriatr Psychiatry 9:400–405, 2001

Omnibus Budget Reconciliation Act of 1987, Pub. L. No. 100-203. Subtitle C: Nursing home reform

Onder G, Liperoti R, Soldato M, et al: Depression and risk of nursing home admission among older adults in home care in Europe: results from the Aged in Home Care (AdHOC) study. J Clin Psychiatry 68:1392–1398, 2007

Orten JD, Allen M, Cook J: Reminiscence groups with confused nursing center residents: an experimental study. Soc Work Health Care 14:73–86, 1989

Oslin DW, Streim JE, Katz IR, et al: Heuristic comparison of sertraline with nortriptyline for the treatment of depression in frail elderly patients. Am J Geriatr Psychiatry 8:141–149, 2000

Oslin DW, Ten Have TR, Streim JE, et al: Probing the safety of medications in the frail elderly: evidence from a randomized clinical trial of sertraline and venlafaxine in depressed nursing home residents. J Clin Psychiatry 64:875–882, 2003

Parmelee PA, Katz IR, Lawton MP: Depression among institutionalized aged: assessment and prevalence estimation. J Gerontol 44:M22–M29, 1989

Parmelee PA, Katz IR, Lawton MP: The relation of pain to depression among institutionalized aged. J Gerontol 46:P15–P21, 1991

Parmelee PA, Katz IR, Lawton MP: Depression and mortality among institutionalized aged. J Gerontol 47:P3–P10, 1992a

Parmelee PA, Katz IR, Lawton MP: Incidence of depression in long-term care settings. J Gerontol 47:M189–M196, 1992b

Phillips CD, Sloane PD, Hawes C, et al: Effects of residence in Alzheimer's disease special care units on functional outcomes. JAMA 278:1340–1344, 1997

Phillips CD, Spry KM, Sloane PD, et al: Use of physical restraints and psychotropic medications in Alzheimer special care units in nursing homes. Am J Public Health 90:92–96, 2000

Politis AM, Vozzella S, Mayer LS, et al: A randomized, controlled, clinical trial of activity therapy for apathy in patients with dementia residing in long-term care. Int J Geriatr Psychiatry 19:1087–1094, 2004

Porsteinsson AP, Tariot PN, Erb R, et al: Placebo-controlled study of divalproex sodium for agitation in dementia. Am J Geriatr Psychiatry 9:58–66, 2001

Rattenbury C, Stones MJ: A controlled evaluation of reminiscence and current topics discussion groups in a nursing home context. Gerontologist 29:768–771, 1989

Ray WA, Federspiel CF, Schaffner W: A study of antipsychotic drug use in nursing homes: epidemiologic evidence suggesting misuse. Am J Public Health 70:485–491, 1980

Ray WA, Taylor JA, Meador KG, et al: Reducing antipsychotic drug use in nursing homes: a controlled trial of provider education. Arch Intern Med 153:713–721, 1993

Reichman WE, Conn DK: Nursing home psychiatry: is it time for a reappraisal? Am J Geriatr Psychiatry 18:1049–1053, 2010

Reichman WE, Coyne AC, Borson S, et al: Psychiatric consultation in the nursing home: a survey of six states. Am J Geriatr Psychiatry 6:320–327, 1998

Risse SC, Cubberley L, Lampe TH, et al: Acute effects of neuroleptic withdrawal in elderly dementia patients. Journal of Geriatric Drug Therapy 2:65–77, 1987

Rosen J, Mulsant BH, Pollock BG: Sertraline in the treatment of minor depression in nursing home residents: a pilot study. Int J Geriatr Psychiatry 15:177–180, 2000

Rovner BW, Kafonek S, Filipp L, et al: Prevalence of mental illness in a community nursing home. Am J Psychiatry 143:1446–1449, 1986

Rovner BW, German PS, Broadhead J, et al: The prevalence and management of dementia and other psychiatric disorders in nursing homes. Int Psychogeriatr 2:13–24, 1990a

Rovner BW, Lucas-Blaustein J, Folstein MF, et al: Stability over one year in patients admitted to a nursing home dementia unit. Int J Geriatr Psychiatry 5:77–82, 1990b

Rovner BW, German PS, Brant LJ, et al: Depression and mortality in nursing homes. JAMA 265:993–996, 1991

Rovner BW, Edelman BA, Cox MP, et al: The impact of antipsychotic drug regulations (OBRA 1987) on psychotropic prescribing practices in nursing homes. Am J Psychiatry 149:1390–1392, 1992

Rovner BW, Steele CD, Shmuely Y, et al: A randomized trial of dementia care in nursing homes. J Am Geriatr Soc 44:7–13, 1996

Ruths S, Straand J, Nygaard HA, et al: Effect of antipsychotic withdrawal on behavior and sleep/wake activity in nursing home residents with dementia: a randomized, placebo-controlled, double-blinded study. The Bergen District Nursing Home Study. J Am Geriatr Soc 52:1737–1743, 2004

Sabin TD, Vitug AJ, Mark VH: Are nursing home diagnosis and treatment inadequate? JAMA 248:321–322, 1982

Saxton J, Silverman M, Ricci E, et al: Maintenance of mobility in residents of an Alzheimer's special care facility. Int Psychogeriatr 10:213–224, 1998

Schneider LS, Pollock VE, Lyness SA: A meta-analysis of controlled trials of neuroleptic treatment in dementia. J Am Geriatr Soc 38:553–563, 1990

Schneider LS, Dagerman KS, Insel P: Risk of death with atypical antipsychotic drug treatment for dementia: meta-analysis of randomized placebo-controlled trials. JAMA 294:1934–1943, 2005

Schnelle JF, Newman DR, White M, et al: Reducing and managing restraints in long-term-care facilities. J Am Geriatr Soc 40:381–385, 1992

Seitz D, Purandare N, Conn D: Prevalence of psychiatric disorders among older adults in long-term care homes: a systematic review. Int Psychogeriatr 22:1025–1039, 2010

Shea DG, Russo PA, Smyer MA: Use of mental health services by persons with a mental illness in nursing facilities: initial impacts of OBRA 87. J Aging Health 12:560–578, 2000

Shorr RI, Fought RL, Ray WA: Changes in antipsychotic drug use in nursing homes during implementation of the OBRA-87 regulations. JAMA 271:358–362, 1994

Siegler EL, Capezuti E, Maislin G, et al: Effects of a restraint reduction intervention and OBRA '87 regulations on psychoactive drug use in nursing homes. J Am Geriatr Soc 45:791–796, 1997

Sink KM, Holden KF, Yaffe K: Pharmacological treatment of neuropsychiatric symptoms of dementia: a review of the evidence. JAMA 293:596–608, 2005

Sloane PD, Mathew LS, Scarborough M, et al: Physical and pharmacologic restraint of nursing home patients with dementia: impact of specialized units. JAMA 265:1278–1282, 1991

Sloane PD, Mitchell CM, Preisser JS, et al: Environmental correlates of resident agitation in Alzheimer's disease special care units. J Am Geriatr Soc 46:862–869, 1998

Smalbrugge M, Jongenelis L, Pot AM, et al: Incidence and outcome of depressive symptoms in nursing home patients in the Netherlands. Am J Geriatr Psychiatry 14:1069–1076, 2006

Smith M, Buckwalter KC, Albanese M: Geropsychiatric education programs: providing skills and understanding. J Psychosoc Nurs Ment Health Serv 28:8–12, 1990

Smyer MA, Shea DG, Streit A: The provision and use of mental health services in nursing homes: results from the National Medical Expenditure Survey. Am J Public Health 84:284–287, 1994

Snow LA, Hovanec L, Brandt J: A controlled trial of aromatherapy for agitation in nursing home patients with dementia. J Altern Complement Med 10:431–437, 2004

Snowden M, Roy-Byrne P: Mental illness and nursing home reform: OBRA-87 ten years later. Omnibus Budget Reconciliation Act. Psychiatr Serv 49:229–233, 1998

Snowden M, Sato K, Roy-Byrne P: Assessment and treatment of nursing home residents with depression or behavioral symptoms associated with dementia: a review of the literature. J Am Geriatr Soc 51:1305–1317, 2003

Stevenson DG, Decker SL, Dwyer LL, et al: Antipsychotic and benzodiazepine use among nursing home residents: findings from the 2004 National Nursing Home Survey. Am J Geriatr Psychiatry 18:1078–1092, 2010

Street JS, Clark WS, Gannon KS, et al: Olanzapine treatment of psychotic and behavioral symptoms in patients with Alzheimer disease in nursing care facilities, a double-blind, randomized, placebo-controlled trial. Arch Gen Psychiatry 57:968–976, 2000

Streim JE, Katz IR: Federal regulations and the care of patients with dementia in the nursing home. Med Clin North Am 78:895–909, 1994

Streim JE, Katz IR: Psychiatric aspects of long-term care, in Comprehensive Textbook of Psychiatry, 9th Edition, Vol II. Edited by Sadock BJ, Sadock VA, Ruiz P. Philadelphia, PA, Lippincott Williams & Wilkins, 2009, pp 4195–4200

Streim JE, Oslin DW, Katz IR, et al: Drug treatment of depression in frail elderly nursing home residents. Am J Geriatr Psychiatry 8:150–159, 2000

Streim JE, Porsteinsson AP, Breder CD, et al: A randomized, double-blind, placebo-controlled study of aripiprazole for the treatment of psychosis in nursing home patients with Alzheimer's disease. Am J Geriatr Psychiatry 16:537–550, 2008

Sunderland T, Silver MA: Neuroleptics in the treatment of dementia. Int J Geriatr Psychiatry 3:79–88, 1988

Sutcliffe C, Burns A, Challis D, et al: Depressed mood, cognitive impairment, and survival in older people admitted to care homes in England. Am J Geriatr Psychiatry 15:708–715, 2007

Swanson E, Maas M, Buckwalter K: Catastrophic reactions and other behaviors of Alzheimer's residents: special unit compared with traditional units. Arch Psychiatr Nurs 7:292–299, 1993

Tariot PN, Podgorski CA, Blazina L, et al: Mental disorders in the nursing home: another perspective. Am J Psychiatry 150:1063–1069, 1993

Tariot PN, Erb R, Podgorski CA, et al: Efficacy and tolerability of carbamazepine for agitation and aggression in dementia. Am J Psychiatry 155:54–61, 1998

Tariot PN, Cummings JL, Katz IR, et al: A randomized, double-blind, placebo-controlled study of the efficacy and safety of donepezil in patients with Alzheimer's disease in the nursing home setting. J Am Geriatr Soc 49:1590–1599, 2001a

Tariot PN, Schneider LS, Mintzer J, et al: Safety and tolerability of divalproex sodium in the treatment of signs and symptoms of mania in elderly patients with dementia: results of a double-blind, placebo-controlled trial. Curr Ther Res Clin Exp 62:51–67, 2001b

Tariot PN, Farlow MR, Grossberg GT, et al: Memantine treatment in patients with moderate to severe Alzheimer disease already receiving donepezil: a randomized controlled trial. JAMA 291:317–324, 2004

Tariot PN, Raman R, Jakimovich L, et al: Divalproex sodium in nursing home residents with possible or probable Alzheimer disease complicated by agitation: a randomized, controlled trial. Am J Geriatr Psychiatry 13:942–949, 2005

Teeter RB, Garetz FK, Miller WR, et al: Psychiatric disturbances of aged patients in skilled nursing homes. Am J Psychiatry 133:1430–1434, 1976

Thapa PB, Gideon P, Cost TW, et al: Antidepressants and the risk of falls among nursing home residents. N Engl J Med 339:875–882, 1998

Tondi L, Ribani L, Bottazzi M, et al: Validation therapy (VT) in nursing home: a case-control study. Arch Gerontol Geriatr 44(suppl):407–411, 2007

Toseland RW, Diehl M, Freeman K, et al: The impact of validation group therapy on nursing home residents with dementia. J Appl Gerontol 61:31–50, 1997

Trappler B, Cohen CI: Using fluoxetine in "very old" depressed nursing home residents. Am J Geriatr Psychiatry 4:258–262, 1996

Trappler B, Cohen CI: Use of SSRIs in "very old" depressed nursing home residents. Am J Geriatr Psychiatry 6:83–89, 1998

van Weert JC, van Dulmen AM, Spreeuwenberg PM, et al: Behavioral and mood effects of snoezelen integrated into 24-hour dementia care. J Am Geriatr Soc 53:24–33, 2005

Wang PS, Schneeweiss S, Avorn J, et al: Risk of death in elderly users of conventional vs. atypical antipsychotic medications. N Engl J Med 353:2335–2341, 2005

Webber AP, Martin JL, Harker JO, et al: Depression in older patients admitted for post-acute nursing home rehabilitation. J Am Geriatr Soc 53:1017–1022, 2005

Wells Y, Jorm FA: Evaluation of a special nursing home unit for dementia sufferers: a randomized controlled comparison with community care. Aust N Z J Psychiatry 21:524–531, 1987

Werner P, Cohen-Mansfield J, Braun J, et al: Physical restraint and agitation in nursing home residents. J Am Geriatr Soc 37:1122–1126, 1989

Wetzels RB, Zuidema SU, de Jonghe JFM, et al: Course of neuropsychiatric symptoms in residents with dementia in nursing homes over 2-year period. Am J Geriatr Psychiatry 18:1054–1065, 2010

Williams-Barnard CL, Lindell AR: Therapeutic use of "prizing" and its effect on self-concept of elderly clients in nursing homes and group homes. Issues Ment Health Nurs 13:1–17, 1992

Winblad B, Kilander L, Eriksson S, et al: Donepezil in patients with severe Alzheimer's disease: double-blind, parallel-group, placebo-controlled study. Lancet 367:1057–1065, 2006

Youssef FA: The impact of group reminiscence counseling on a depressed elderly population. Nurse Pract 15:32–38, 1990

Zerhusen JD, Boyle K, Wilson W: Out of the darkness: group cognitive therapy for depressed elderly. J Psychosoc Nurs Ment Health Serv 29:16–21, 1991

Zhong KX, Tariot PN, Mintzer J, et al: Quetiapine to treat agitation in dementia: a randomized, double-blind, placebo-controlled study. Curr Alzheimer Res 4:81–93, 2007

Zimmer JG, Watson N, Treat A: Behavioral problems among patients in skilled nursing facilities. Am J Public Health 74:1118–1121, 1984

Suggested Readings

American Geriatrics Society, American Association for Geriatric Psychiatry: The American Geriatrics Society and American Association for Geriatric Psychiatry recommendations for policies in support of quality mental health care in U.S. nursing homes. J Am Geriatr Soc 51:1299–1304, 2003

Bharucha AJ, Dew MA, Miller MD, et al: Psychotherapy in long-term care: a review. J Am Med Dir Assoc 7:568–580, 2006

Centers for Medicare and Medicaid: State Operations Manual, Appendix PP: Guidance to Surveyors for Long Term Care Facilities. Baltimore, MD, Centers for Medicare and Medicaid, 2007. Available at: http://www.cms.hhs.gov/manuals/Downloads/som107ap_pp_guidelines_ltcf.pdf. Accessed December 31, 2007.

Sink KM, Holden KF, Yaffe K: Pharmacological treatment of neuropsychiatric symptoms of dementia: a review of the evidence. JAMA 293:596–608, 2005

Snowden M, Sato K, Roy-Byrne P: Assessment and treatment of nursing home residents with depression or behavioral symptoms associated with dementia: a review of the literature. J Am Geriatr Soc 51:1305–1317, 2003

Streim JE, Katz IR: Federal regulations and the care of patients with dementia in the nursing home. Med Clin North Am 78:895–909, 1994

Index

*Page numbers printed in **boldface** type refer to figures or tables.*

Clorazepate, 280
Clozapine, 274–275
  adverse effects of, 63–64, 275
  in bipolar disorder, 156
  dosage of, 275
  for psychosis in Lewy body disorders, 170, 275
  receptor blockade of, **275**
  for schizophrenia, 169, 274–275
CMS (Centers for Medicare and Medicaid Services), 361–362, 363
Cognitive assessment, 5, 39, 54, 55–56
  in depression, 135, **135**
  neuropsychological testing, 75–85
Cognitive-behavioral social skills training (CBSST), 169
Cognitive-behavioral therapy (CBT), 320
  for anxiety disorders, 178, 179–180, 183, 323–324
    pharmacotherapy and, 181
  for complicated bereavement, 200–201, 203
  for depression, 136, 320–322
    dialectical behavior therapy, 321–322
    exercise therapy, 321
    in groups, 321–323
    individual, 320–321
    problem-solving therapy, 136, 321
  for insomnia, 215–216, 217
  in nursing homes, 356
  for personality disorders, 326–327
  for substance use disorders, 234, 325–326
Cognitive effects
  of drugs, 257
    benzodiazepines, 182, 280
    citalopram, 262
    clozapine, 275
    gabapentin, 279
    lithium, 154, 277
    mirtazapine, 268
    olanzapine, 274
    risperidone, 272
    tricyclic antidepressants, 269
  of electroconvulsive therapy, 139, 140, 308, 311
Cognitive enhancers, 281–283
  cholinesterase inhibitors, 35–36, 116–117, 281, **282**

key points related to, 284
  memantine, 281–283
Cognitive function
  age-related changes in, 35, 76–78
  in schizophrenia, 164
Cognitive impairment
  anxiety and, 178–179
  delirium, 93–104, 249–250
  dementia, 78–84, 107–120
    Alzheimer's disease, 78–79, **80, 83,** 167
    in Creutzfeldt-Jakob disease, **82**
    dementia with Lewy bodies, **80,** 82–84, 114
    due to hydrocephalus, **81**
    frontotemporal lobar degeneration, 79, **80,** 82, 114–115
    in geriatric depression, **82**
    in Huntington's disease, **81**
    in Parkinson's disease, **81,** 82, 113
    in progressive supranuclear palsy, **81**
    vascular dementia, 79, **81**
  depression and, 127, 132, 134
  disturbances of thought content, 53
  disturbances of thought progression, 53–54
  electroconvulsive therapy–induced, 139, 140
  environmental factors and, 17
  mild, 78, **80, 83, 108,** 109
    prevalence of, **7,** 8
  neuropsychological assessment of, 75–85
  not dementia, **108**
  in nursing home residents, 352–354
  prevalence of, 6–8, **7**
  vascular, 109
Cognitive stimulation therapy, 327–328, 355
Cognitive therapy
  for anxiety disorders, 179
  for complicated bereavement, 200
  in nursing homes, 356
Colon, 29
Combativeness, 250
Communication
  nonverbal, 60
  with older adults, 59–60
    and their families, 340–341
  strategies to reduce agitation, 247–248
Complementary and alternative medicine, for anxiety disorders, 181

Neurofibrillary tangles, 112
Neuroimaging, 68–70.
   See also specific imaging modalities
  in bipolar disorder, 152–153
  computed tomography, 68–69
  in delirium, 94–96, 100
  in dementia, 69, 110
  in dementia with Lewy bodies, 114
  before electroconvulsive therapy, 139
  indications for, **69**
  magnetic resonance imaging, 69–70
  plain film radiography, 68
  positron emission tomography, 70
  single-photon emission computed
    tomography, 70
  for suspiciousness or paranoia, 245
  in vascular dementia, 113
  in vascular depression, 131
Neurological disorders
  anxiety and, 176, 177–178
  delirium and, 96, **97**
  dementia and, 109
  electroconvulsive therapy and, 309
  mania and, 150, 151–152
Neurological examination, 39, 135
Neurological soft signs, 135
Neuropathic pain
  duloxetine for, 264
  gabapentin for, 279
  pregabalin for, 279
Neuropathology
  of Alzheimer's disease, 112
    with psychosis, 167
  of dementia, 107–108
  of frontotemporal lobar degeneration, 79,
    82, 115
  of vascular dementia, 79
  of vascular depression, 131
Neuropsychiatric Inventory, 359
Neuropsychological assessment, 75–85
  of delirium, 96
  of dementia, 78–84, 110
    Alzheimer's disease, 78–79, **80, 83,** 85
    in Creutzfeldt-Jakob disease, **82**
    due to hydrocephalus, **81**
    frontotemporal lobar dementia, 79, **80,**
    82, 85

    in Huntington's disease, **81**
    Lewy body dementia, **80,** 82–84, 85
    in Parkinson's disease, **81,** 82–83, 85
    in progressive supranuclear palsy, **81**
    vascular dementia, 79, **81**
  domains evaluated by, 76
  of geriatric depression, **82,** 84, 85
  in geriatric settings, 75–76
  indications for, 75–76, 84–85
  interpreting results of, 76
  key points related to, 85
  of mild cognitive impairment, **80, 83**
  of normal aging, 76–78, **80,** 85
  tests for, 76, **77**
Neuroticism, depression and, 131
Neurotransmitters
  in delirium, 96
  in depression, 130
Neutropenia, mirtazapine-induced, 269
Nifedipine, 34
Night sweats, 215
Nightmares, cholinesterase inhibitor–induced,
  281
Nitrazepam, 280
Nocturia, 214–215
Nonsteroidal anti-inflammatory drugs
  (NSAIDs), 34
  delirium induced by, 98, **99**
  drug interactions with
    lithium, 153, 277
    selective serotonin reuptake inhibitors,
    262, 283
Norepinephrine, 30
  in delirium, 96
  in depression, 130
North Carolina Established Populations for
  Epidemiologic Study of the Elderly
  cohort, 128
Nortriptyline
  for complicated bereavement, 199, 201
  for depression, 127, 137, 269, 322
    in nursing home residents, 359
  dosage of, 137, **138**
  therapeutic plasma levels of, 269
NSAIDs.
  See Nonsteroidal anti-inflammatory drugs
Nursing Home Reform Act, 361, 363, 367